For Jeff and David,
aka husbands of awesome

Our health and this book would not be
possible without your love and support.

Interior design by Yordan Terziev and Boryana Yordanova

Recipe photography by Alaena Haber, except for the following:

Sarah Ballantyne (Lettuce Soup)

Meagan Klementowski (Peach & Kale Summer Salad, Beef or Pork Carnitas)

Portrait photography by Dawn Brewer and Meagan Klementowski

Printed in the U.S.A.

RRD 0216

contents

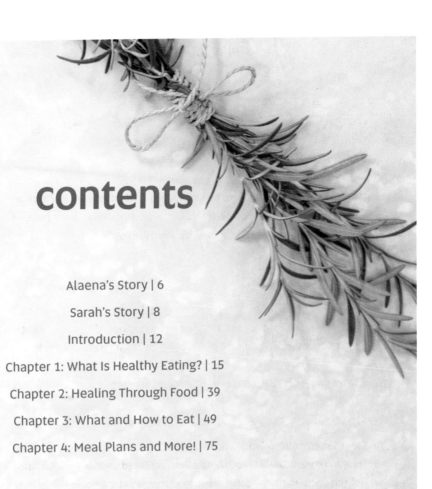

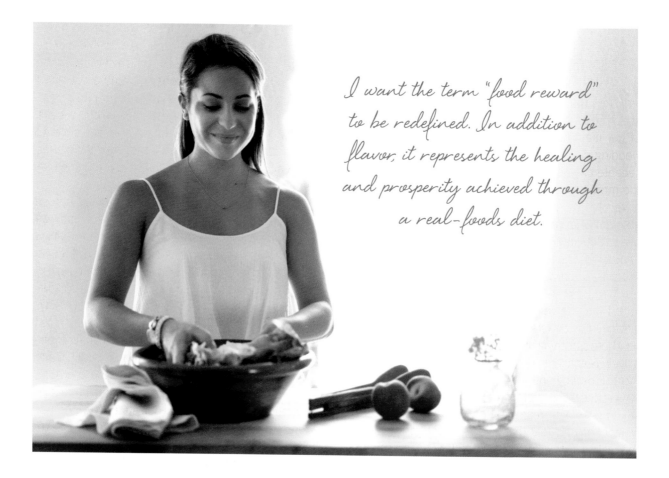

I want the term "food reward" to be redefined. In addition to flavor, it represents the healing and prosperity achieved through a real-foods diet.

Alaena's story

You can probably tell by flipping through this book that I am a complete veggie-holic, I prefer mineral-rich fresh herbs to the dried stuff, and I believe that a healing diet doesn't have to be a time-consuming one. Most of all, I am dedicated to using food as medicine in a miraculous way that really isn't a miracle at all.

I firmly believe that preparing and enjoying a large variety of nutrient-rich foods is what gives us the physical and mental energy to achieve the goals we each deem meaningful. I've seen this in my own life: in my short twenty-seven years, I have had a number of what I call "health hiccups" that most people go through only in their later years, and I've experienced how changing the way we eat can change our health completely.

I was born in Montreal, the first in a set of twins, in August 1988. My parents have told me that I came out kicking, screaming, and wailing my head off, while my sister, Olivia, arrived into this world like a "peaceful angel." Not much has changed. I've been a high-energy girl from the beginning, and it got me in trouble during school. I talked too much, wanted to play all the time, and thought I had figured out life by age six while all of the adults were too busy following the rules. In conferences with my parents, my teachers praised my eagerness to help others but added that doing other students' assignments for them wasn't as helpful as I thought. Whoops. I guess you *can* have too much of a good thing. I also wanted to excel from a young age. Second place may as well have been last, and 95 percent on a math test left room for improvement. These self-set high expectations followed me through my adolescence, and with them came inevitable disappointment and stress.

I truly believe that my journey with autoimmune disease has more than a little something to do with these overachieving tendencies. A typical nineteen-year-old in her sophomore year of college shouldn't be diagnosed with Hashimoto's thyroiditis and go through the scariest thyroid storm she could imagine. Bouts of fevers, rashes, and digestive sickness shouldn't be how one remembers year twenty-three of her life. And a young woman shouldn't fear her wedding day because she's worried that an unforeseeable case of facial and hand swelling could ruin the moment her husband tries to fit the ring on her finger. So why does a young, active girl develop an autoimmune disease that expresses itself in some pretty debilitating ways? There's obviously a genetic component, as there is with many diseases, but without an environmental trigger, the genetic predisposition shouldn't be expressed. I truly believe physical stress and not managing life's daily stressors triggered my development of Hashimoto's.

There's nothing like a full-on thyroid flare to stop a lively teenager in her tracks. I wasn't invincible anymore. I lost my energy, my zest, my personality, and my fearlessness. Instead, I lived in fear. Fear that it would get worse, fear that I would never lose all the weight I gained, fear that I would never gain back all the weight I then lost due to malnourishment, fear that my emotions would stay flat and stunted and I would never burst out into a belly laugh ever again. It sounds dramatic, but when you have a disease that affects every cell in your body, you start to feel a little hopeless when things don't change or only change for the worse.

At the peak of my disease at age twenty-four, I finally found a doctor (after going to *many*) who agreed with my feeling that diet could influence healing. He introduced me to the Paleo diet, and in my all-or-nothing way, I went home and threw out all the whole-grain pasta, steel-cut oats, and low-fat cheese in my apartment. And I never looked back. The daily headaches I'd had since age three were no longer my normal, and the intense lower-back pain I'd experienced in the evenings suddenly disappeared. I realized that I'd likely been gluten-intolerant for most of my childhood—there had never been an explanation for all of the infections, eczema, rashes, and digestion problems I had throughout my youth, and finally, here it was.

The traditional Paleo diet cleared up about half of my nagging daily symptoms, but my drastic weight loss and wrenching intestinal pain kept me up late searching for an answer online. I eventually stumbled upon the Autoimmune Protocol, and that led me to Sarah's website, where she had a flurry of articles on her version of the protocol, which she called the Paleo Approach. I only needed to read a couple of them before I rid my fridge and pantry of all eggs, nuts, seeds, coffee, and nightshades. Within weeks, my stomach pain disappeared, my digestion became regulated, and my mood stabilized. Over the course of a year, my hormonal health was restored and I regained the weight I had lost due to my illness.

But as the change in my diet started to improve my symptoms, I realized that I would never get 100 percent better unless I addressed the stress I put on myself to be perfect. I started allowing myself to be imperfect in every way—with my relationships, my body, my writing, and my career. And then I rediscovered joy in what had always mattered most: my family, my dog, my friends, and helping others. Once I focused on combining diet with stress management, my well-being improved drastically and I could finally say I reached a true state of health, inside and out. I encourage you to learn from my story that no matter how much good food is on your plate, if you do not address the emotional stress in your life, you can't be fully healed.

So is there a happy ending for all this? Yes! I am symptom-free of all those life-stalling problems that riddled my early and mid-twenties. My creativity in the kitchen has exploded as I'm discovering all of the amazing ways you can turn Mother Earth's simplicities into delectable, nourishing dishes. The best part is that the Paleo diet has allowed me to understand my body on a very deep level. I know which foods make me feel best, and I know which can put me back on the couch for a few days straight. That knowledge will take me a long way in preventing disease and maintaining health.

Each of the more than 175 recipes in this book was designed to help you the same way—to show you how food can help you feel better and, when combined with stress management, activity, and other lifestyle changes, lead you to optimal health. So I encourage all of you to explore this book with an open mind. Remember when I said that I am helpful to a fault? I didn't write these recipes for *me*, I wrote them for *you*. Let the abundance and vibrancy of a whole-foods lifestyle fill your kitchen, and may you live each day without fear and with the ability to achieve anything you desire.

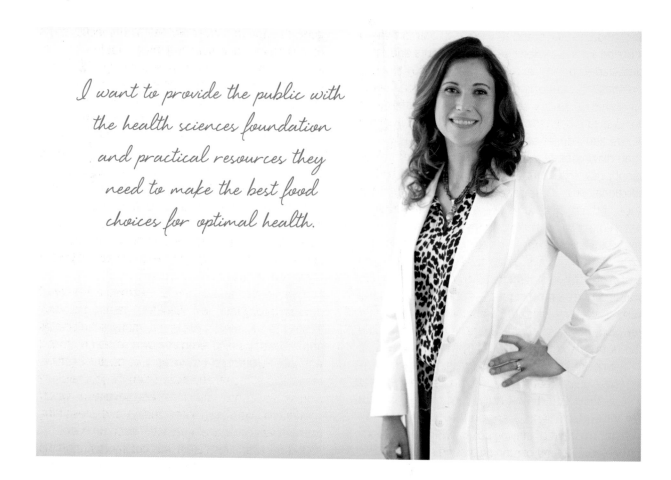

I want to provide the public with the health sciences foundation and practical resources they need to make the best food choices for optimal health.

Sarah's story

Passionate is a word that most people would use to describe me (along with some other choice words, like *geek, nerd,* and *nerdy geek*). Two of my biggest passions are improving scientific literacy and improving public health, which I believe go hand in hand. I see the biggest barrier to changing the epidemic of chronic illness in our society as the fact that most of us don't have the foundation of scientific knowledge needed to truly understand what the best choices are and to be motivated to implement them. And it's become my *raison d'être* to help people regain their health by providing health education rooted in science.

This passion originates from my personal history of health struggles and my own scientific education—which I didn't even think to apply to my health until it got bad enough to compel me to give up my career in science.

I was the kid who fell asleep in the car every time we drove anywhere more than a few miles away. I always liked waking up to discover we were already at our destination, and both my family and I didn't think it was anything more than my "just being a sleeper." But sleeping a lot wasn't my only symptom. I started getting teased for being the "fat kid" at seven years old; I hit puberty extremely early, just after my tenth birthday, when I also stopped growing; I battled constipation for most of my life and dealt with mild depression and anxiety throughout my teens and twenties; and I was morbidly obese by my twentieth birthday, my heaviest weight being close to 300 pounds in my late twenties. And from age seven on, I was always getting sick with whatever was going around, or strep throat if nothing was going around. From puberty on, I always had dry skin, acne, crazy dandruff, thin hair, eyebrows that would cyclically thin out and then grow back in, and random rashes and allergic reactions to things I touched. I don't remember when my joints and muscles started aching and feeling stiff, but by my late twenties, I had repetitive strain injuries, carpel tunnel syndrome, and early arthritis. I developed infrequent but debilitating migraines at the age of eighteen and severe adult-onset asthma at the age of twenty-five. I had diagnoses of irritable bowel syndrome, gastro-esophageal reflux disease, eczema, psoriasis, and an additional skin condition called *lichen planus*. Yet none of these symptoms or conditions was severe. It was a collection of annoyances, some things my doctors would dismiss (or just treat with painkillers, steroids, bronchodilators, or laxatives) and many things I didn't even think to mention to my doctors. My blood pressure was borderline high, my blood sugar levels were borderline diabetic, and my LDL cholesterol was just above the normal range. Nothing was off the charts, but I wasn't healthy by any metric.

Being tired and prone to illness throughout my formative years kept me out of trouble like no threat of grounding could. I willingly went to bed at eight p.m. on school nights, slept on the bus on the way to school instead of playing poker with the other kids my age, and instead of running around or hanging out with the smokers at recess, I preferred to find a quiet place to do my homework. Being too tired for mischief, combined with some innate geekiness and ambition, meant that my energy was focused on schoolwork and on playing the violin. Because I didn't know any different, I worked hard despite not feeling energetic or physically comfortable most of the time. In fact, not feeling great somehow translated to a stubborn drive to work harder, determination to do whatever I needed to do to succeed at everything I set my mind to, and a habit of breaking molds along the way.

I started my academic career in physics, earning an honors bachelor of science degree with distinction from the University of Victoria, Canada, in 1999. I went on to earn a doctorate degree in medical biophysics at the University of Western Ontario, Canada, in 2003, at the age of twenty-six, and spent the next four years doing medical research as a postdoctoral fellow, first in the cardiology department at St. Michael's Hospital in Toronto and then in the Department of Cell Biology at the University of Arizona.

During my training and research career, I switched fields repeatedly, moving from physics to medical biophysics to physiology to cell biology, with focuses ranging from immunology to vascular health to gene therapy to cancer biology. The specific goals of my research also spanned the gamut from simply increasing basic scientific understanding of a particular system to more medically based research that included preclinical and clinical trial work. Yes, I like to make unconventional and fairly dramatic career shifts. Normally, each step in an academic career builds on the knowledge and experience learned in the previous steps. The way I did it, each time I moved on to a new degree or position, I had experience to draw on but had to teach myself an entire bachelor's degree worth of knowledge, plus learn new lab and experimental techniques in order to continue to do high-quality research at the level I expected of myself.

Despite that added hurdle, I earned a variety of awards throughout my academic career, including awards for research excellence, many scholarships and fellowships, and even my own research grant. I was prolific during these years too, publishing fourteen papers in peer-reviewed scientific journals (including seven first-author papers, several of which continue to be widely cited today) and presenting twenty-five abstracts at international conferences.

But my academic career was cut short. Although I didn't yet know it, I suffered from Hashimoto's thyroiditis and fibromyalgia in addition to the two secondary autoimmune diseases that affect my skin (psoriasis and lichen planus). By the time my first daughter was born when I was thirty years old, at the end of my second postdoctoral research fellowship, my body couldn't keep up with the demands of my burgeoning academic career. I was sick and incapable of finding balance between my ambitions as a scientist and my ambitions as a mother. I made the decision to stay home with my baby and put my academic career on hold. Yes, another unconventional choice.

Staying home with my daughters (I had a second one three years later) gave me the space I needed to focus on my health. I lost a hundred pounds, got fit, and lived happily ever after—er, or not. I did lose a hundred pounds and became physically active, but while my blood sugar levels and blood pressure improved, everything else did not. In fact, the frustration of getting thinner and thinner while feeling worse and worse—my energy levels tanked, my headaches grew more frequent, my joints felt stiff and sore every morning, and my skin continued to look worse and worse with its plethora of conditions—motivated me to start digging deeper. I finally began to apply my scientific background and broad knowledge base to the problem of my health—and that brought me to the Paleo diet and the Autoimmune Protocol.

Within two weeks of adopting a Paleo diet, I was able to discontinue six prescription medications, one of which I had been taking for twelve years. The further refinement of my diet with the adoption of the Autoimmune Protocol allowed me to put my autoimmune diseases into remission. My weight stabilized, my skin improved, my energy levels soared, my body stopped hurting all the time, and symptoms that I had endured for nearly three decades melted away. Needless to say, my rapid health turnaround convinced me of the healing power of the right foods.

Finding a solution to my health problems—a solution as simple as changing the foods I was eating—lit a fire under me. I couldn't sit back and simply enjoy better health myself; I had to tell the world and help others who were going through the same thing I did. I found my voice through my blog, *The Paleo Mom*, where I could combine all my interests: science,

health, cooking, and art. It became my mission to effectively communicate that some foods can support health by providing a wealth and diversity of essential and nonessential nutrients while others undermine health by disrupting the gut microbiome, dysregulating hormones, or instigating inflammation. I needed to help people understand how sleep, stress, and activity affect the health equation. And, perhaps more important, I needed to create resources so people could actually implement the choices they made to improve their health.

And so enters *The Healing Kitchen*, my third book that deals with the Paleo Autoimmune Protocol. The goal of this book is to make healthy eating as straightforward, budget-friendly, quick, and easy as possible. And I couldn't have asked for a better coauthor and partner in this project. Alaena and I have created a masterpiece that neither of us could have accomplished on our own, one that I know you will love not just for the good health the recipes promote but also for their flavor.

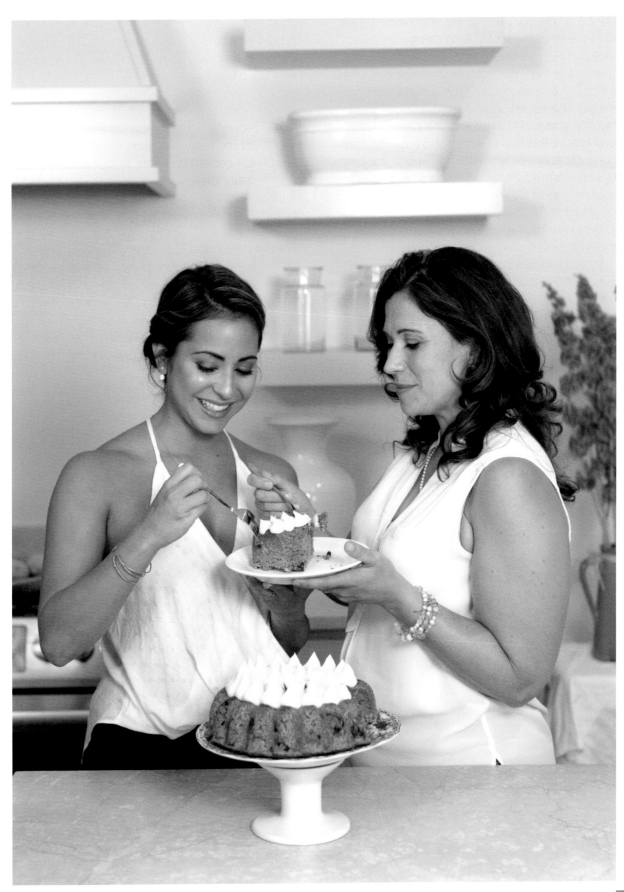

introduction

Chronic illness is epidemic in our society. More than half of all Americans take two or more prescription drugs, and about one-fifth of us take at least *five* different daily medications prescribed by our doctors. This isn't normal. We're not supposed to be so sick that we need multiple medications to get us through each day. We're not supposed to be this unhealthy.

Not that long ago, people were substantially healthier. Incidences of just about every chronic health problem—things like cardiovascular disease, obesity, diabetes, asthma, allergies, autoimmune disease, and even cancer—are on the rise and have been for several decades. Rates of chronic health problems are so high that nowadays more of us are unhealthy than are healthy. So what's changed?

The answer is, a lot. The food we eat today is not the same as what people ate fifty years ago, not by a long shot. Our food is more refined, more manipulated, more prepackaged, and more addictive than ever—all while being less nutritious. We spend less time cooking our own food and consume substantially more calories than we used to. And we tend to choose foods based on palatability, not nutritive value. We're also more stressed, we sleep less, we're sedentary, and we spend more time indoors than at any time in human history. All of these things contribute to poor health. But step back and think about that for a moment. These are all things we have control over. We can choose different foods. We can be proactive in terms of our lifestyle choices. And by making slightly different choices, we can turn the tide of health in our homes and our society.

It's easy to feel that our own health is beyond our control—we blame our genetics or our environment, we say it runs in our family, our doctors tell us that it's just bad luck and that no one knows why one person gets a particular disease while the next one remains healthy. But in truth, we *do* have control: our health is almost entirely within our power to change and improve. And it starts when we make one healthy choice at a time.

Making healthy choices does not need to be hard, and it doesn't have to mean that you feel deprived of your favorite foods. (This book will see to that!) You don't have to get up at five a.m. to work out, nor do you have to quit your job to de-stress. Good health comes from a collection of small changes, each one contributing its own tiny bit to an overall big improvement. It still might feel like a diet and lifestyle overhaul by the time you total up all those small changes, but it will be one that fits into your life, rather than the other way around. And there's no law saying that you can't tackle this journey one small change at a time.

The first thing is to understand what the best options are for your health. We're stuck in a society in which most of us make choices every day that are undermining our health, to the point that we need drugs to keep us going. But what those bad choices are might surprise you. It's easy to recognize that sitting on the couch all day and eating nothing but fried chicken and candy bars are poor health choices. It's harder to think of choices that fall under the category of "that's just life" as being unhealthy, things like skipping breakfast to run out of the house in the morning, having a long commute to work, buying a salad and sandwich from the drive-through on the way home from soccer practice, or staying up late to watch *Game of Thrones* once the kids are finally in bed. But none of those are choices conducive to good health. They all create stress in our bodies and contribute to inflammation and irregular hormones, both of which can lead to disease, and while that salad and sandwich on multigrain bread might make us feel like we're on the right track, they aren't providing our bodies with the nutrients they actually need. But if it's a challenge to wrap our minds around the idea that these everyday choices can be bad for us, it's mind-numbingly difficult to realize that things we've been told will make us healthier, like eating whole grains and low-fat yogurt and training to run that marathon, are contributing to the current rise in chronic illness. There are few things more frustrating than realizing that most of what we're told about how to lose weight, get fit, and live a happier, healthier, and longer life is just plain wrong.

> *Good health comes from a collection of small changes, each one contributing its own tiny bit to an overall big improvement.*

> *There are few things more frustrating than realizing that most of what we're told about how to lose weight, get fit, and live a happier, healthier, and longer life is just plain wrong.*

Getting healthy requires two things: understanding what to do and then actually doing it. Most of us think we know what to do but just find it too hard to do it. But the truth is that what we're told to do to be healthy isn't optimal for our bodies, and probably one of the biggest reasons we're finding it so hard to follow that advice is that it isn't effective. Why keep doing something difficult if it doesn't make us feel better?

This book tackles both sides of that problem.

using this book

First, before we get into the recipes, the beginning of this book will explain why what we're taught is healthy eating actually isn't, and what a truly healthy, nutrients-first approach means. No, we won't be going into a lot of scientific detail (you can read Sarah's book *The Paleo Approach* for that!), but it's important to have a basic understanding of why these food choices are necessary for good health. Then we'll look at the best food choices for someone battling chronic illness and explain how diet can actually promote healing.

Finally, we'll explore what making healthy food choices means day to day. One of the biggest barriers to changing how we eat is that it means dedicating more time to shopping and cooking. But the fact is that preprepared foods, whether we're talking about the drive-through window or the deli counter at the grocery store, are rarely the best options (when you're in a bind, see page 62 for help). *The Healing Kitchen* will help you get organized, plan ahead, and navigate the complexities of this way of eating and living. We've included twelve meal plans, complete with shopping lists, and you'll find dozens of helpful charts, lists, tips, and tricks throughout this book, all designed to help make eating healthy easy, practical, and affordable.

And of course, there are more than 175 mouth-watering recipes to choose from in the second part of this book. We've put special care into making sure that these recipes are simple to make, quick to prepare, and budget conscious, and they use everyday ingredients that you can find at most grocery stores—all while never skimping on flavor. The biggest part of sticking to a healthy eating plan is enjoying the food you're eating, and we're taking care of that!

The recipes in this book are simply organized by type of dish: Kitchen Basics, Breakfast Favorites, Soups & Salads, Easy-Peasy Mains, Simple Sides, Satisfying Snacks, Thirst Quenchers, and Timeless Treats. But we've also labeled the recipes with the handy icons below so you can easily find those that are especially quick and easy.

 5 ingredients or less

 20 minutes or less

 No cook

 One pot

 Leftovers reinvented

For each recipe, you'll see the number of servings, the average prep time and cook time, and the total time needed, so you can plan ahead. You'll also see suggestions for recipe pairings because, let's face it, some things just taste amazing together. And throughout the recipes you'll find tips, make-ahead suggestions, serving ideas, storing and reheating instructions, and ideas for "changing it up" with different ingredients.

But before we get into our Healing Kitchens, let's start by looking at what healthy eating actually is. Once we have a more thorough understanding of what the healthiest options are, then we get to see just how powerful the right foods can be in helping us regain our health!

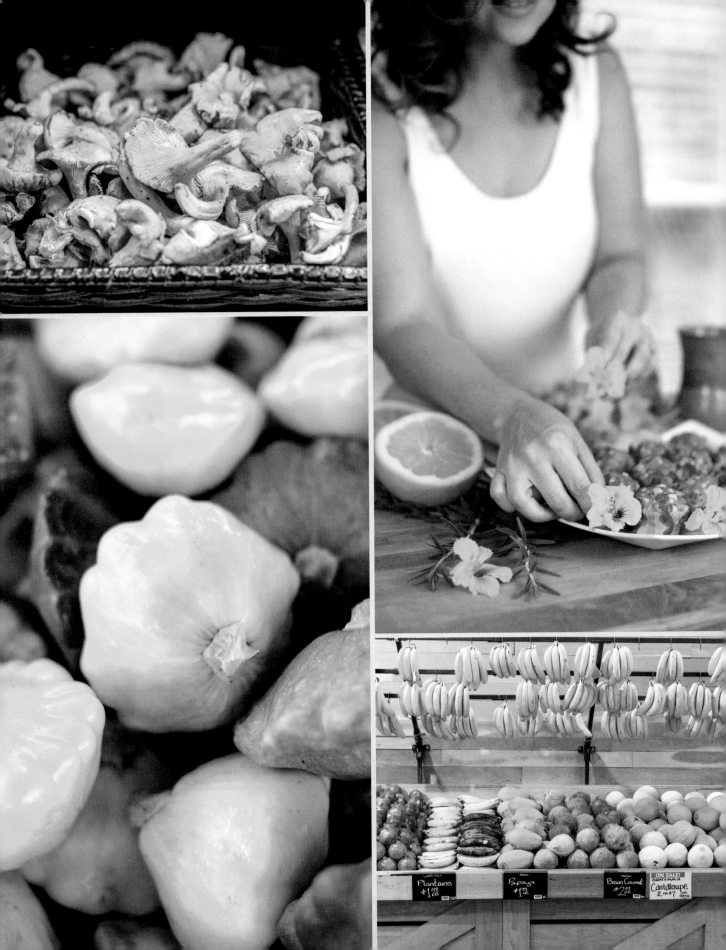

CHAPTER 1

what is healthy eating?

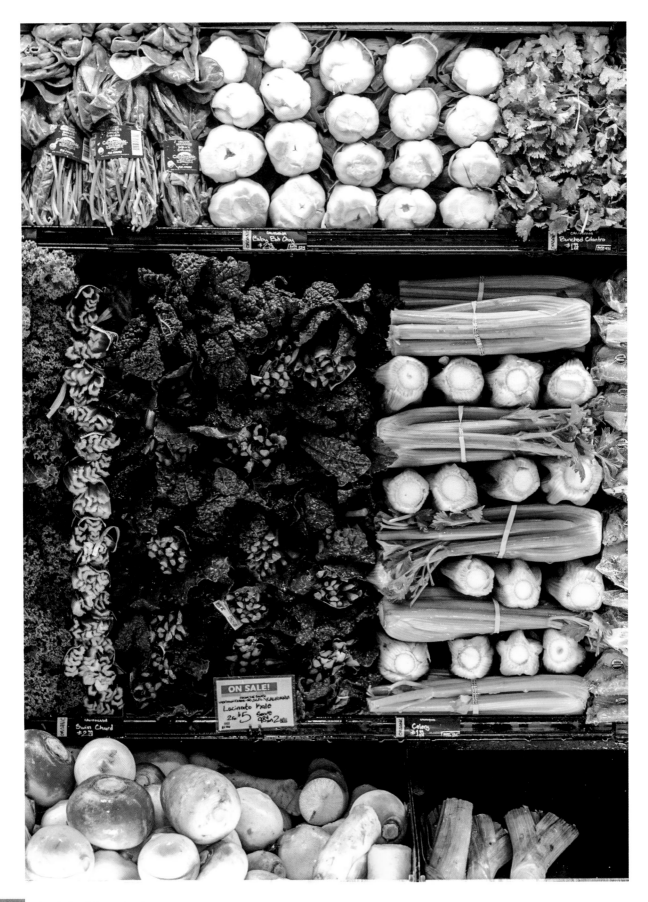

what is healthy eating?

We're fairly used to thinking about how food is related to weight: eat too much of the wrong things and you become overweight; eat the right amount of the right things and you lose weight. But health is about so much more than whether you could stand to lose a few pounds. And food has a much more profound impact on health than whether you've got a spare tire around your middle.

Food provides all of the building blocks used to make every cell, tissue, organ, and structure in our bodies. Food provides all of the raw materials for the millions of chemical reactions happening inside our bodies in every moment. And food provides the energy needed to sustain life. When you think about it this way, it's easy to see how eating the right foods is so important for health: without all the building blocks, raw materials, and energy that our bodies need to operate normally (and healthily!), how can we expect them to stay free of disease?

When we make our food choices based on what provides the best raw materials for our bodies, we have what's called a *micronutrient dietary focus*. Micronutrients are chemicals in foods that are essential for life and health, but we need only relatively small amounts of them. These include vitamins, minerals, phytochemicals (antioxidants and vitamin-like chemicals found in plant foods), essential amino acids (the building blocks of proteins), and essential fatty acids (the building blocks of fats, but they're also used to make essential structures in every cell, like the outer cell membrane). In contrast, macronutrients

> *Without all the building blocks, raw materials, and energy that our bodies need to operate normally (and healthily!), how can we expect them to stay free of disease?*

are the constituents of food that provide the energy that we need in larger amounts: carbohydrates, protein, and fat. The hallmark of any healthy diet is micronutrient sufficiency. That means every day we're getting all of the building blocks and raw materials that our bodies need. There's more than one way to accomplish micronutrient sufficiency, and nowhere is this more evident than in hunter-gatherer and traditional cultures.

Depending on where in the world these groups of people live, their traditional diets vary dramatically, and thus so do the ratios of protein, fat, and carbohydrate in their diets—in other words, the proportion of animal foods and plant foods. But these cultures are typically extremely healthy, with none of the chronic illnesses that plague us in first-world countries (like cardiovascular disease, cancer, and diabetes). For example, the Kitavans, who live on one of the islands of Papua New Guinea and eat a diet rich in starchy tubers, fruit, coconut, and seafood, have virtually no incidence of ischemic heart disease or stroke, despite the fact that nearly 80 percent of them smoke! The Inuit have a vastly different traditional diet from the Kitavans—theirs is rich in animal foods and saturated fats—yet they also boast an extraordinarily low prevalence of cardiovascular disease. One of the major contributors to this good health is micronutrient sufficiency. These cultures demonstrate that the human body can thrive on a wide range of macronutrient proportions, so long as we're getting plenty of the full complement of micronutrients.

the problems with the US dietary guidelines

Historically, government dietary guidelines have not focused on micronutrients. In fact, current recommendations for a healthy diet fall far short of the mark.

Instead of dividing foods into groups based on the micronutrients they contain, the guidelines base the food groups on how the foods are produced. For example, vegetables, which vary widely in the vitamins, minerals, phytochemicals, and fiber they contain, all get lumped together based on both farming practices to grow them and very broad botanical classifications. And until 1992, vegetables were lumped together with fruit, even though fruit typically comes from entirely different kinds of plants and different kinds of fruit vary just as widely in nutrients! After the guidelines lump all these foods into one or two food groups, they recommend that we "eat the rainbow." The concept of eating a variety of fruits and vegetables of different colors is an excellent one—the pigments that give plants their colors are also micronutrients, so eating many different-colored vegetables and fruits is a great way to make sure that you're getting the full complement of nutrients that plant foods can provide. But what would make far more sense from a public health perspective is to divide fruits and vegetables by color into four groups: blue and purple, green and yellow, red and orange, and white. Eating one to three servings daily from each color group would result in a vastly superior micronutrient intake.

The US dietary guidelines also group together meat, fish, eggs, legumes, nuts, and seeds based on the fact that they all contain protein. While it's great that nutrients are being considered, protein is a macronutrient, and it would make much more sense to focus on micronutrients. Plant-based proteins are very difficult to digest and don't contain all of the amino acids our bodies need (that's why they're referred to as *incomplete proteins*), yet they get equal playing time with meat, fish, and eggs, which are much more useful to our bodies. This nod to vegetarians is extremely respectful and kind from a social perspective, but it implies that kidney beans provide the same sort of nutrition to your body as a steak. They don't. And for those who are not following vegetarian diets for ethical or religious reasons, this is important information. In addition, all vegetarians need to make sure they're eating specific combinations of foods to get all twenty amino acids, and this grouping of foods isn't taken into account. And finally, these foods provide many, many nutrients other than protein, and they absolutely do not provide them equally. From a micronutrient perspective, it would make far more sense for this food group to be divided into at least four groups: meat and eggs, fish and shellfish, nuts and seeds, and legumes. Organ meat could possibly be celebrated as its own food group—it's one of the most micronutrient-dense foods available in the modern food supply, and it has a very different nutrient profile from other meats.

Grains enjoy their own food group despite the fact that they don't contribute much more than calories to our diets. Our food system is abundant in calories (the United States produces about six thousand calories' worth of food per person per day), but the standard American diet is deficient in most of the essential vitamins and minerals that our bodies need to be healthy. This is the opposite of what we need from our food—more nutrients and fewer calories—and a large contributor to this mismatch is the fact that whole grains are touted as being the foundation of a healthy diet. The fact is, vegetables and fruit contain up to ten times more vitamins and minerals than grains, just as much fiber, and only a fraction of the amount of sugar, plus they have high amounts of health-promoting phytochemicals. There is absolutely no need for grains in a diet that contains vegetables and fruit. Given that so many grain-based products also contribute a disproportionately high amount of blood-sugar-spiking, too-easily-digested carbohydrates (a contributor to obesity and diabetes) as well as high amounts of the most inflammatory fatty acids, they most likely belong in the same food group as candy, fast food, and other junk.

Dairy is the only food group that focuses on a micronutrient: calcium. This group includes all foods made from milk as well as calcium-fortified beverages made from milk alternatives like soy. Of course, there are plenty of other amazing sources of calcium that are not included in this food group. Not only do fruits, vegetables, nuts, seeds, and seafood contain substantial amounts of calcium, there is scientific evidence that we actually absorb more calcium from cruciferous vegetables like kale than we do from dairy! In fact, several studies show that fruit and vegetable intake correlates much more strongly with bone health than dairy intake—yes, to prevent osteoporosis and look after your bones, eat your veggies!

How did the government's dietary guidelines become so misguided? Since their earliest beginnings in 1894, various United States Department of Agriculture (USDA) nutrition guidelines have been criticized as not accurately representing scientific information about optimal nutrition and as being inappropriately influenced by the agricultural industries. The earliest guidelines justifiably focused on avoiding malnutrition and starvation, problems that were rampant in many areas of the US at that time. The 1916 guidelines introduced food groups, and their recommendation to liberally consume foods from all five groups— milk and meat, cereals, vegetables and fruits, fats and fatty foods, and sugars and sugary foods—successfully targeted the issue of gross malnutrition.

In 1943, the USDA updated its guidelines with what was called the "Basic 7," which, flawed as it was, represents the best (and perhaps only) attempt at creating food groups based on micronutrients. The scientific understanding of essential nutrients was in its infancy in the early 1940s: the roles of many minerals in the human body, as well as the very existence of many of the vitamins that we now know are necessary for survival, had yet to be discovered. Yet the Basic 7 guidelines were on the right track with a partial shift away from the previous focus on energy and toward a focus on micronutrients. While some of the earlier food groups remained, vegetables and fruits were divided into three different categories, based on the few micronutrients that were known at the time. For example, oranges, tomatoes, grapefruit, salad greens, and cabbage formed one food group based on their high levels of vitamin C. Butter got its own food group

> *" Whether dietary guidelines are distilled to recommended servings from four food groups or twenty, what's missing isn't a fancy graphic but the reasons behind the recommendation. ""*

thanks to its vitamin A content. While we certainly would come up with different micronutrient-based food groups now, the Basic 7 was a good effort and a move in the right direction.

Unfortunately, the Basic 7 was met with public skepticism and confusion. Policymakers decided that, in order to be successful, dietary guidelines needed to be simplified. And with the newly established Recommended Dietary Allowances providing a target for daily dietary intake of each micronutrient we need, it was simpler to stop basing food groups on nutrients. The pinnacle of dietary guideline simplicity was achieved in the next update to USDA dietary recommendations with the "Basic 4," which enjoyed the longest reign of all the USDA dietary recommendations, from 1956 until 1992. When the Basic 4 was finally revamped for subsequent USDA dietary guidelines, including the Food Guide Pyramid, MyPyramid, and most recently MyPlate, vegetables and fruits were divided into their own food groups. Yet the only appreciable differences among all the dietary recommendations of the last sixty years are the number of servings suggested from each food group and the way that the information is presented visually.

Since the public's rejection of the Basic 7, the idea of basing dietary recommendations on micronutrient content has been lost. Yet the last sixty years of steadily increasing rates of chronic disease have proven that distilling dietary recommendations to a simple set of rules is not an effective strategy to support public health. One major problem is that these rules are presented with very little explanation about why one food is a better choice than another. If we're expected to follow a set of rules about what we eat, they had better be well founded. Whether dietary guidelines are distilled to recommended servings from four food groups or twenty, what's missing isn't a fancy graphic but the reasons behind the recommendation.

a better way to eat

Nutritional science has come a long way since the first half of the twentieth century, when its primary focus was identifying micronutrients and establishing their recommended daily intakes. Now, our understanding of how nutrients (both those deemed essential and those currently considered nonessential) and other compounds in food act in the body to promote or to undermine health spans many disciplines of science. There are tens of thousands of scientific articles on the topic, each examining one small piece of the human health puzzle as it pertains to diet. And while we still don't have all the pieces, when we put together what we do know, we find that an optimal human diet is very far from the average American diet.

So let's change what we eat. Let's focus on foods that support our health. Let's start making better food choices right now. Whether you suffer from a chronic illness or simply want to experience the best health possible, a diet that is abundant in all the micronutrients and that simultaneously omits foods known to be problematic for health is your best bet. What does this diet look like? Its foundation is the most micronutrient-dense foods available to us, including organ meat, seafood, and a huge variety and copious quantities of vegetables, with other quality meats and fruit to round it out. At the same time, it omits foods known to be inflammatory, to disrupt hormones, or to negatively impact the health of the gut, including all grains, legumes, dairy products, nuts, seeds, and nightshades (see pages 33 to 35).

That may seem overwhelming. Policymakers in the past have decreed that nutrition guidelines with too many rules are too complicated to be effective. However, when nutrition guidelines are oversimplified, they lose their scientific validity, which causes them to be ineffective. We don't want to give you just a new set of rules. We want to explain why meat, seafood, vegetables, and fruit form a diet for optimal health and wellness. While the detailed science behind why these foods are the best choices to support health is beyond the scope of *The Healing Kitchen* (see Sarah's book *The Paleo Approach* for that information), it's still important to provide some explanations. It is immeasurably easier to make a better food choice when we understand why one food is superior to another.

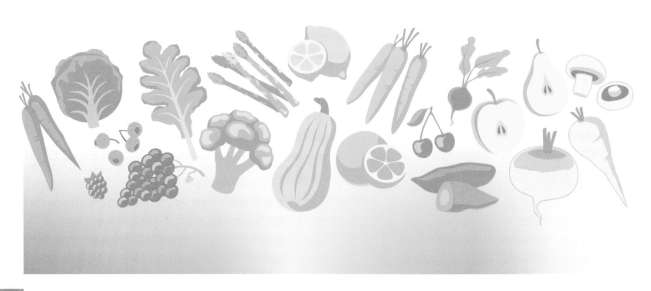

Eat

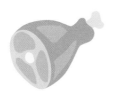
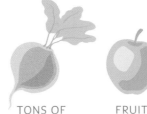

| MEAT | SEAFOOD | TONS OF VEGETABLES* | FRUIT |

*except nightshades

Don't Eat

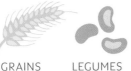
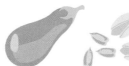

| GRAINS | LEGUMES | DAIRY | PROCESSED & REFINED FOODS | NIGHTSHADES (see page 55) | NUTS & SEEDS | EGGS | ALCOHOL |

wait! is this the caveman diet?

If that list of foods to avoid rings a bell, there's a good reason. This way of eating—variously called the Paleo diet, ancestral diet, or caveman diet; it's also closely related to the primal diet and the Weston A. Price Foundation Diet—is derived from what biology, physiology, health sciences, and nutritional sciences tell us the human body is designed to thrive on. More specifically, this book follows a variation of the Paleo diet called the Paleo Autoimmune Protocol (AIP; described in detail in *The Paleo Approach*), which is designed to be exceptionally nutrient-dense and anti-inflammatory, to promote hormone and gut health, and to enable immune-system regulation and overall healing.

> *People who try out the Paleo diet find that once they've adjusted to this new way of eating, continuing to follow it is satisfying and really quite easy.*

The Paleo diet is a nutrient-dense whole-foods diet that's based on eating a variety of quality meats, seafood, eggs, vegetables, fruits, nuts, and seeds. It provides balanced and complete nutrition while avoiding processed and refined foods and empty calories. It has gained phenomenal traction in recent years as the number of people committing to the Paleo lifestyle has grown exponentially. By some estimates, in America there are more people following a version of the Paleo diet—more than six million people in 2014—than there are vegetarians and vegans. This may be because people who try out the Paleo diet find that once they've adjusted to this new way of eating, continuing to follow it is satisfying and really quite easy. Another likely contributor is that, because the Paleo diet can mitigate such a wide range of health concerns, Paleo followers see improvements in their health, and that's a tremendous motivator to continue!

The Autoimmune Protocol is a specialized version of the Paleo diet, with an even greater focus on nutrient density and even stricter guidelines for which foods should be eliminated. Foods can be viewed as having two kinds of constituents within them: those that promote health (like nutrients!) and those that undermine health (like inflammatory compounds). (While there are constituents that neither promote nor undermine health, they are not used to evaluate the merit of an individual food.) Some foods are obvious wins for a health-promoting diet because they have tons of beneficial constituents and very few or no constituents that undermine health—good examples of these superfoods are organ meats, seafood, and most vegetables. Other foods are obvious fails because they have a relative lack of health-promoting constituents and are rife with problematic compounds—good examples are gluten-containing grains, peanuts, and most soy products. But most foods fall into the amorphous world of gray in between these two extremes. Tomatoes, for example, have some exciting nutrients, but they also contain several compounds that are so effective at stimulating the immune system that they have been investigated for use in vaccines as adjuvants (the chemicals in vaccines that enhance your immune response to whatever you're getting immunized against).

> *While the term* Paleo *refers to the Paleolithic era, the Paleo diet these days can be more accurately described as a contemporary approach to nutrition based on insight gleaned from a comprehensive collection of scientific research.*

The biggest difference between a standard Paleo diet and the Autoimmune Protocol is where we draw the line between "yes" foods and "no" foods in order to get more health-promoting compounds and fewer detrimental compounds in our diet. Those who are typically quite healthy can tolerate more less-optimal foods than those who aren't. You can think of the Autoimmune Protocol as a pickier version of the Paleo diet; it accepts only those foods that are clear winners.

As such, the Autoimmune Protocol places greater emphasis on the most nutrient-dense foods in our food supply, including organ meat, seafood, and vegetables. And the Autoimmune Protocol eliminates foods allowed on the typical Paleo diet that have compounds that may stimulate the immune system or harm the gut environment, including nightshades (like tomatoes and peppers; see page 55), eggs, nuts, seeds, and alcohol. The goal of the Autoimmune Protocol is to flood the body with nutrients while simultaneously avoiding any food that might be contributing to disease (or at the very least interfering with our efforts to heal). It is an elimination diet strategy, cutting out the foods that are most likely to be holding back our health. After a period of time, many of the excluded foods, especially those that have nutritional merit despite also containing some (but not too many) potentially detrimental compounds, can be reintroduced (see pages 44 and 45).

While the Paleo diet is sometimes labeled as a fad diet, its health benefits are supported by scientific research. The body of research pitting Paleo against other dietary strategies is in its infancy, but the studies that have been performed overwhelmingly support Paleo. They prove that it beats out other recommended diets, even the Mediterranean diet, for weight loss, management of diabetes, improvement of cardiovascular disease risk factors, and reversal of metabolic syndrome. Studies have also shown that it has therapeutic potential for the debilitating autoimmune disease secondary progressing multiple sclerosis. And while anecdotal stories cannot be used to validate any dietary approach, the fact that tens of thousands (and counting!) of people have successfully used variations of the Paleo diet, including the Autoimmune Protocol, to mitigate and even completely reverse their diseases is compelling.

So yes, this could be called the caveman diet or the Paleo diet or the Paleo Autoimmune Protocol, but the reasons for choosing these types of foods are far more profound than a simple desire to reenact history. While the original tenets of this nutritional approach were derived from evolutionary biology and anthropological data, the diet is justified by the scientific understanding of the roles that food and individual constituents of food play in human health. While the term *Paleo* refers to the Paleolithic era, the Paleo diet these days can be more accurately described as a contemporary approach to nutrition based on insight gleaned from a comprehensive collection of scientific research.

a nutrients-first approach

There are two elements of healthy eating. The first is nutrient sufficiency, meaning that you consume an ample amount of all the nutrients your body needs. The second is avoidance of problematic foods, meaning any food that has the capacity to undermine your health, whether by increasing inflammation, damaging the gut, negatively affecting hormones, or creating other undesirable effects.

Nutrient sufficiency is arguably the most important quality that any dietary approach can have. Every cell, tissue, organ, and system in the human body needs specific amounts of specific nutrients in order to function efficiently and effectively. Nutrients are used not only in the formation of the components of our bodies but also in the millions of chemical reactions that occur in our bodies in every moment. We are made of nutrients, and our bodies need them to do even basic things like breathing. Every tiny detail of every function of every part of the human body requires nutrients, and it isn't just macronutrients—protein, fat, and carbohydrates—that supply the energy that fuels the complex functions of life. Micronutrients— vitamins, minerals, plant phytochemicals, and other compounds—are necessary resources that get used up, too, and our micronutrient stores must be continuously topped up from the foods we eat. Being even slightly deficient in a single essential nutrient can have negative consequences for our health.

Unfortunately, getting all of our required nutrients from food is easier said than done. Many of the staple foods of the typical American diet have very little nutritional value. Even worse, the more a food is refined and processed and manufactured, the more the nutrients inherent to the raw ingredients are leached out, removed, or degraded. Processed foods, refined foods, fast food, and junk food all contribute next to no nutrients to our diets (plus, as we'll get to, they're often problematic for our health in other ways). But even foods that many of us think are healthy, like whole grains and low-fat dairy, are pretty weak when it comes to essential nutrients. And every time a nutritionally weak food displaces a nutritional powerhouse, the overall nutritional value of our diet suffers.

Generally, a nutrients-first approach to eating focuses on micronutrients. Once we're getting all of the essential amino acids, essential fatty acids, vitamins, minerals, and plant phytochemicals that our bodies need to thrive, it's nearly impossible not to be consuming sufficient macronutrients.

Micronutrients can be categorized as essential and nonessential. *Essential* means that you'll die without them. *Nonessential* means that you'll go on living without them, though you may not be particularly healthy—and indeed, many micronutrients that are considered nonessential are known to improve health. Often, a micronutrient is called nonessential simply because we don't really understand exactly what it does in our bodies to support health—we just know that when we consume more of it, our risk of disease decreases. This is the case for most phytochemicals and many vitaminlike compounds. There are thousands of plant phytochemicals, and our understanding of their roles in health is so rudimentary that the most we can typically say about them is that they have antioxidant activity (that is, they help prevent damage to molecules in our body from oxidation). Yet we know that the more plant phytochemicals in your diet, the lower your risk of chronic disease. When you think about it in these terms, it's easy to realize that even nonessential nutrients are pretty darned important.

vitamins and minerals

We do know the roles that all of the known vitamins and many minerals play in the human body, however. These micronutrients are considered essential, and when we examine more closely how the body uses these chemicals, it quickly becomes obvious why we can't experience good health without the full complement of essential nutrients—for details, see the descriptions of vitamins and minerals on the following pages.

essential vitamins and minerals for health

Vitamin A (Retinol): Not to be confused with beta-carotene (which is a vitamin A precursor, not vitamin A itself!), this vitamin is essential for bone growth, tooth remineralization, skin health, vision, reproduction, and immune function. Retinol is found only in animal foods, including liver, eggs, dairy products, and seafood (especially shrimp, salmon, sardines, and tuna).

Vitamin B1 (Thiamin): Important for energy metabolism, cellular function, and a wide variety of organ functions. Sources include organ meat, pork, seeds, squash, fish (especially trout, mackerel, salmon, and tuna), and legumes.

Vitamin B2 (Riboflavin): Helps in the production of two other B vitamins (B3 and B6) and serves an important role in energy metabolism. It also acts as an antioxidant. Rich sources include organ meat, mushrooms, leafy green vegetables, eggs, legumes, and squash.

Vitamin B3 (Niacin): Helps improve circulation, aids the body in manufacturing various stress- and sex-related hormones, and suppresses inflammation. Excellent sources include organ meat, poultry, fish and shellfish, red meat (including beef and lamb), mushrooms, and leafy green vegetables.

Vitamin B5 (Pantothenic Acid): Along with assisting in energy metabolism (like all B vitamins), vitamin B5 plays a role in manufacturing red blood cells, sex hormones, and stress hormones. It also helps maintain a healthy digestive tract and allows the body to use vitamin B2. Vitamin B5 is found in organ meat, mushrooms, oily fish, avocados, red meat (especially beef and lamb), and seeds.

Vitamin B6 (Pyridoxine): Important for cell metabolism and the production of hemoglobin, which carries oxygen in the blood. It's also vital for producing the key neurotransmitters GABA, dopamine, and serotonin. Sources include a wide variety of plant and animal foods, including leafy and root vegetables, bananas, red meat, poultry, and seeds (especially sunflower and pumpkin).

Vitamin B9 (Folate): Plays an important role in methylation (the process of adding a methyl group to different molecules), making it a key player in methylation-dependent processes like detoxification and neuron signaling. Folate is also crucial for cardiovascular health, reproductive function (especially protecting against neural tube defects), and red blood cell production. Rich sources include organ meat, green vegetables (both leafy and non-leafy), legumes, beets, avocados, and certain fruits, such as papayas, strawberries, and pomegranates.

Vitamin B12 (Cobalamin): Involved in energy metabolism, like the other B vitamins, but also plays a unique role in DNA production. It's vital for maintaining cardiovascular, brain, and nervous system health. Because vitamin B12 is manufactured exclusively by microorganisms, it's found mostly in animal foods that concentrate bacterially produced B12 in their cells, such as fish (especially sardines, salmon, tuna, and cod), shellfish such as shrimp and scallops, organ meat, beef, eggs, and poultry. Some fermented soy products like tempeh also contain vitamin B12.

Biotin: A B-complex vitamin involved in many metabolic pathways, especially fat and sugar metabolism. It also helps maintain skin and hair health. Foods high in biotin include eggs, liver, nuts such as almonds and walnuts, root vegetables, and tomatoes.

Choline: Plays an essential role in building cell membranes. It also serves as the backbone for a neurotransmitter called acetylcholine, which is involved in heart health, gut motility, and muscle movement. Choline is abundant in foods such as fish and shellfish, liver, eggs, poultry, and green vegetables (both leafy and non-leafy).

Vitamin C: A potent antioxidant that's necessary for immune system function and the function of several enzymes (like some that help make collagen, which is why vitamin C deficiency causes scurvy). Foods rich in vitamin C include bell peppers, leafy dark green vegetables, citrus fruits, and other fruits such as papaya, cantaloupe, guava, and berries. Some organ meats are also good sources of vitamin C.

Vitamin D: A fat-soluble vitamin that assists in calcium absorption, immune system function, bone development, modulation of cell growth, neuromuscular function, and the reduction of inflammation. Although vitamin D can be produced when the sun's UV rays hit the skin and trigger vitamin D synthesis, it can also be obtained from foods, including oily fish (such as salmon, tuna, and mackerel), mushrooms, fish roe, liver, and eggs.

Vitamin E: Actually a group of eight fat-soluble antioxidants, the most well-known of which is alpha-tocopherol. All forms of vitamin E help protect against free-radical damage, reduce the harmful oxidation of LDL cholesterol particles in the bloodstream, and boost cardiovascular health. Foods high in vitamin E include nuts, seeds, leafy green vegetables, fatty fish, organ meat, and oily plant foods like avocados and olives.

Vitamin K: Central to maintaining bone health and critical for making important proteins in the body that are involved in blood clotting and metabolism (in fact, that's where the "K" comes from—the German word for blood clotting, koagulation). Vitamin K exists in the forms of K1, K2, and K3, and, in the form of K2, boosts cardiovascular health. The richest sources of vitamin K include cruciferous vegetables (such as broccoli, cauliflower, cabbage, and Brussels sprouts) and leafy dark green vegetables (such as spinach, collard greens, parsley, and Swiss chard), as well as asparagus. Vitamin K2, specifically, is found in natto (a fermented soybean product), eggs, fish, butter, and liver.

Boron: Supports bone health and is essential for the utilization of vitamin D and calcium in the body. Food sources include nuts, avocados, leafy green vegetables, legumes, and a variety of other vegetables and fruits, such as apples, carrots, broccoli, pears, and olives.

Calcium: In addition to forming bone, calcium is essential to many processes within cells, as well as neurotransmitter release and muscle contraction (including the beating of your heart!). Foods rich in calcium include dark green vegetables, whole sesame seeds, dairy products, whole sardines (bones included), and squash.

Chlorine: Required for the production of hydrochloric acid in the stomach and important for electrolyte balance and fluid balance in the body. Foods high in chloride ions include seaweed, tomatoes, olives, celery, and lettuce, although most foods contain at least small amounts.

Chromium: Important for sugar and fat metabolism and particularly critical for blood sugar control. Chromium is found in small amounts in every food group but is most abundant in foods such as oysters, liver, broccoli, green beans, leafy green vegetables, mushrooms, and tomatoes.

Copper: Involved in the absorption, storage, and metabolism of iron and the formation of red blood cells. It's also important for building strong tissue and producing cellular energy. Excellent sources include oysters and other shellfish, legumes, nuts, organ meat, and mushrooms.

Iodine: A constituent of thyroid hormones, iodine thus has diverse essential roles in the body. It is also important for lactation and plays a part in supporting the immune system. Sources include sea vegetables (especially brown varieties such as kelp and wakame), fish, shellfish, eggs, and dairy products.

Iron: A key component of hemoglobin, the protein in the blood that binds to oxygen and transports it throughout the body. It's also important for supporting energy production and proper metabolism in muscles and active organs. You can find iron in foods such as liver, dark leafy greens, red meat, legumes, and olives.

Magnesium: Necessary for cell life. More than 300 different enzymes need magnesium to work, including every enzyme that uses or synthesizes ATP (the basic energy molecule in a cell) and enzymes that synthesize DNA and RNA. It also enhances control of inflammation and maintains nervous system balance. Foods rich in magnesium include green vegetables, nuts and seeds, fish, legumes, and avocados.

Manganese: Necessary for enzymes that protect the body from and repair damage caused by free radicals. This mineral is important for bone production, skin integrity, and blood sugar control. Foods high in manganese include fish and shellfish, nuts and seeds, legumes, leafy dark green vegetables, and cruciferous vegetables (such as broccoli, cauliflower, cabbage, kale, Brussels sprouts, and turnip greens).

Molybdenum: Necessary for activity of key enzymes that perform detoxification functions in the liver and plays an important role in nervous system metabolism. It is found in foods such as legumes, eggs, tomatoes, lettuce, and a variety of other vegetables, including celery, fennel, and cucumbers.

Phosphorus: Plays a role in every metabolic reaction in the body and is important for the metabolism of fats, carbohydrates, and proteins. It also serves a central function in bone support. Phosphorous is abundant in protein-rich foods such as dairy products, fish, shellfish, seeds, and legumes.

Potassium: Critical for the function of every cell; it is necessary for nerve function, cardiac function, and muscle contraction. As an electrolyte, it helps conduct electrical charges in the body. Rich sources include leafy dark green vegetables, cruciferous vegetables, some fruits (such as bananas and cantaloupe), legumes, and many orange vegetables (such as carrots, squash, and sweet potatoes).

Sodium: Necessary for electrolyte balance; for regulating blood pressure, volume, and pH; for controlling the movement of fluids across cell membranes; and for neuron function. Along with any food doused in table salt or cured in salt, such as olives and some meats, natural sources of sodium include seaweed, celery, turnips, artichokes, and some leafy green vegetables, such as spinach and collard greens. Too much sodium isn't a good thing, so it's preferable to get your sodium from whole food sources and conservative use of unrefined sea salt.

Selenium: Required for the activity of 25 to 30 different enzymes that protect the brain and other tissues from oxidative damage. It also helps support normal thyroid function. Good sources include red meat, poultry, fish and shellfish, Brazil nuts, and mushrooms.

Silicon: Required for the formation of connective tissues and bone and supports the health of hair, nails, and skin. Foods featuring this mineral include bananas, string beans, legumes, apples, and cabbage.

Sulfur: Widely used in biochemical processes, sulfur is a structural component of many proteins and is necessary for the function of many enzymes and antioxidants. Sulfur is abundant in cruciferous vegetables (including cabbage, broccoli, cauliflower, and Brussels sprouts), alliums such as onions and garlic, eggs, and other protein-rich animal foods, such as fish, meat, and poultry.

Zinc: Important for nearly every cellular function, from protein and carbohydrate metabolism to cell division and growth. It also plays a role in skin health and maintaining sensory organs (that's why zinc deficiency is associated with loss of smell and taste) and is a vital nutrient for immune system function. The richest source of zinc is oysters, but other good sources include red meat, poultry, nuts and seeds, and legumes.

When we consider the foods richest in essential vitamins and minerals, certain foods keep coming up again and again as powerhouses of nutrition, especially liver and other organ meat, seafood (especially shellfish), and vegetables of all kinds, but notably leafy greens and vegetables from the cruciferous family (which includes cabbage, broccoli, and kale). One of the best things we can do to ensure that our diet is abounding with micronutrients is to eat these foods liberally!

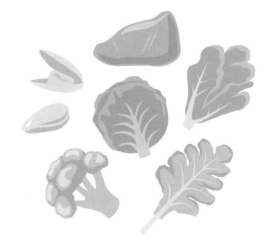

amino acids

Vitamins and minerals aren't the only essential micronutrients, however. Amino acids are the basic building blocks of protein, which forms a substantial percentage of our bodies. Nine of the twenty amino acids that our bodies use to make proteins are considered *nutritionally indispensable,* meaning that we absolutely have to get them from food—our bodies can't make them. A further six amino acids are considered *conditionally indispensable,* meaning that while other amino acids can be converted into these, the process is so inefficient that most of the time we still need to get these from food. The remaining five amino acids are considered *nutritionally dispensable,* meaning that our bodies can make them in sufficient quantities provided there's enough protein in our diets. While technically we only need to get the nine essential amino acids through diet—our bodies can create the remaining eleven—it is far preferable from a health standpoint to get all of the amino acids from foods. That way, we don't have to rely on oftentimes inefficient conversion processes for the amino acids our bodies need to make all the various proteins in our cells and tissues.

Complete proteins provide sufficient quantities of all nine essential amino acids, and for the most part, these come from animals—meat, eggs, seafood, and dairy, for instance, are all complete proteins. Most plant foods are not complete proteins, and it's not usually easy for our bodies to fully digest and break down plant proteins in order to absorb the amino acids they include. All proteins from animal foods are easier to digest than proteins from plant foods, and the easiest-to-digest protein is found in fish and shellfish, followed by meat and poultry. While plant foods are extremely important for health, it's misleading to think of them as a good protein source—even legumes, nuts, and seeds, which technically contain way more protein than fruits and vegetables, are not as rich in protein as animal foods. Animal foods contain all twenty amino acids and are also the only sources of some other key nutrients, including vitamin B12, creatine (see page 32), taurine, and carnosine (while these last three are not considered essential, they are very important and help promote health). Therefore, a micronutrient-sufficient diet must include fish and shellfish at the very least, if not a wide variety of meats.

fatty acids

There are also two essential fatty acids, the building blocks of fats, which are used not only for energy but also for many basic structures in the human body, such as the outer membrane of every single cell. The rather-arbitrarily-assigned-yet-officially-deemed-essential fatty acids are alpha-linolenic acid (ALA; the smallest omega-3 polyunsaturated fatty acid) and linoleic acid (LA; the smallest omega-6 polyunsaturated fatty acid).

The term *essential* is misleading here. The fatty acids with the most profound roles in the human body are arachidonic acid (AA), an omega-6 polyunsaturated fatty acid, and eicosapentaenoic acid (EPA) and docosahexaenoic acid (DHA), both omega-3 polyunsaturated fatty acids. Our bodies can convert any omega-6 polyunsaturated fatty acid to any other omega-6 polyunsaturated fatty acid, and similarly, we can convert any omega-3 polyunsaturated fatty acid to any other omega-3 polyunsaturated fatty acid—which means that we can make EPA and DHA from ALA and AA from LA. But that conversion can be extremely inefficient, so it's important to get these from food. While ALA and LA are abundant in plant foods, AA, EPA, and DHA are found in seafood, meat, and poultry.

It's also worth noting that the body does best when the ratio of omega-6 fatty acids to omega-3 fatty acids in our diets is somewhere in the range of 3:1 to 1:1. This is one of the exceptions to the "more is always better" approach to micronutrients. Achieving this ideal ratio of omega-6 to omega-3 requires a fair bit of attention to food choices. Omega-6s are abundant in grains, legumes, nuts, seeds, processed "vegetable" oils (like safflower oil or canola oil), poultry (even organic!), and industrially produced meat (the kind that doesn't say "grass-fed" or "pasture-raised" on the package). On the other hand, the extremely important omega-3s DHA and EPA are found in substantial quantities only in grass-fed meat and seafood (mainly fish and shellfish, but sea vegetables and algae also contain some DHA). Balancing the intake of these fats requires both lowering the amount of omega-6-rich foods in our diets and conscientiously including more seafood.

Study after study shows that increasing consumption of DHA and EPA, whether via diet or short-term intervention with fish oil supplements, reduces disease severity and symptoms—for instance, it reduces the symptoms of rheumatoid arthritis—and lowers the risk of developing certain diseases, such as cardiovascular disease.

the problems with supplements

But why is it important to get micronutrients from foods? Can't we just take a good multivitamin and a fish oil supplement to cover all our bases and then eat whatever we want? Unfortunately, no. There are several reasons why you can't supplement your way out of a bad diet.

First, the micronutrients in supplements tend to be poorly absorbed, and some synthetic forms of vitamins can't even be readily used by our bodies. In the case of fish oil, the process of extracting the oils can damage them, and studies show that they only benefit health for a fairly short time, about four to six weeks, beyond which they either no longer provide a benefit or may even be detrimental. Second, supplements contain only nutrients that have been identified as the most essential and don't include other extremely important (although maybe not technically essential) nutrients. Given how little we really know about what each nutrient does in our bodies, it seems a bit premature to be trying to extract them into pill form.

Another issue to consider is that many nutrients work synergistically: they need to be consumed in specific combinations in order to be most effective at enhancing health. At the same time, some nutrients compete with each other, either for absorption or for use (this competition is an important way that the body regulates certain chemical reactions), so consuming those nutrients together in the same supplement means you benefit from none of them. Our understanding of these relationships between nutrients is still limited, but one thing we do know is that whole foods tend to have the right combinations of nutrients to be most effective. It is always better to get nutrients from whole foods. And it is always better to choose those foods that are abundant in nutrients.

going beyond the basics

Even following a standard Paleo diet is not a guarantee that you're getting all of the micronutrients that you need to be healthy. And while the foods endorsed by the Paleo diet represent the most nutrient-dense foods in our food supply, reaching micronutrient sufficiency still requires commitment. In fact, analyses of typical Paleo food choices reveal that biotin (especially abundant in liver and root vegetables), calcium (especially abundant in its most bioavailable form in dark leafy greens like kale, as well as in whole fish like sardines) and chromium (especially abundant in dark leafy greens, oysters, and liver) are commonly deficient on the Paleo diet. While the Paleo diet far outstrips other dietary approaches in terms of micronutrient sufficiency, if you just stick to the stereotypical meat and veggies, you may be missing out on important nutrients for optimal health.

Taking a nutrients-first approach to diet means eating organ meat, other high-quality meats, seafood, a wide variety of vegetables in large portions, and some fruit. When those foods form the foundation of our diets, we guarantee that we're consuming all the nutrients our bodies need to thrive.

functional foods

Functional foods provide health benefits beyond basic nutrition. In a way, the entire Paleo diet is focused on functional foods. As soon as we focus on micronutrient-rich foods, we're talking about foods that benefit health beyond basic nutrition. Functional foods include all those rich in the following:

· **Plant phytochemicals,** which support the immune system and fight aging

· **Dietary fiber,** including prebiotics and resistant starch, which improves digestion, regulates hormones, and supports a healthy gut microbiome, thereby supporting immune health

· **Functional lipids,** like omega-3 fatty acids and conjugated linoleic acid, which have many beneficial effects on human health, such as supporting immune health, bone health, brain health, and cardiovascular health

· **Vitamins and minerals,** which are crucial for the health of every cell and every system

Sound familiar? Yep, we're talking about seafood, vegetables, fruit, meat, eggs, nuts, and seeds—all foods that provide a range of health benefits thanks to so many great micronutrients and other health-promoting compounds. Go, Paleo!

There are a variety of diet programs, meal replacement bars and beverages, and multivitamins that focus on providing 100 percent of the recommended dietary allowance of all the essential micronutrients. While this is, of course, extremely important, it's also a myopic approach to nutrition. If we focus only on those nutrients currently known to be essential, we miss out on the huge variety of nonessential yet amazingly important nutrients that we've already identified, as well as any nutrients that haven't been discovered yet.

In many ways, the importance of functional foods is another endorsement for a whole foods–based diet. When we eat foods as they appear in nature, unprocessed and without manipulation other than cooking, we benefit from their vast array of nutrients.

It's also another endorsement for eating a variety of vegetables, which are fantastic functional foods. As we examine the nutrients in functional foods, how they relate to our health, and what foods are abundant sources of them, we start to see a strong pattern emerging: vegetables are an essential part of any healthy diet. In fact, study after study shows that higher vegetable consumption (at least five servings a day) reduces the risk of disease, everything from diabetes to osteoporosis to diseases of the gastrointestinal tract to cardiovascular disease to autoimmune disease to cancer. There are three likely reasons. First, vegetables tend to be rich in very important vitamins and minerals, including the most absorbable form of calcium. Second, vegetables contain plenty of fiber to support a healthy diversity of gut microorganisms. Third, vegetables are rich in thousands of different beneficial plant phytochemicals. Phytochemicals abound in antioxidant, anti-inflammatory, and other health-promoting properties, and this giant class of chemicals forms a large proportion of the known micronutrients in functional foods.

The micronutrients that make functional foods such important contributors to better health aren't considered essential, yet study after study shows that they lead to better health. We might not die if we don't eat them, but we certainly can't thrive without them.

Again, there are some functional foods superstars. Cruciferous vegetables (such as cabbage, broccoli, kale, cauliflower, and Brussels sprouts) find their way onto functional-food lists over and over again. Other foods that shine are leafy greens; highly pigmented fruits like berries (think fruits that stain your clothes); seafood of all kinds, including fish, shellfish, and sea vegetables; and grass-fed meat.

It should be comforting to know that focusing on micronutrient-rich whole foods is a strategy that delivers not only all of the essential nutrients but also the full range of other health-promoting nutrients. And it certainly reinforces the idea that a diet based on seafood, quality meats, tons of vegetables, and some fruit is the way to go!

what's in functional foods

CAROTENOIDS: These potent antioxidants play an important role in immune system function. The specific carotenoids outlined here also have different health benefits. Foods rich in carotenoids include anything red, orange, or yellow (like tomatoes, carrots, beets, sweet potatoes, and bell peppers) or dark green (like kale, spinach, collard greens, and broccoli). All carotenoids are best absorbed when eaten with some fat.

Beta-carotene: Helps neutralize free radicals, boosts antioxidant defenses, and can be converted to vitamin A by the body. Excellent sources include orange foods like carrots, sweet potatoes, and cantaloupe, as well as leafy green vegetables like Swiss chard, spinach, and beet greens.

Lycopene: Helps support prostate health, including potentially protecting against prostate cancer. The best sources are tomatoes (especially tomatoes that have been cooked or crushed, which makes the lycopene more bioavailable), watermelon, papaya, and red or pink grapefruit.

Lutein and Zeaxanthin: Vital for eye health and vision (they're abundantly concentrated in the retina) and may decrease the risk of age-related macular degeneration. Rich sources include leafy dark green vegetables (especially kale, spinach, and collards), eggs, orange bell peppers, citrus fruits, and broccoli.

DIALLYL SULFIDE: A compound released by crushing garlic and other alliums. It has potent antimicrobial effects (including acting against the stomach ulcer bacteria *H. pylori*), reduces risk of cardiovascular disease, and may be responsible for the protective effect that garlic has against colorectal cancer. Foods containing diallyl sulfide include garlic, onions, chives, shallots, scallions, and leeks.

DITHIOLETHIONES: A class of cancer-protective compounds that also induce detoxification. Sources of dithiolethiones include cruciferous vegetables such as broccoli, collard greens, kale, and cabbage.

POLYPHENOLS: A class of chemical compounds with antioxidant properties, helping prevent cell damage from free radicals and potentially reducing the risk of heart disease and other chronic diseases. Rich sources include berries, citrus fruits, brightly colored vegetables, dark chocolate, and plums.

Lignans: A type of polyphenol that can be metabolized by intestinal bacteria into enterodiol and enterolactone, which may play a role in preventing osteoporosis, cardiovascular disease, and hormone-associated cancers (breast, endometrial, ovarian, and prostate). Foods high in lignans include flax seeds, sesame seeds, legumes, and cruciferous vegetables.

PLANT STEROLS AND STANOLS: With a similar chemical structure to animal cholesterol, these compounds can block the absorption of cholesterol in the small intestine and reduce levels of LDL ("bad") cholesterol in the blood without altering levels of HDL ("good") cholesterol. Sources of plant sterols and stanols include nuts, legumes, and most fruits and vegetables.

ISOTHIOCYANATES: Sulfur-containing plant chemicals with strong anticancer properties due to their ability to help suppress tumor formation and eliminate carcinogens from the body. Foods with isothiocyanates include cruciferous vegetables such as broccoli, cabbage, cauliflower, kale, and Brussels sprouts, especially when eaten raw.

Sulforaphane: A type of isothiocyanate that works by increasing the body's natural defenses against oxidative stress, inflammation, and DNA damage. Along with potent antioxidant and anticancer properties, it has the potential to assist in cardiovascular health by improving blood cholesterol and reducing high blood pressure. Its main sources are cruciferous vegetables, including broccoli (the richest source), cabbage, Brussels sprouts, and cauliflower.

FLAVONOIDS: A class of more than 6,000 compounds with a range of health effects, including reducing inflammation, protecting against smoking-related cancers, and reducing cardiovascular disease risk. They also have antibacterial properties. Foods rich in flavonoids include parsley, berries (especially blueberries), citrus fruits, peanuts with the skin on, and cocoa.

Anthocyanins: A type of flavonoid responsible for red, purple, and blue pigments in plant foods. They may help protect against liver injuries, reduce blood pressure, maintain vision and eye health, counteract compounds in cooked food that cause DNA mutation, and suppress the proliferation of cancer cells. Foods containing anthocyanins include berries (especially blueberries, cranberries, blackberries, and raspberries), grapes, red cabbage, cherries, and eggplant.

Flavanols: Also called *flavan-3-ols,* these are a type of flavonoid that may reduce risk of certain chronic diseases and help maintain the elasticity of blood vessels, which helps support normal blood flow. Foods rich in flavanols include apples, bananas, berries, peaches, and pears.

Proanthocyanidins: A class of flavanols that act as antioxidants while also making other antioxidants more effective (for instance, they prolong the shelf life of vitamin C). Proanthocyanidins are found in grapes, cranberries, black currants, and elderberries.

Procyanidins: A class of flavanols (and subtype of proanthocyanidins) that play a potential role in preventing cancer and cardiovascular disease and may be partly responsible for the protective effects of red wine. Sources include grapes and other dark-skinned fruits (like black currants and elderberries), apples, cranberries, and chocolate.

Flavonols: A category of flavonoids that may help reduce the risk of cardiovascular disease, cancer, and stroke due to their antioxidant effects. Sources include onions, apples, tomatoes, sweet potatoes, and almonds.

Kaempferol: A type of flavonol with a wide range of potential health effects, including reducing inflammation, reducing the risk of type 2 diabetes, reducing cardiovascular disease mortality, and interrupting the growth of a variety of cancers (breast, ovarian, bladder, prostate, colorectal, lung, gastric, pancreatic, and leukemia). It also exhibits antimicrobial activity. Foods containing kaempferol include cruciferous vegetables (such as broccoli, cabbage, and kale), apples, grapes, tomatoes, and onions.

Myricetin: A type of flavonol with the potential to protect cells from carcinogenic mutations, protect neurons from oxidative stress, reduce osteoporosis risk, reduce inflammation, and inhibit the activity of a number of viruses, including HIV. Myricetin is found in cruciferous vegetables (such as broccoli, cabbage, and kale), chia seeds, garlic, peppers, and guava.

Quercetin: A type of flavonol that may suppress inflammation in the brain, reduce high blood pressure, and protect neurons from oxidative stress. Sources include onions, watercress, cilantro, capers, and radicchio.

Flavonones: One of the largest subgroups of flavonoids, these may play a role in protecting against or treating cardiovascular disease and cancer, as well as maintaining bone health and neurological health. Foods high in flavonones include oranges, lemons, tomatoes, and grapefruit.

UBIQUINOL: A reduced, more bioavailable form of the vitaminlike compound coenzyme Q10. It is a potent antioxidant and may be helpful in treating or preventing heart and blood vessel conditions, diabetes, gum disease, muscular dystrophy, chronic fatigue syndrome, and breast cancer. Foods containing ubiquinol include beef, pork, mackerel, yellowtail fish, and chicken, and in smaller amounts it's also found in vegetables like broccoli and parsley.

FIBER: A carbohydrate present in plant cell walls that our bodies can't digest. It provides us a variety of benefits by:

- feeding beneficial probiotic bacteria in our digestive tracts

- binding with toxins, hormones, bile salts, cholesterol, and other substances in the gut

- stimulating the release of some hormones (like the hunger hormone ghrelin, which signals satiety to the brain) and some neurotransmitters (like melatonin, which helps control sleep)

- adding bulk to the stool, which improves the quality of bowel movements

Diets rich in fiber reduce the risk of cardiovascular disease and of many cancers (especially colorectal cancer, but also liver cancer, pancreatic cancer, and others), and promote overall lower inflammation. In fact, the higher your intake of fiber, the lower your inflammation. If you have kidney disease or diabetes, a high-fiber diet reduces your risk of mortality. High fiber intake can even reduce your chances of dying from an infection. Fiber is broadly categorized as soluble or insoluble (that is, whether or not it dissolves in water), and each class of fiber has different health benefits. In general, foods that are high in fiber include fruit (especially berries), vegetables (especially leafy green vegetables, root vegetables, and cruciferous vegetables), legumes, and nuts and seeds.

Soluble Fiber: This type of fiber forms a gel-like material in the gut and tends to slow the movement of material through the digestive system. Soluble fiber is typically readily fermented by the bacteria in the colon (although not all soluble fibers are fermentable), producing gases and physiologically active by-products (like short-chain fatty acids, which yield a variety of health benefits and vitamins). Soluble fiber also has cholesterol-lowering properties. Rich sources include apples, berries, pears, citrus fruits, and legumes.

Insoluble Fiber: This type of fiber tends to speed up the movement of material through the digestive system. Fermentable insoluble fibers also produce gases and physiologically active by-products (like short-chain fatty acids and vitamins). Unfermentable insoluble fiber increases stool bulk by absorbing water as it moves through the digestive tract, which is believed to be very beneficial in regulating bowel movements and managing constipation. Insoluble fiber reduces inflammation. It also binds to toxins and surplus hormones in the gastrointestinal tract, facilitating their elimination from the body. Foods high in insoluble fiber include leafy green vegetables, bell peppers, cruciferous vegetables (such as broccoli, bok choy, cauliflower, and Brussels sprouts), celery, and carrots.

GLYCINE: A conditionally indispensable amino acid that plays a number of beneficial roles in the body and may help improve sleep quality, enhance memory, regulate bile acids, and assist in the synthesis of several extremely important proteins. It may also help reverse age-related damage to fibroblasts, a type of cell in connective tissues that produces collagen, and as a result, may have antiaging effects. Foods containing glycine include high-protein animal products (fish, meat, poultry, and dairy), spinach, legumes, squash, and cruciferous vegetables.

GLUTAMINE: A conditionally indispensable amino acid that can help improve intestinal barrier function and reduce intestinal permeability (which may be associated with many chronic diseases), treat mood disorders, prevent disease-related weight loss, and reduce infection risk. Rich sources include high-protein animal products (fish, meat, poultry, and dairy), legumes, spinach, beets, and parsley.

ALANINE: A nutritionally dispensable amino acid that's involved in sugar and acid metabolism and can potentially increase exercise capacity, help build lean muscle mass, and improve immunity. Foods high in alanine include animal products (fish, meat, poultry, and dairy), legumes, nuts, and seeds.

ARGININE: A conditionally indispensable amino acid that plays a vital role in cell division, wound healing, hormone release, and immune function. Arginine is found in both plant and animal foods, including dairy products, meat, poultry, seafood, nuts, and legumes.

PROLINE: A conditionally indispensable amino acid that's used in collagen production and helps maintain healthy skin, joints, tendons, and cardiac muscle. Foods high in proline include dairy products, meat, poultry, eggs, and seafood, as well as some vegetables like broccoli and cabbage.

CREATINE: Helps supply energy to cells, especially muscle cells. It may help increase muscle strength, boost functional performance, and reduce DNA mutation. Foods high in creatine include animal products like meat, dairy, eggs, poultry, and seafood.

DHA (Docosahexaenoic Acid): An omega-3 fatty acid that's abundant in the brain and retina and that plays a role in maintaining normal brain function, treating mood disorders, and reducing risk of heart disease (or improving outcomes for people who already have it). The richest sources are shellfish and fatty fish, such as salmon, mackerel, tuna, herring, and sardines.

EPA (Eicosapentaenoic Acid): An omega-3 fatty acid that plays a role in anti-inflammatory processes and the health of cell membranes and may help reduce symptoms of depression. Sources include fatty fish (such as salmon, mackerel, tuna, herring, and sardines), shellfish, purslane, and algae.

CLA (Conjugated Linoleic Acids): A family of fatty acids that exhibit strong anticancer effects and may improve bone density and increase muscle mass. CLAs are found in ruminant meat, such as beef, lamb, elk, and goat, as well as dairy from grass-fed animals.

MONOUNSATURATED FATTY ACIDS (MUFA): A type of fat that may help reduce LDL ("bad") cholesterol while potentially increasing HDL ("good") cholesterol and that may help improve blood sugar control. Foods rich in MUFA include olives, tree nuts like almonds, avocados, and seeds.

the dark side of foods

There are some micronutrient-rich foods that are not included in either the Paleo diet or the Autoimmune Protocol. It seems counterintuitive at first, but some foods that contain compelling amounts of beneficial nutrition are not great choices for those battling chronic illnesses. The problem usually comes down the food's indigestibility and therefore the body's inability to access the beneficial nutrients it contains, and/or the presence of a few chemicals that may actually undermine health.

Foods can be difficult to digest in two ways: the molecular structure of compounds in the food may be incompatible with our body's digestive enzymes, or the food may contain compounds that block our digestive enzymes from working. Digestive enzymes are produced in the mouth, stomach, and pancreas and do their work of breaking down carbohydrates into simple sugars, proteins into amino acids, and fats into fatty acids in the small intestine, liberating vitamins, minerals, and phytochemicals along the way. As we've discussed, many plant proteins are difficult for our body to digest, and this is because their amino acid structures are simply not compatible with our digestive enzymes. This is especially true of legumes and grains. We can't access the nutrients in foods we can't digest, and beyond that, undigested or incompletely digested foods can cause the wrong types or amounts of bacteria to grow in our digestive tracts. Plus, some plants—like legumes, grains, nuts, and seeds—contain relatively high amounts of digestive enzyme inhibitors, compounds that block the activity of our digestive enzymes, thereby inhibiting digestion, and that can damage the gut. Furthermore, compounds called *antinutrients* that block absorption of essential nutrients are present in many of these same plant foods. Beyond supporting health with adequate nutrition, any health-promoting diet must exclude foods that can be problematic for our health. Most of us aren't used to thinking of foods in these terms. Certainly, we understand that fast food and junk food might make us gain weight or raise our cholesterol levels, but we don't typically think of

> *A healthy diet isn't just about eating more of the good; it's also about avoiding the bad.*

them as contributing to our diagnosed health conditions. Type 2 diabetes is likely the only exception: most of us recognize that diabetes is linked to our food choices (although probably not the extent to which the link truly exists). The fact is, there is an alarming number of compounds in common foods that are known to negatively impact our health. And unfortunately, they are not considered in most diets or nutrition guidelines.

This may be one of the biggest differences between the Paleo diet and other dietary approaches that focus on micronutrient sufficiency. The Paleo diet goes beyond making sure that our bodies have the resources they need to be healthy to also omit problematic foods—meaning any food that has the capacity to undermine our health, whether by increasing inflammation, damaging the gut, negatively affecting hormones, or causing other problems. A healthy diet isn't just about eating more of the good; it's also about avoiding the bad.

foods that cause inflammation

As we'll discuss in more detail in chapter 2, inflammation is a contributor to all chronic illnesses and sometimes is even the outright cause of the illness. Resolving inflammation is key in mitigating and reversing these conditions. Plenty of things in our lives cause inflammation, from infection and toxin exposure to more mundane things like staying up late and being under a lot of stress, so the last thing we need is for the foods we eat to be adding fuel to the fire.

Some foods are inherently inflammatory. It's actually quite surprising just how many different ways foods can cause inflammation. Processed foods, fast food, foods made with processed "vegetable" oils, grains, and legumes are all high in omega-6 fatty acids, which control cell signaling that turns on inflammation (via the production of specific paracrine and autocrine cell-signaling molecules). We discussed the ideal ratio of omega-6 to omega-3 in our diets on page 27, and when that ratio is off balance—as it often is when we eat these rich sources of omega-6s—omega-3s can't effectively counteract the inflammatory effect of omega-6s by producing different, less-inflammatory cell-signaling molecules.

In addition, both high blood sugar and high insulin levels in the blood propel inflammation, so any food that is high in refined carbohydrates, sugars, and starches that hit the bloodstream quickly (owing to the absence of compounds in the food that slow the digestion of carbohydrates) is inflammatory. These foods also negatively impact many hormones, thanks to all the effects that insulin has in the body. Insulin is a hormone that affects many other hormones and organ systems in the human body, and having insulin in the happy-medium range is critical for health. Excess refined carbohydrates also negatively impact two other important hormones: leptin and ghrelin. These hormones help control our appetite, metabolism, and immune systems.

Okay, so there go processed foods, fast food, and junk food. But then, those foods were already on the blacklist because they don't possess any nutritionally redeeming properties. What's less commonly known is that many foods considered to be healthy, like multigrain bread and low-fat dairy products, also spike blood sugar and insulin levels, and several compounds found in grains (even whole grains), legumes, and nightshades (see page 55) are inflammatory. Compounds called *agglutinins* (particularly wheat germ agglutinin, kidney bean lectin, soybean lectin, tomato lectin, and peanut lectin) and *glycoalkaloids* (found in nightshades such as tomatoes, potatoes, eggplants, and peppers) are such potent inducers of inflammation and stimulators of the immune system that several of these compounds have been investigated for use in chemotherapy or for use in vaccines as adjuvants, chemicals added to vaccines to ramp up the immune system. They're a necessary aspect of how vaccines work, but not a desirable property of food!

foods that damage the gut

Some foods are inherently damaging to the gut, usually because they either harm the beneficial microorganisms that live in the digestive tract or damage or alter the cells that form the gut barrier, whose job is to transport nutrients to the bloodstream while stopping everything else from getting in.

The microorganisms that live in our gut are essential to our health. They help us digest food, they produce chemicals that improve the health of the cells that form our gut barrier (thus promoting gut barrier health), they directly regulate our immune system, and they can even influence brain health by producing neuroactive chemicals that are absorbed into the bloodstream and travel to the brain. A healthy diversity of the right kinds of microorganisms in the gut is one of the most fundamental aspects of good health. Beyond eating plenty of fiber to support their growth, it's also important to avoid foods that promote the growth of the wrong kinds of bacteria. Grains, dairy, legumes, nightshades, and alcohol are all known to contain compounds that can hinder the growth of beneficial strains of bacteria while supporting the growth of undesirable strains of bacteria, like *E. coli*. When too many of the wrong types of bacteria grow in our guts, a situation called *gut dysbiosis*, digestion is hindered, the health and function of the gut barrier becomes impaired, and the immune system is stimulated.

There are two main ways foods directly damage the gut barrier: by adversely affecting the health of the cells that form the gut barrier or by interfering with how those cells bond together. Both of these cause the barrier to become permeable, or "leaky" (hence *leaky gut syndrome*, the umbrella term for chronic diseases associated with this problem). Many compounds that are supposed to stay inside the gut (like toxins, waste products, and even otherwise beneficial microorganisms) are able to pass into the body, where they can stimulate the immune system, 80 percent of which resides in the tissues surrounding the gut and whose job it is to attack foreign invaders like these. But an immune system that's chronically stimulated can end up attacking not just invaders but also body tissues, which can contribute to many chronic illnesses and result in autoimmune disease. (These mechanisms, as well as other ways certain foods can undermine your health and many related topics, are described in much more detail in Sarah's book *The Paleo Approach*.)

Grains, legumes, dairy, nuts, seeds, and nightshades all contain substances that increase the permeability of the gut either directly, by damaging the cells that form the gut barrier or opening up the bonds between them, or indirectly, by feeding the wrong kinds of microorganisms in the gut. These harmful substances include prolamins (like gluten) and agglutinins, digestive enzyme inhibitors, glycoalkaloids, and phytic acid.

How harmful these substances are probably varies greatly from individual to individual. Certainly, your genetics, your nutrient sufficiency, how much sleep you get, how much stress you're under, and how active you are all affect how strongly your body responds to these foods and how quickly you recover after eating them. However, with only a few exceptions, these foods aren't making the lists of micronutrient-rich and functional foods. If you're battling chronic illness, you may benefit substantially from removing these foods from your diet. If you're simply in search of optimal health, you have nothing to lose from cutting out these foods.

weighing the good against the bad

This may be an oversimplification, but we can lump together all the health-promoting nutrients in foods as "Good Stuff" and all the health-undermining compounds in foods as "Bad Stuff." When evaluating the merits of an individual food, we can weigh how much Good Stuff is in that food versus how much Bad Stuff. Some foods have tons of Good Stuff and no Bad Stuff—these are the definite "yes" foods! We can eat plenty of them with no guilt. Other foods have tons of Bad Stuff and very little Good Stuff—these are the definite "no" foods and should be avoided the vast majority of the time.

But what about the many foods that fall somewhere in the middle? How much Bad Stuff can be tolerated for the sake of the Good Stuff in a food? And how much Good Stuff does there need to be in a food to compensate for the presence of some Bad Stuff? How do our health histories affect where we draw the line? Is genetic makeup a significant factor? Might some foods be okay if we reserve them for special occasions? And how strict do we need to be in order to mitigate chronic health problems?

Hard-and-fast answers to these questions are extremely difficult to pinpoint. The Paleo diet definitely focuses on foods that have lots of Good Stuff and little or no Bad Stuff. Yet there are plenty of foods included in the Paleo diet that fall into the gray area in between the "yes" foods and the "no" foods, such as grass-fed dairy, nuts, seeds, wine, chocolate, coffee, unrefined and natural sugars, nightshades (including tomatoes, potatoes, and peppers), and eggs. The Autoimmune Protocol is stricter about foods to avoid, eliminating all of those gray-area foods, and simultaneously requires an even greater focus on the most nutrient-dense foods. If you're pretty healthy, you'll likely prefer to start with a standard Paleo diet and see how you do before considering tweaking it. If you're struggling with chronic health problems, you may want to jump into the Autoimmune Protocol and give it a 100 percent commitment for a few months.

The Autoimmune Protocol is designed to give you the best chance of improving your health by making the vast majority of the foods you eat the most health-promoting foods available. But we are all individuals. It is quite possible that you'll do very well with some of the eliminated foods. It's even possible that you're sensitive to one of the included foods. This dietary strategy to improve health and mitigate disease should be viewed as a starting place, not a life sentence! Once you've been following the Autoimmune Protocol strictly for at least a month, we encourage you to experiment by reintroducing certain foods. The best way to do this is summarized on pages 44 and 45 (and discussed in detail in Sarah's book *The Paleo Approach*).

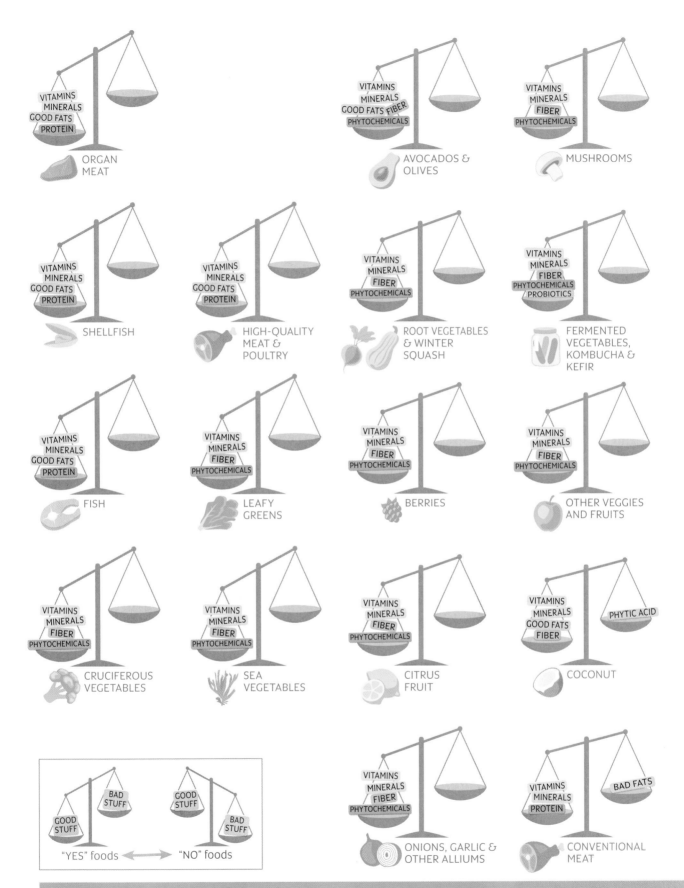

VITAMINS
MINERALS
GOOD FATS
PROTEIN
ORGAN MEAT

VITAMINS
MINERALS
GOOD FATS FIBER
PHYTOCHEMICALS
AVOCADOS & OLIVES

VITAMINS
MINERALS
FIBER
PHYTOCHEMICALS
MUSHROOMS

VITAMINS
MINERALS
GOOD FATS
PROTEIN
SHELLFISH

VITAMINS
MINERALS
GOOD FATS
PROTEIN
HIGH-QUALITY MEAT & POULTRY

VITAMINS
MINERALS
FIBER
PHYTOCHEMICALS
ROOT VEGETABLES & WINTER SQUASH

VITAMINS
MINERALS
FIBER
PHYTOCHEMICALS
PROBIOTICS
FERMENTED VEGETABLES, KOMBUCHA & KEFIR

VITAMINS
MINERALS
GOOD FATS
PROTEIN
FISH

VITAMINS
MINERALS
FIBER
PHYTOCHEMICALS
LEAFY GREENS

VITAMINS
MINERALS
FIBER
PHYTOCHEMICALS
BERRIES

VITAMINS
MINERALS
FIBER
PHYTOCHEMICALS
OTHER VEGGIES AND FRUITS

VITAMINS
MINERALS
FIBER
PHYTOCHEMICALS
CRUCIFEROUS VEGETABLES

VITAMINS
MINERALS
FIBER
PHYTOCHEMICALS
SEA VEGETABLES

VITAMINS
MINERALS
FIBER
PHYTOCHEMICALS
CITRUS FRUIT

VITAMINS
MINERALS
GOOD FATS
FIBER
PHYTIC ACID
COCONUT

BAD STUFF / GOOD STUFF
GOOD STUFF / BAD STUFF
"YES" foods ⟷ "NO" foods

VITAMINS
MINERALS
FIBER
PHYTOCHEMICALS
ONIONS, GARLIC & OTHER ALLIUMS

VITAMINS
MINERALS
PROTEIN
BAD FATS
CONVENTIONAL MEAT

"Yes" foods

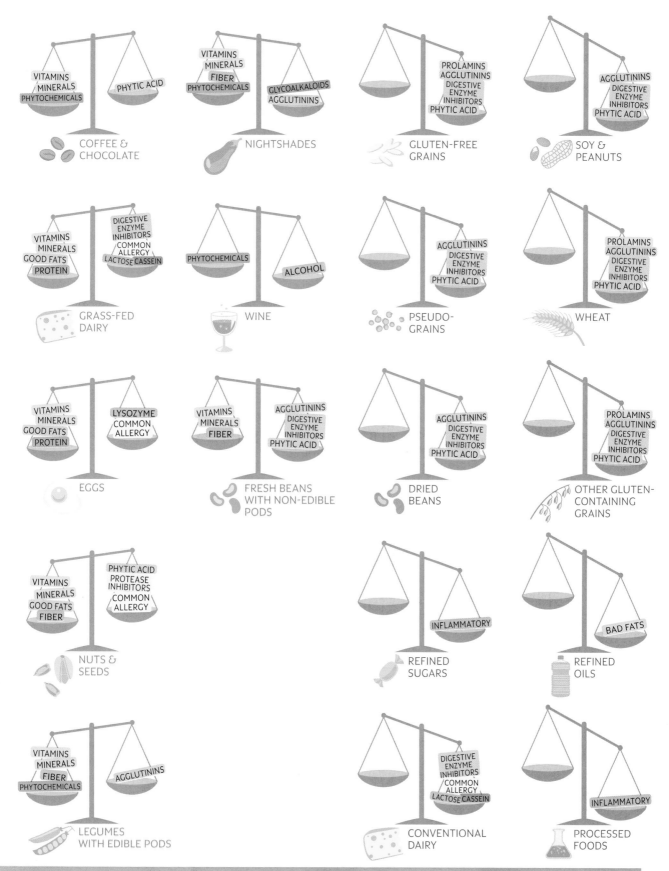

VITAMINS
MINERALS
PHYTOCHEMICALS
PHYTIC ACID
COFFEE &
CHOCOLATE

VITAMINS
MINERALS
FIBER
PHYTOCHEMICALS
GLYCOALKALOIDS
AGGLUTININS
NIGHTSHADES

PROLAMINS
AGGLUTININS
DIGESTIVE
ENZYME
INHIBITORS
PHYTIC ACID
GLUTEN-FREE
GRAINS

AGGLUTININS
DIGESTIVE
ENZYME
INHIBITORS
PHYTIC ACID
SOY &
PEANUTS

VITAMINS
MINERALS
GOOD FATS
PROTEIN
DIGESTIVE
ENZYME
INHIBITORS
COMMON
ALLERGY
LACTOSE CASSEIN
GRASS-FED
DAIRY

PHYTOCHEMICALS
ALCOHOL
WINE

AGGLUTININS
DIGESTIVE
ENZYME
INHIBITORS
PHYTIC ACID
PSEUDO-
GRAINS

PROLAMINS
AGGLUTININS
DIGESTIVE
ENZYME
INHIBITORS
PHYTIC ACID
WHEAT

VITAMINS
MINERALS
GOOD FATS
PROTEIN
LYSOZYME
COMMON
ALLERGY
EGGS

VITAMINS
MINERALS
FIBER
AGGLUTININS
DIGESTIVE
ENZYME
INHIBITORS
PHYTIC ACID
FRESH BEANS
WITH NON-EDIBLE
PODS

AGGLUTININS
DIGESTIVE
ENZYME
INHIBITORS
PHYTIC ACID
DRIED
BEANS

PROLAMINS
AGGLUTININS
DIGESTIVE
ENZYME
INHIBITORS
PHYTIC ACID
OTHER GLUTEN-
CONTAINING
GRAINS

VITAMINS
MINERALS
GOOD FATS
FIBER
PHYTIC ACID
PROTEASE
INHIBITORS
COMMON
ALLERGY
NUTS &
SEEDS

INFLAMMATORY
REFINED
SUGARS

BAD FATS
REFINED
OILS

VITAMINS
MINERALS
FIBER
PHYTOCHEMICALS
AGGLUTININS
LEGUMES
WITH EDIBLE PODS

DIGESTIVE
ENZYME
INHIBITORS
COMMON
ALLERGY
LACTOSE CASSEIN
CONVENTIONAL
DAIRY

INFLAMMATORY
PROCESSED
FOODS

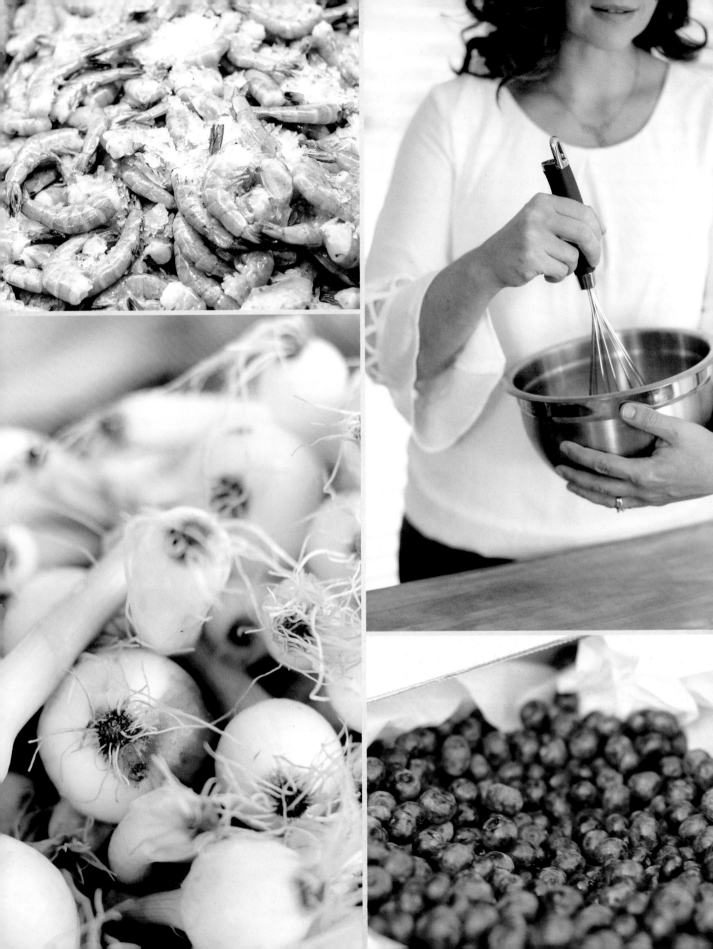

healing through food

The food we eat is one of many factors that affect our health, but it's one that permeates every aspect of it. Our bodies simply cannot function efficiently and effectively without all the nutrients our systems need to form tissues and do their jobs, and the only way to get all those nutrients is to choose micronutrient-dense functional foods. Neither can we be healthy if the foods we eat cause inflammation, disrupt our hormones, or damage our guts. It's preposterous that we even call substances that undermine our health to this extent "food." Grains and grainlike seeds (like buckwheat and quinoa), legumes, nightshades, dairy, refined sugars, processed "vegetable" oils, and processed foods are not doing us any favors.

So, once you flood your body with micronutrients and eliminate the problematic foods from your diet, does that mean you can completely reverse a chronic illness?

The answer is, it depends. First, poor diet is only one contributor to chronic illness. The other contributors, which include stress, poor sleep, and inactivity (see pages 45 to 47), also need to be addressed. Genetics, while they certainly don't doom us to chronic illness (most of the time), are a factor, too, and one that we can't control. And then there are confounding factors—extra things you may be dealing with that are barriers to healing. These can include anything from toxin exposure to infection to hormone issues to medications. Some diseases cause permanent damage to tissues in the body, and while changing your diet and lifestyle may halt the disease, there's a limit to how much the body can regenerate damaged tissues. Some diseases are just plain incurable, but these can typically still go into remission, which means that you don't suffer any symptoms of the disease (and that feels pretty much the same as a cure!).

Inflammation is a factor in all chronic illnesses, and this is one area where the foods we eat can make a huge difference (as we'll talk about in detail in a moment). In some cases, an immune system that isn't regulating itself properly directly causes the illness; in others, inflammation is merely an element of the illness or a contributor to how the illness came about—but it is always a player and a problem. What this means is that reducing inflammation and giving the immune system the resources it needs, as well as the opportunity to regulate itself, can help in every single chronic illness. This is important because inflammation is strongly influenced by what we eat, how well we sleep, how stressed we are, and how active we are. And this is why chronic illness can respond so positively to changes in diet and lifestyle.

So food does have therapeutic potential for every chronic illness—but that's not the same thing as calling food a cure. Depending on the illness you're struggling with, how long you've had it, how aggressive the disease is, and what confounding factors you're dealing with, dietary changes may get you as far as a complete reversal of your disease, or they may slow the progress of your illness, or they may simply improve your quality of life. These are all successes worth celebrating. Good food may not be the miracle cure you're hoping for, but it's pretty darn powerful all the same.

But seeing improvement can be a long road. While some people notice massive improvements to their symptoms within a couple of days of a diet revamp, a few months is a more typical timeline. This is because the body has to heal significantly before you can really see and feel the changes. Confounding factors like poor gut health (typical if you have symptoms of irritable bowel syndrome or a diagnosed pathology of the gut, like celiac disease or inflammatory bowel disease) can mean that you aren't absorbing all the amazing nutrients you're consuming. In this case, your gut has to heal substantially before enough nutrients can make it to other tissues for them to benefit, too. Once you crest this hill, however, improvement can be rapid and

> *There are no guarantees, but that doesn't mean dietary changes aren't worthwhile. The fact is, you won't know just how far healthy eating can get you until you give it a good all-in try.*

wonderful! Other times, a delay in seeing improvements has more to do with your particular condition. For instance, the skin is generally the body's lowest-priority organ, so if your illness affects your skin, your body will first heal extensively internally before it starts directing resources toward healing your skin. All this is to say that patience may be required—but if you are frustrated with your progress, find a health-care professional who is familiar with the Paleo diet to help you troubleshoot.

There are no guarantees, but that doesn't mean dietary changes aren't worthwhile. The fact is, you won't know just how far healthy eating can get you until you give it a good all-in try. And the recipes in this cookbook mean that you can commit to the Autoimmune Protocol without spending all day in the kitchen, without breaking the bank, and, most importantly, without missing out on flavor and joy from food!

how can food reduce inflammation?

Inflammation is part of the pathology of every chronic illness. It might not be the cause of the illness, but it contributes, every single time. When we're told that we have a chronic illness related to inflammation, it's accompanied either by a what-can-you-do shrug or a prescription for a medication geared at reducing inflammation. But how much inflammation we have is a direct result of how we eat, how much we sleep, how active we are, and how much stress we're under, so rather than masking symptoms with drugs that don't address the underlying problem (that doesn't include necessary, sometimes lifesaving medication, which is awesome!), it makes more sense to change our diet and lifestyle to reduce inflammation.

The immune system has two main jobs. The first is attacking whatever foreign invader is causing problems, be it a virus, bacteria, a parasite, or even dirt (like what might get into a cut or scrape)—that results in inflammation, but it's the good kind that's a necessary defense against invaders. The second job is keeping the entire system reined in and, once the foreign invader is vanquished, turning off the cells that attack invaders. We don't give enough credit to the types of cells that do the latter job, but they're essential. Without them, your immune system would turn on when you get a cold and never turn off again!

Most of the time, different types of cells are doing these jobs simultaneously; some cells are attacking that flu virus while others are making sure that things don't get out of hand. But in the case of chronic illness, the immune system is out of control, and our own tissues are innocent bystanders that are affected—or, worse, there's a simultaneous failure on the part of the immune system that's supposed to make sure that the attacking cells don't mistake our own tissues for foreign invaders, so the immune system targets our own tissues. How does the immune system break down this badly? There are many factors.

Genetics certainly play a role in disease, but it only accounts for about one-quarter to one-third of our risk for autoimmune disease and most other chronic illnesses. Unlike with genetic diseases like cystic fibrosis or sickle cell anemia, which are directly caused by a single gene mutation, your specific genetic makeup only makes you more or less susceptible to developing nongenetic chronic illnesses, like cardiovascular disease, diabetes, obesity, and autoimmune disease. Having some of the gene mutations that have been identified to increase risk of nongenetic chronic illnesses is considered having a genetic predisposition, which really just means that our bodies are not resilient to suboptimal nutrition, lifestyle choices, and environment. That makes understanding how the immune system is affected by nutrition and lifestyle even more important.

First, the immune system is a nutrient hog. It uses micronutrient resources like no other system in the human body. And it needs a vast array of nutrients, including essential fatty acids, essential amino acids, vitamins, minerals, and plant phytochemicals, to do its jobs effectively. When the body is low on these nutrients, the first part of the immune system that suffers is the regulatory part, the part responsible for turning off inflammation when the job is done. When we're deficient in nutrients, our immune system doesn't do a good job of regulating itself and has a tendency to get easily turned on and stay on.

Second, when you compound an immune system that isn't regulating itself well due to nutrient deficiency with things that stimulate inflammation, things aren't going to turn out well. We've already talked a bit about how some foods can cause inflammation (see page 33), but foods are only the tip of the iceberg. Stress causes inflammation. Not getting enough sleep causes inflammation. Being too sedentary causes inflammation. Participating

immune system superheroes

While every nutrient plays some role in the immune system, a few nutrients stand out as especially important. It's particularly vital to get enough of these Immune System Superheroes in your diet!

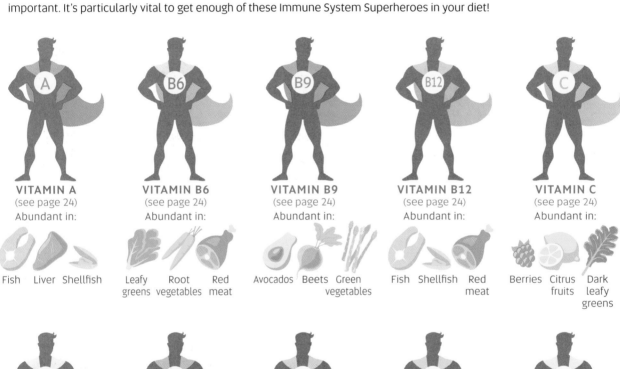

VITAMIN A
(see page 24)
Abundant in:

Fish   Liver   Shellfish

VITAMIN B6
(see page 24)
Abundant in:

Leafy greens   Root vegetables   Red meat

VITAMIN B9
(see page 24)
Abundant in:

Avocados   Beets   Green vegetables

VITAMIN B12
(see page 24)
Abundant in:

Fish   Shellfish   Red meat

VITAMIN C
(see page 24)
Abundant in:

Berries   Citrus fruits   Dark leafy greens

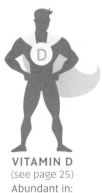

VITAMIN D
(see page 25)
Abundant in:

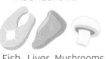

Fish   Liver   Mushrooms

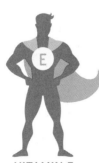

VITAMIN E
(see page 25)
Abundant in:

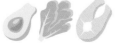

Avocados   Leafy greens   Fish

VITAMIN K2
(see page 25)
Abundant in:

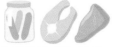

Fermented vegetables   Fish   Liver

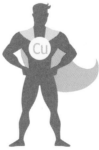

COPPER
(see page 25)
Abundant in:

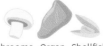

Mushrooms   Organ meats   Shellfish

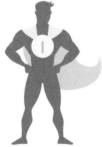

IODINE
(see page 25)
Abundant in:

Fish   Shellfish   Sea vegetables

in extremely intense sports causes inflammation. Eating too much or too frequently causes inflammation. Exposure to toxins causes inflammation. Chronic and acute infections cause inflammation (a problem if your immune system doesn't regulate itself well). Not getting enough sleep further hinders the regulatory arm of the immune system. Too much stress hinders the regulatory arm of the immune system. It may feel like we don't have any control over these things (and some of them we genuinely can't control), but many of them are within our power to change, and that can mean great improvements to our health. Combine getting enough sleep, managing stress, and avoiding inflammatory foods with a super-nutrient-dense approach to food choices, and now we're talking about creating an internal environment that primes the immune system for success!

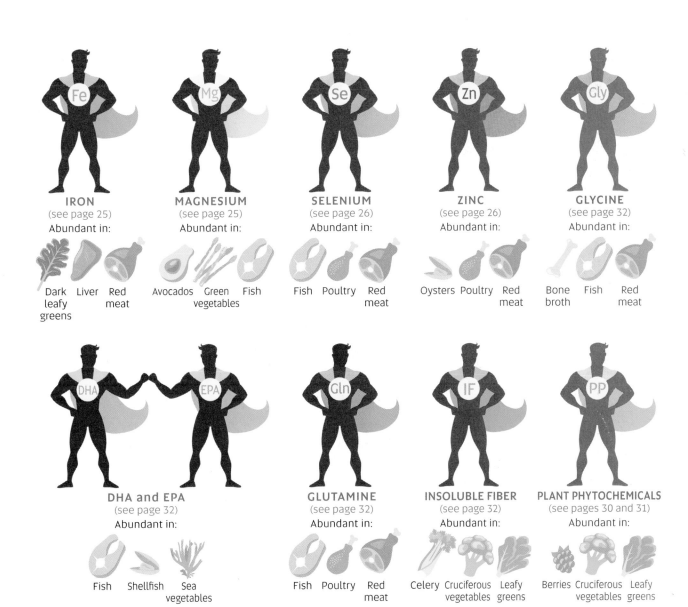

IRON
(see page 25)
Abundant in:
Dark leafy greens · Liver · Red meat

MAGNESIUM
(see page 25)
Abundant in:
Avocados · Green vegetables · Fish

SELENIUM
(see page 26)
Abundant in:
Fish · Poultry · Red meat

ZINC
(see page 26)
Abundant in:
Oysters · Poultry · Red meat

GLYCINE
(see page 32)
Abundant in:
Bone broth · Fish · Red meat

DHA and EPA
(see page 32)
Abundant in:
Fish · Shellfish · Sea vegetables

GLUTAMINE
(see page 32)
Abundant in:
Fish · Poultry · Red meat

INSOLUBLE FIBER
(see page 32)
Abundant in:
Celery · Cruciferous vegetables · Leafy greens

PLANT PHYTOCHEMICALS
(see pages 30 and 31)
Abundant in:
Berries · Cruciferous vegetables · Leafy greens

elimination and reintroduction

The Paleo diet and its stricter, more specific version, the Autoimmune Protocol, can be thought of as nutritional interventions for a diet gone badly awry, overabundant in calories and relatively lacking in vital nutrients. But how well an individual tolerates suboptimal foods—whether we're talking about something like tomatoes, which are included in the Paleo diet but eliminated on the Autoimmune Protocol, or something like grains, which are not included in either nutritional approach—depends on nutrient status, stress, sleep, activity level, genetics, and health history. As we improve as many of these as possible with diet and lifestyle changes, it's fairly common to see tolerance of certain foods increase. The Autoimmune Protocol is an elimination diet at its core, designed to cut out the most likely food culprits while flooding the body with nutrients. And the best part about an elimination diet is that eventually you get to reintroduce foods that you've been avoiding.

How long is eventually? Ideally, you'd wait to reintroduce foods until you're feeling amazing, but as long as you're seeing improvements thanks to your diet and lifestyle changes, you can try some reintroductions after three to four weeks. The full protocol for reintroductions, including which foods are best to try reintroducing first, is detailed in Sarah's book *The Paleo Approach*, but a basic outline is on the following page. In general, reintroduce only one food every five to seven days and spend that time monitoring yourself for symptoms.

Symptoms of a reaction aren't always obvious, so keep an eye out for the following:

- Symptoms of your disease returning or worsening
- Gastrointestinal symptoms: tummyache, heartburn, nausea, constipation, diarrhea, change in frequency of bowel movements, gas, bloating, undigested or partly digested food particles in stool
- Reduced energy, fatigue, or energy dips in the afternoon, or a second wind in the late evening that makes it hard to go to bed at a good time
- Cravings for sugar, fat, or caffeine
- Pica (craving minerals from nonfood items like clay, chalk, dirt, or sand)
- Trouble falling asleep or staying asleep, or just not feeling well rested in the morning
- Headaches (mild to migraine)
- Dizziness or lightheadedness
- Increased mucus production: phlegm, runny nose, or postnasal drip
- Coughing or increased need to clear your throat
- Itchy eyes or mouth
- Sneezing
- Aches and pains: muscle, joint, tendon, or ligament
- Changes in skin: rashes, acne, dry skin, little pink bumps or spots, dry hair or nails
- Mood issues: mood swings, feeling low or depressed
- Feeling anxious, less able to handle stress

The procedure for reintroductions, taken from the procedure used to challenge food allergies and sensitivities, is as follows:

1. Select a food to challenge. Be prepared to eat it two or three times in one day, then avoid it completely again for a few days.

2. The first time you eat the food, eat half a teaspoon or even less (one teensy little nibble). Wait fifteen minutes.

3. If you have any symptoms, don't eat any more. If you don't, eat one teaspoon of the food (a small bite). Wait fifteen minutes.

4. If you have any symptoms, don't eat any more. If you don't, eat one and a half teaspoons of the food (a slightly bigger bite).

5. That's it for now. Wait two to three hours and monitor yourself for symptoms.

6. Now eat a normal-sized portion of the food—either by itself or as part of a meal.

7. Do not eat that food again for five to seven days and don't reintroduce any other foods during that time. Monitor yourself for symptoms.

8. If you have no symptoms during the challenge day or at any time in the next five to seven days, you may reincorporate this food into your diet.

It's best not to be in a hurry to reintroduce foods. Generally, the longer you wait, the more likely you are to be successful. But when you introduce particular foods is ultimately your choice. How you feel is the best gauge, and only you will know if you are ready. A word of caution, though: don't let cravings influence you. Your decision should be based on how good you feel and how much improvement you're seeing in your disease. And to help you out with cravings until you're ready for this phase, we've created some amazing comfort food and treat recipes, so you won't feel like you're missing out!

the other important stuff

We've mentioned it a few times: the food you eat isn't the only important thing to address in order to get healthy. Of course, this is a cookbook, so we've got a built-in focus on food, but as you transition to a new way of eating, don't forget about the other important stuff that affects your health. Even though these small lifestyle changes seem easy, we often put them off (and off, and off) because we don't realize the big impact they can have. So, while you dive into the recipes and meal plans, keep these lifestyle factors in mind. If you aren't seeing the improvement you're hoping for with changes in your diet, chances are one of these areas needs some work.

> *Even though these small lifestyle changes seem easy, we often put them off (and off, and off) because we don't realize the big impact they can have.*

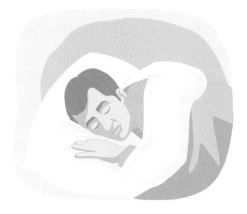

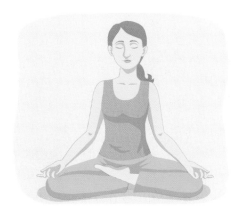

Sleep. Studies show that adults need seven to nine hours of sleep every single night. Getting enough sleep reduces the effects of stress on our bodies and has a tremendous positive impact on our hormones, metabolisms, and insulin sensitivity. On the other hand, shortchanging your sleep by even a small amount, even a few times a week, can have terrible consequences for your health. The regulatory arm of our immune systems works primarily while we're sleeping, so just plain not getting enough sleep causes inflammation. The importance of adequate and consistent sleep cannot be underestimated. And while seven hours may seem like a doable minimum, if you're battling a chronic illness, chances are your body needs more than that.

The single best thing that you can do to prioritize sleep is to have a regular bedtime—and make sure that bedtime is early enough that you can get at least eight hours of sleep (or more, if eight hours isn't enough for you to wake up feeling refreshed and energetic). Having a bedtime is such a simple thing, but it's one of the hardest things for adults to implement. Everything seems to be more important than sleep: going out with coworkers after work, watching that amazing new television show, checking Facebook, doing the laundry . . . But sleep needs to come first, and not just in the initial healing phase of our health journeys but for the rest of our lives.

What else can you do to make sure you get good sleep? Spend some time outside during the day and keep your indoor lighting dim in the evenings—this helps maximize production of melatonin, the hormone that regulates sleep, in the evenings. Sleep in a cool, dark, quiet room. And avoiding anything stimulating (work, exhaustive exercise, arguments, and emotionally intense, scary, or suspenseful television shows and movies) in the last two hours before bed. It can also be helpful to avoid evening snacking.

Stress Management. Stress has a direct impact on immune system function. Being under chronic stress (the kind that most of us struggle with) both increases inflammation and undermines the regulatory arm of the immune system. Stress is a major contributor to chronic illness, and when stress is out of control, it worsens your prognosis. When it comes to stress management, there are two factors: stress reduction and resilience.

Reducing stress simply means removing things from your life that are causing stress. Even if individual responsibilities aren't causing undue stress on their own, the sheer number of them on your plate may be creating stress. Whenever you can, say no, or ask for help. And there are as many ways to reduce stress as there are stressed people—it's up to you to figure out what works for you. Have a critical look at everything you do and how it impacts your stress level, and determine where you can make small changes (or big ones!) to reduce stress.

Resilience refers to how your body responds to stressors in your life. This is different from reducing stress—instead, it's about implementing strategies so that the stressful aspects of your life just don't get to you as much. Activities that improve resilience include getting enough sleep, being active, meditating, social bonding, connecting with nature, laughing, and playing. Making time for these things can have a direct impact on both your health and your sense of well-being.

Activity. We all know that we're supposed to exercise, but what is much less well known is that gentle movement throughout the day and daily weight-bearing exercise (like walking!) has a bigger impact on your overall health than a sweaty session at the gym five times per week. Yes, building muscle has all kinds of health benefits, and including some exercise sessions in

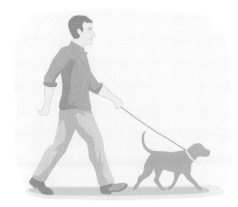

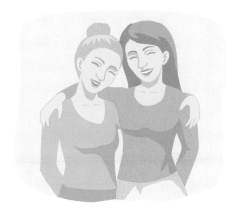

your week definitely has benefits, but when it comes to the immune system, it's most important to simply avoid being sedentary. That means not sitting all day!

There are lots of ways to add movement to your day, but the simplest strategy is to set a timer to go off every twenty minutes during the part of your day where you typically sit (at work and in front of the television, for most of us) and then, whenever the timer goes off, get up and move around for two minutes. You can jump rope, do some push-ups, stand and stretch, or do some yoga poses—whatever works for you! Yes, studies show that just two minutes of movement for every twenty that you're sitting is all it takes. Of course, you can ramp this up with treadmill desks and bicycle desks if you have access to those sorts of things.

There are also tremendous health advantages to one of the simplest and most accessible activities out there: walking. Walking helps build muscle, improves cardiovascular health, strengthens bones, helps improve resilience to stress, improves brain health (everything from mood to memory to cognition) and reduces risk of problems like dementia, improves hormone health, and can even help you sleep better! If all you do is make time for a thirty-minute walk every day (in addition to moving every twenty minutes throughout the day), you are doing great!

More intense activity is awesome, too. If you love to lift weights, participate in a sport, or get your groove on at the gym, those activities are all worthwhile. It's important to emphasize, though, that even the hardest workout can't make up for damage sitting all day does to your health. Even if you sweat up a storm for a couple of hours each day, moving around every twenty minutes is still essential for health. And another word of caution: exhaustive, strenuous, and overly intense exercise can actually undermine your health by harming your immune system, gut health, and hormone health.

Connection. An often-underrated lifestyle factor that directly impacts our health is community. Connecting with others, whether a spouse, child, friend, family member, or pet, helps regulate hormones and neurotransmitters that directly impact inflammation. Plus, this social bonding improves resilience to stress and generally improves mood, which makes every other change you're working on seem a bit easier.

There's a practical aspect to connection as well. When we have people in our lives whom we can depend on and ask for help, we have resources to help us reduce stress and put other priorities, like getting enough physical activity and sleep, at the top of our to-do lists. And having a companion for your health journey, whether it's a walking buddy, a friend to meet up with at the farmers market, someone to watch your kids while you do whatever it is you need to do, or a family member to batch cook with on weekends, having support while you tackle the job of healing is better than Mary Poppins's spoonful of sugar.

For some people, making community a priority requires effort and dedication. It can be easy to let social media sites provide us with the illusion of connection without having actual, meaningful interactions with our friends and family. It also can be easy to let every other item on our to-do lists supplant quality time with the people we care about. If you're struggling to find time for connection, see where you can combine social interaction with other activities, like exercise, play, shopping, and even cooking!

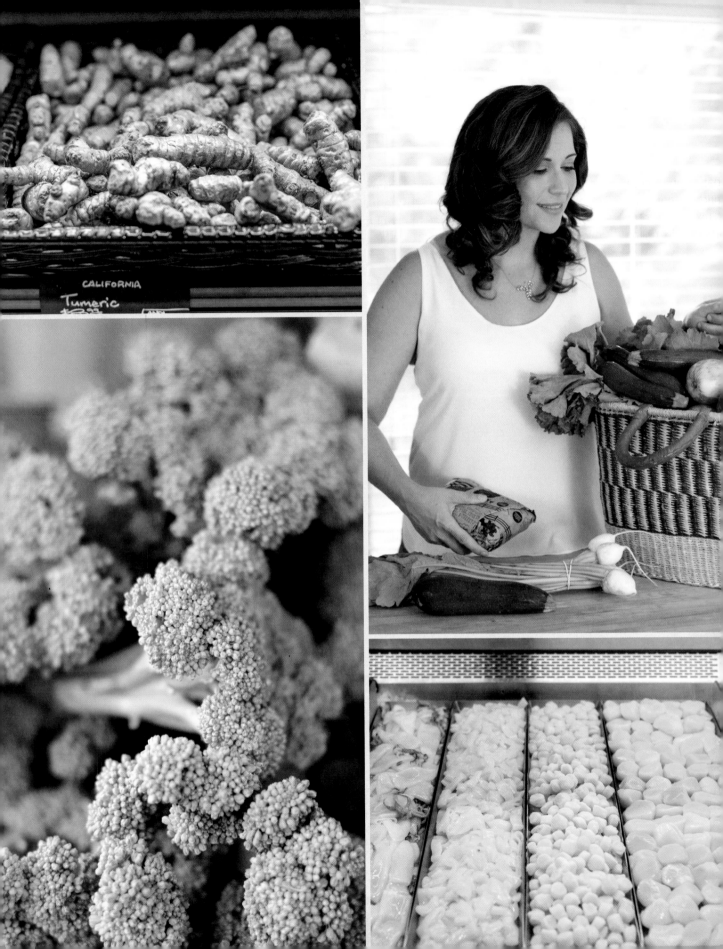

CHAPTER 3

what and how to eat

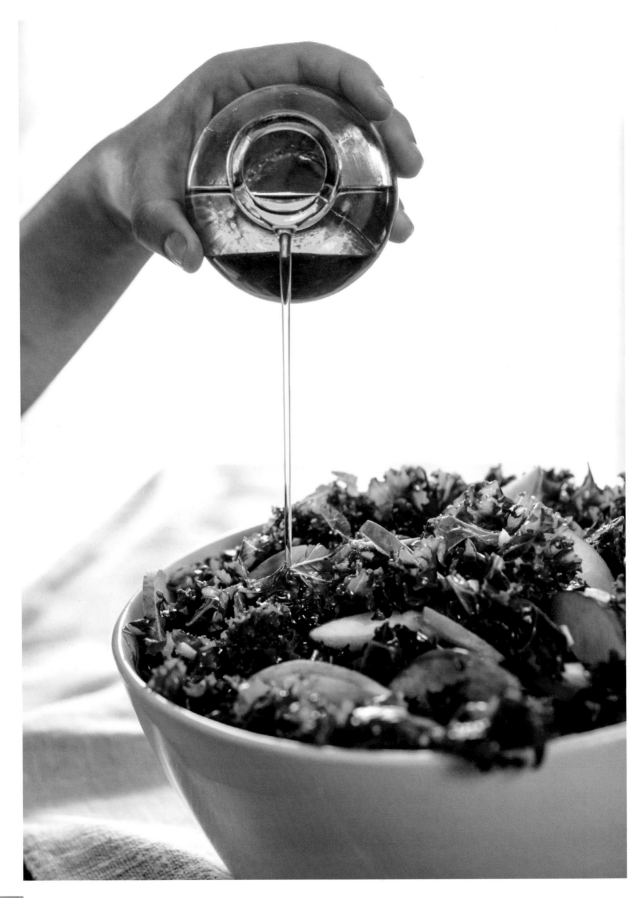

Following the Paleo and Autoimmune Protocol ways of eating is certainly more challenging than choosing foods simply based on whether you like the taste, but as we've discussed in the past few chapters, these approaches have their foundation in science. There are sound biological reasons why focusing on quality meats and seafood, as many vegetables as you can eat, and some fruit, with fresh herbs and mineral-rich unrefined sea salt (pink or gray) to add both flavor and nutrients, contributes to our health, and why the eliminated foods are best avoided.

As you pursue healthy eating with these guidelines, it will help to keep two ideas in mind. First, the greater the variety of foods you eat, the better, in terms of both nutrients and quality of life (eating the same thing day in and day out gets boring!). Different nutrients are found in different foods, and even foods that are closely related (green cabbage and red cabbage, for example) can vary substantially in the nutrients they contribute to your diet—one isn't necessarily better than the other, but it's good to sometimes choose one variety and sometimes another to get the most nutrients possible.

Second, the higher the quality of your food, the better, in terms of both nutrients and flavor. Grass-fed meats, wild-caught seafood, and local, organic, in-season produce all represent the height of food quality. Grass-fed beef has substantially more nutrition than conventionally grown beef, for example, and carrots grown on the farm down the road have substantially more nutrition than those bagged baby carrots from the grocery store. That said, if you don't have access to a bountiful variety of high-quality foods—whether they aren't available where you live or they don't fit into your food budget—don't despair: the greatest health impact comes from simply choosing these types of foods. Yes, you get even more benefit from higher-quality versions, but they aren't typically necessary in order to see improvements to your health.

Here's a statistic to keep in mind as you venture forth into your own Healing Kitchen: 60 percent of people will still choose to eat a food they know is bad for them. Unfortunately, steering clear of tempting foods can be extremely difficult, but for those of us who struggle with chronic health problems, "cheating" can be akin to taking two giant steps backward. As you contemplate satisfying that craving for an old favorite or indulging in some treat before you, think about the effort you've put into changing your diet and how frustrated you would feel with a setback in your health. Choose to be part of the 40 percent who stay on the plan despite the lure of poor-choice foods. This gets easier over time. We suspect that a major factor behind the 60 percent statistic is that what people are told are healthy foods actually don't help us get healthier, and it's a lot harder to stick to a diet plan if you don't notice a difference in how you feel. Once you start to enjoy the benefits of true healthy eating, choosing from the "yes" foods list becomes easier and easier and those old favorites lose their hold. And hey, if enough of us choose to be part of that 40 percent, we can change that statistic altogether!

> **Once you start to enjoy the benefits of true healthy eating, choosing from the "yes" foods list becomes easier and easier and those old favorites lose their hold.**

the healing kitchen food groups

The first criterion for choosing foods is nutritional merit. Eating a wide variety of foods from all of these food groups, as well as other vegetables and fruits, is the best strategy to make sure that your diet is micronutrient sufficient.

Organ Meat

Complete protein	Phosphorus
Healthy fats	Proline
Alanine	Selenium
Arginine	Sulfur
Biotin	Ubiquinol
Calcium	Vitamin A
Chlorine	Vitamin B1
Choline	Vitamin B2
Chromium	Vitamin B3
CLA (when grass-fed)	Vitamin B5
Cobalt	Vitamin B7
Copper	Vitamin B9
Creatine	Vitamin B12
DHA and EPA (when grass-fed)	Vitamin C
Glycine	Vitamin D
Iron	Vitamin E
Molybdenum	Vitamin K
	Zinc

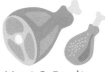

Meat & Poultry

Complete protein	Proline
Healthy fats	Selenium
Alanine	Sulfur
Arginine	Ubiquinol
CLA (when grass-fed)	Vitamin B1
	Vitamin B2
Creatine	Vitamin B3
DHA and EPA (when grass-fed)	Vitamin B5
	Vitamin B6
Glycine	Vitamin B12
Iron	Zinc
Phosphorous	

Fish

Complete protein	Proline
Healthy fats	Selenium
Alanine	Sulfur
Arginine	Ubiquinol
Calcium	Vitamin A
Choline	Vitamin B1
Creatine	Vitamin B2
DHA and EPA	Vitamin B3
Glycine	Vitamin B5
Iodine	Vitamin B6
Iron	Vitamin B9
Magnesium	Vitamin B12
Manganese	Vitamin D
Phosphorus	Vitamin E
Potassium	Zinc

Shellfish

Complete protein	Potassium
Healthy fats	Proline
Alanine	Selenium
Arginine	Sulfur
Calcium	Ubiquinol
Choline	Vitamin A
Cobalt	Vitamin B1
Copper	Vitamin B2
Chromium	Vitamin B3
Creatine	Vitamin B6
DHA and EPA	Vitamin B9
Glycine	Vitamin B12
Iodine	Vitamin C
Iron	Vitamin D
Magnesium	Zinc
Manganese	Trace minerals
Phosphorus	

Sea Vegetables

Fiber (more soluble)	Manganese
Calcium	Phosphorus
Carotenoids	Vitamin B1
Chlorine	Vitamin B2
Copper	Vitamin B3
DHA and EPA	Vitamin B5
Glycine	Vitamin B9
Iron	Vitamin C
Iodine	Vitamin E
Magnesium	Vitamin K
	Trace minerals

Leafy Greens

Fiber (more insoluble)

Boron

Calcium

Carotenoids

Chlorine

Choline

Chromium

Copper

Flavonoids

Iron

Magnesium

Manganese

Molybdenum

Plant sterols and stanols

Potassium

Polyphenols

Vitamin B2

Vitamin B3

Vitamin B6

Vitamin B9

Vitamin C

Vitamin E

Vitamin K

Cruciferous Vegetables

Fiber (more insoluble)

Boron

Calcium

Carotenoids

Choline

Chromium

Dithiolethiones

Flavonoids

Glycine

Isothiocynates

Magnesium

Manganese

Molybdenum

Plant sterols and stanols

Polyphenols

Potassium

Proline

Silicon

Sulfur

Ubiquinol

Vitamin B6

Vitamin B9

Vitamin C

Vitamin K

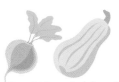

Root Vegetables & Winter Squash

Slow-burning starchy carbohydrates

Fiber (more soluble)

Biotin

Calcium

Carotenoids

Copper

Flavonoids

Glycine

Magnesium

Manganese

Phosphorous

Plant sterols and stanols

Polyphenols

Potassium

Vitamin B1

Vitamin B2

Vitamin B3

Vitamin B5

Vitamin B6

Vitamin B9

Vitamin C

Vitamin K

Mushrooms

Fiber (more insoluble)

Chromium

Copper

Phosphorous

Plant sterols and stanols

Potassium

Selenium

Vitamin B1

Vitamin B2

Vitamin B3

Vitamin B5

Vitamin B6

Vitamin C

Vitamin D

Berries

Fiber (more soluble)

Copper

Flavonoids

Iron

Magnesium

Manganese

Plant sterols and stanols

Polyphenols

Potassium

Vitamin B3

Vitamin B6

Vitamin B9

Vitamin C

Vitamin E

Vitamin K

Zinc

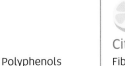

Citrus Fruit

Fiber (about equal proportions of soluble and insoluble)

Calcium

Carotenoids

Flavonoids

Plant sterols and stanols

Polyphenols

Potassium

Vitamin B1

Vitamin B5

Vitamin B6

Vitamin B9

Vitamin C

Olives & Other High-Fat Fruits

Fiber (more insoluble)

Healthy fats

Boron

Chlorine

Choline

Copper

Iron

Magnesium

Manganese

MUFA

Phosphorous

Potassium

Vitamin B1

Vitamin B2

Vitamin B3

Vitamin B5

Vitamin B6

Vitamin B9

Vitamin C

Vitamin E

Vitamin K

Zinc

Onions, Garlic & Other Alliums

Fiber (more soluble)

Choline

Diallyl sulfide

Flavonoids

Manganese

Phosphorus

Plant sterols and stanols

Potassium

Sulfur

Vitamin B1

Vitamin B6

Vitamin B9

Vitamin C

Other Fruits & Veggies

Nutrients vary, but these are all great choices!

"Yes" foods

Here are some ideas from each of the major food Paleo Autoimmune Protocol food groups!

Organ Meat
bone broth
heart
kidney
liver
tongue

Meat & Poultry
beef
bison
chicken
lamb
mutton
pork
turkey
wild game

Fish
anchovies
catfish
cod
halibut
herring
mackerel
mahi mahi
salmon
sardines
snapper
tilapia
trout
tuna

Shellfish
clams
crab
crawfish
lobster
mussels
octopus
oysters
prawns
scallops
shrimp
squid

Sea Vegetables
arame
dulse
kombu
nori
wakame

Leafy Greens
arugula
beet greens
bok choy
carrot tops
collard greens
dandelion greens
endive
herbs
kale
lettuce
mustard greens
napa cabbage
spinach
Swiss chard
turnip greens
watercress

Cruciferous Vegetables
arugula
broccoli
Brussels sprouts
cabbage
cauliflower
collard greens
kale
kohlrabi
mustard greens
napa cabbage
radishes
radicchio
turnips
watercress

Root Vegetables & Winter Squash
arrowroot
beets
carrots
cassava (tapioca, yuca)
jicama
pumpkins
squash
rutabagas
sweet potatoes
taro
yams

Berries
blackberries
blueberries
cranberries
currants
grapes
raspberries
strawberries

Citrus Fruit
clementines
grapefruit
lemons
limes
Mandarin oranges
oranges

Olives & Other High-Fat Fruits
avocados
black olives
coconuts
green olives

Onions, Garlic & Other Alliums
chives
garlic
leeks
onions
scallions
shallots
spring onions

Other Fruits & Veggies

apples	celery	kiwis	pineapples
apricots	cherries	mangoes	plantains
artichokes	coconuts	nectarines	plums
asparagus	cucumbers	okra	pomegranates
bananas	dates	papayas	watermelons
cantaloupes	figs	peaches	zucchini
capers	honeydew melons	pears	

Yes, you get to add herbs, spices, and other ingredients to prepare these foods in delicious ways! See page 68.

"No" foods

Alcohol
Beer, wine (okay for cooking), spirits

Eggs

Coffee
Except for perhaps an occasional cup

Grains
Barley, corn, durum, fonio, Job's tears, kamut, millet, oats, rice, rye, sorghum, spelt, teff, triticale, wheat (all varieties, including einkorn and semolina), wild rice

Grainlike Seeds
Amaranth, buckwheat, chia, quinoa

Dairy
Butter, buttermilk, butter oil, cheese, cottage cheese, cream, curds, dairy-protein isolates, ghee, heavy cream, ice cream, kefir, milk, sour cream, whey, whey-protein isolate, whipping cream, yogurt

Legumes
Adzuki beans, black beans, black-eyed peas, butter beans, calico beans, cannellini beans, chickpeas (garbanzo beans), fava beans (broad beans), great Northern beans, green beans, Italian beans, kidney beans, lentils, lima beans, mung beans, navy beans, peanuts, peas, pinto beans, runner beans, split peas, soybeans (including edamame, tofu, tempeh, other soy products, and soy isolates, such as soy lecithin)

Processed Vegetable Oils
Canola oil (rapeseed oil), corn oil, cottonseed oil, palm kernel oil, peanut oil, safflower oil, soybean oil, sunflower oil

Processed Food Chemicals & Ingredients
Acrylamides, artificial food color, artificial and natural flavors, autolyzed protein, brominated vegetable oil, emulsifiers (carrageenan, cellulose gum, guar gum, lecithin, xanthan gum), hydrolyzed vegetable protein, monosodium glutamate, nitrates or nitrites (naturally occurring are okay), olestra, phosphoric acid, propylene glycol, textured vegetable protein, trans fats (partially hydrogenated vegetable oil, hydrogenated oil), yeast extract, any ingredient with a chemical name that you don't recognize

Problematic Sugars & Sweeteners
Agave, agave nectar, barley malt, barley malt syrup, brown rice syrup, brown sugar, cane crystals, cane sugar (refined), caramel, corn sweetener, corn syrup, corn syrup solids, crystalline fructose, dehydrated cane juice, demerara sugar, dextrin, dextrose, diastatic malt, evaporated cane juice, fructose, fruit juice, fruit juice concentrate, galactose, glucose, glucose solids, golden syrup, high-fructose corn syrup, invert sugar, inulin, lactose, malt syrup, maltodextrin, maltose, monk fruit (luo han guo), panela, panocha, refined sugar, rice bran syrup, rice syrup, sorghum syrup, sucrose (saccharose), syrup, treacle, turbinado sugar, yacon syrup

Sugar Substitutes
Acesulfame potassium (acesulfame K), aspartame, erythritol, mannitol, neotame, saccharin, sorbitol, stevia, sucralose, xylitol

Nuts & Seeds
Almonds, Brazil nuts, cashews, chestnuts, flax seeds, hazelnuts, hemp seeds, macadamia nuts, pecans, pine nuts, pistachios, poppy seeds, pumpkin seeds, sesame seeds, sunflower seeds, walnuts, any flours, butters, oils, or other products derived from nuts or seeds

Nightshades & Spices Derived from Nightshades
Ashwagandha, bell peppers (sweet peppers), cayenne peppers, cape gooseberries (ground cherries, not to be confused with regular cherries, which are okay), eggplant, garden huckleberries (not to be confused with regular huckleberries, which are okay), goji berries (wolfberries), hot peppers (chili peppers and chili-based spices), naranjillas, paprika, pepinos, pimentos, potatoes (sweet potatoes are okay), tamarillos, tomatillos, tomatoes (Note: Some curry powders contain nightshade ingredients.)

Spices Derived from Seeds
Anise, annatto, black caraway (Russian caraway, black cumin), celery seed, coriander, cumin, dill, fennel, fenugreek, mustard, nutmeg

food quality

In general, it's best to consume whole and fresh foods, which means foods made from unprocessed, unmanipulated ingredients and foods in their most natural state and as close to harvest as possible. Both processing and storing foods depletes their nutrients. It's still okay to stock your pantry and have a variety of flavoring ingredients in the door of your fridge, but the vast majority of the foods you cook with should look as close as possible to how they look while growing or roaming in the wild. And when farm-fresh isn't an option, buying frozen is typically just as good.

The higher the quality of your foods, the more nutrients they contain. While eating solely from the pinnacle of food perfection is not typically necessary to see great improvements in health, knowing what the best options are is still important.

For red meat and poultry, high-quality means grass-fed if the animal is an herbivore (like a cow, buffalo, or lamb), pasture-raised if the animal is an omnivore (like a pig, turkey, or chicken), or wild if the animal is a game animal (like deer or boar). For all these animals, high-quality sourcing means leaner and more vitamin- and mineral-rich meat with healthier fats (most notably, a better ratio of omega-6 to omega-3 fatty acids, but also some other health-promoting fats, like conjugated linoleic acid) that's never been treated with antibiotics or hormones.

For seafood, high-quality ideally means wild-caught from the ocean or from unpolluted lakes, rivers, and streams. However, farmed fish is still a great option (and far better than not eating fish at all); it provides high levels of beneficial omega-3 fatty acids (DHA and EPA), highly digestible protein, and a plethora of vitamins and minerals that are essential for thyroid and immune function.

For produce, high-quality ideally means fresh, locally grown, organic, and in-season vegetables, fruits, and herbs. This may not be practical where you live, but whatever produce you can source from local farmers or grow in your backyard will be more nutrient-dense than even organic produce purchased from a grocery store. Frozen organic vegetables and fruits are the next best thing to fresh, since they are frozen very soon after being harvested and are harvested ripe at the peak of the season. For mushrooms, wild is best, and for dried herbs and spices, the best choice is organic.

Animal fats like lard or tallow should come from grass-fed or pasture-raised animals or wild game. Plant fats like coconut oil and olive oil should be cold-pressed, ideally completely unrefined, and as fresh as possible.

Eating the best-quality foods that you can source is very important, but if you can't afford these high-quality ingredients or you don't have access to them where you live, it's not a nonstarter. Even conventionally grown and raised food from the grocery store will have you feeling better once you start eating healthy.

> *The higher the quality of your foods, the more nutrients they contain.*

shopping

If you're intrigued by the extra benefits that come from the best-quality foods, you may be wondering where you can find them.

Local farmers (farmers markets, farmstands, pick-your-own farms, farm shares, community-supported agriculture, and co-ops): Sourcing food from local farmers is one of the best ways to maximize the quality of your food and can be a vital tool for getting high-quality food on a tight budget. It's also a great way to get organ meat, buy a half or whole butchered animal, and find vegetables and fruits that you might not be familiar with.

Specialty stores (health-food stores, natural-food stores, supplement stores, cultural food markets, and co-ops): From big-chain natural-food stores to mom-and-pop cultural food markets, these stores can be a boon to seekers of unusual ingredients and high-quality foods. Even supplement stores and small health-food stores often stock local produce. Cultural food markets are a great place to find unusual fruits and vegetables, although they're typically imported unless there's a large ethnic community to cater to, in which case they may be locally grown.

Online: Frozen high-quality meat and seafood, farm-fresh produce, and the full range of pantry ingredients used in this cookbook are all available online. In fact, these foods are often cheaper online than in stores (though not always, so make sure to compare prices!). And there's something about the convenience of having foods delivered to your door that can't be beat. Some of our favorite online vendors to check out are:

- Amazon.com
- Barefoot Provisions, barefootprovisions.com
- Farmbox Direct, farmboxdirect.com
- Grass-Fed Traditions, grassfedtraditions.com
- One Stop Paleo Shop, onestoppaleoshop.com
- US Wellness Meats, grasslandbeef.com

Regular ol' grocery stores: Never fear if the above food vendors are beyond your reach, either geographically or budgetwise. More and more grocery stores are stocking grass-fed meat, free-range chicken, wild-caught fish and shellfish, and organic vegetables and fruits. Most of the pantry ingredients used in this cookbook can be found pretty easily in most grocery stores, and if your grocery store has an organic food aisle, gluten-free aisle, or vegan/vegetarian food aisle (these are often combined into one space), and/or a cultural/international foods aisle, these can be great places to find some of the more unusual pantry ingredients. When in doubt, ask someone at the store—while not all grocery stores are willing to special-order foods, if a store perceives a market for an ingredient it doesn't usually carry, it may hop on the bandwagon.

But don't worry if your local grocery store doesn't carry anything more than the industrially produced basics or if the higher-quality options are simply beyond your budget. You can still see substantial improvements in your health! Simply choose fresh or frozen plain meats, vegetables, seafood, and fruits—that's really all there is to it. And for additional strategies for revamping your diet without expanding your budget, see page 60.

For more great places to shop online, see page 325.

navigating your grocery store

One of the biggest changes you may see in your shopping is how you navigate your grocery store. You'll likely never go down many of the interior aisles that used to be your go-to aisles for every trip to the store.

Grocery stores are all laid out slightly differently, but in general, here's the path you'll likely take through your grocery store and what you'll find where.

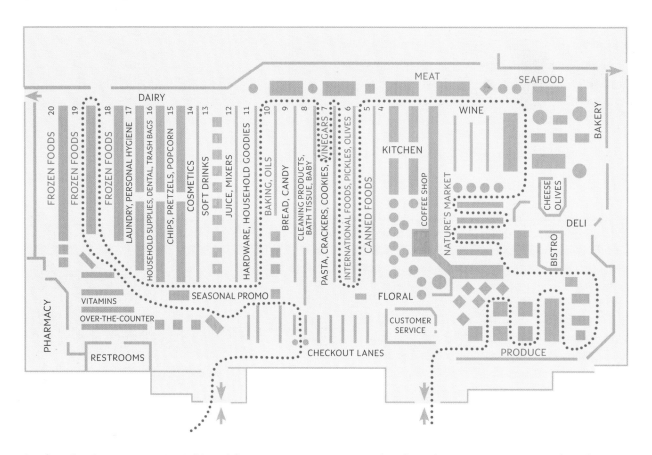

Produce Section
Fresh vegetables

Fresh herbs

Fresh fruit

Meat Section
Fresh meat

Bacon

Seafood Counter
Fresh fish

Fresh shellfish

Baking Aisle
Avocado oil

Coconut oil

Dried fruit

Dried herbs

Olive oil

Sea salt

Spices

Unsweetened shredded coconut

International Foods Aisle
Coconut aminos

Coconut milk

Fish sauce

Nori wraps

Olives

Nature's Market (organic/gluten-free)
Arrowroot starch

Tapioca starch

Carob powder

Palm shortening

Plantain chips

Sweet potato chips

Frozen Foods Aisles
Frozen broccoli

Frozen carrots

Frozen chicken breast

Frozen salmon

Frozen shrimp

Canned Foods Aisle
Canned fish

Canned pumpkin

Coconut milk

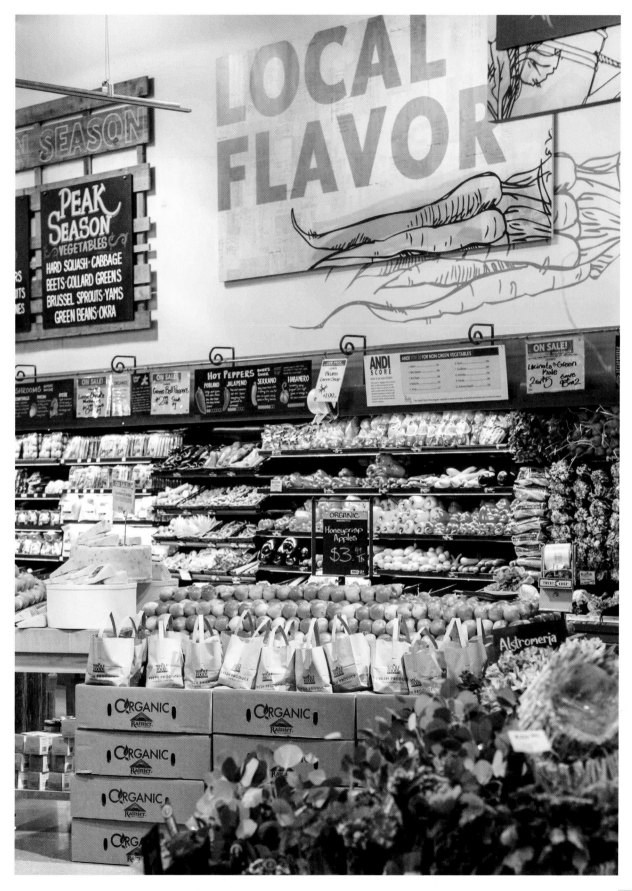

eating on a budget

Savings strategies

- Know the average prices for foods and shop around.
- Clip coupons.
- Shop sales.
- Buy in bulk.
- Haggle or barter.
- Grow your own.

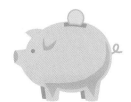

Longcuts to save money
(not shortcuts, but worth the effort)

- Buy bigger cuts of meat, which are typically cheaper per pound, and butcher them yourself.
- Buy tough cuts of meat that take longer to cook.
- Buy veggies in bulk rather than washed and chopped in packages.
- Buy meat, seafood, veggies, and fruit when heavily discounted and freeze them yourself.

Cheapest options

Beef: chuck roast, ground beef, sirloin, tri-tip, liver, heart, kidney, bones

Pork: Boston butt, picnic, shoulder, ground pork, belly, loin

Chicken: whole chicken, chicken thighs, ground chicken, liver, heart

Seafood: canned, frozen, cod, farmed salmon, tilapia

Vegetables: carrots, cucumbers, kale, lettuce, onions, spinach, sweet potatoes

Fruit: apples, avocados, bananas, frozen berries, olives, plantains

Frozen foods: veggies, fruit, seafood, meats (frozen is usually much cheaper than fresh)

Surprising ways healthy food and lifestyle choices will save you money

- You'll no longer eat at fast food joints, deli counters, or restaurants.
- You'll be cutting out expensive beverages like soda, coffee, beer, wine, and spirits.
- Walking or cycling more will save money on gas.
- You'll reduce the need for medications and doctor visits.

Cheap veggies that stretch a meal

| Butternut squash | Cabbage | Collard greens | Kale | Plantains | Sweet potatoes | Turnips and rutabagas |

Foods that give you a bang for your buck (and your health)

| Avocados | Canned seafood (wild salmon, mussels, oysters, sardines) | Chicken livers (preferably pastured and organic) | Frozen organic berries | Leafy greens (kale, Swiss chard, spinach, dandelion greens) | Sea salt |

getting back into the kitchen

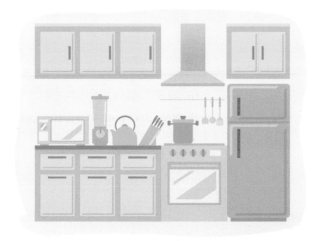

One effect of dramatically changing how you eat that many people find difficult at first is that convenience foods are mostly a thing of the past. No longer are you able to quickly pick something up from a drive-through or dial a number to have a meal delivered to your door (with a few exceptions, depending on where you live). Even grabbing a box or can of something preprepared for a microwave meal that is just three minutes on high away is no longer an option (unless that preprepared meal is one that you prepared yourself!).

Yet preparing your own food is one of the most important aspects of changing your diet. When you shop and cook your food yourself, you have complete control over which ingredients are used and the quality of those ingredients. You also have the opportunity to cater to your own taste buds! You can think of your food choices in terms of the nutrition your body needs and plan your meals to ensure that you're getting the full complement of nutrients throughout the week.

Preparing your own food is also the best way to ensure that you don't accidentally expose yourself to a food that might set you back (gluten, for instance).

When you eat at home (or eat meals that you packed and took with you), it's far, far easier to stay on track and eat only foods that you feel good about eating. Preparing your own food means that nothing will get into your food that might make you feel ill or hinder your progress toward better health.

The amount of time we spend cooking has decreased dramatically over the last fifty years, correlating with the rise in chronic disease. Cooking more means choosing more fresh foods, which naturally have way more nutrition than anything prepackaged or manufactured. Simply embracing home cooking is a sneaky way to make better food choices!

Spending more time in the kitchen doesn't need to be a hardship. As you revamp both your diet and your lifestyle, you might find that food preparation becomes an opportunity to unwind or visit with your spouse or your kids. Maybe you'll use the time to catch up on your favorite podcast or audiobook or talk to a far-off friend on the phone. Maybe it will be an opportunity to fit some activity into your day (lunges while the meat is browning, squats while the food processor is running, wall push-ups or dips using the kitchen counter between chopping vegetables). Maybe it will become a time to be in your own thoughts, to contemplate and reflect and appreciate. Maybe it'll just be about the food and the enjoyment of creating delicious, nourishing meals. The point is that cooking is only a chore if you approach it as one.

And spending more time in the kitchen doesn't mean that you have to spend your whole life in the kitchen! We've gone to great efforts to make sure that the recipes in *The Healing Kitchen* are simple to make while full of complex and delicious flavors, and they're quick to prepare so that you can minimize your time spent cooking and go out and do all the other things you'd rather do. So yes, you will have to cook, but no, you won't have to slave over a hot stove.

eating on the go

Another common obstacle to healthy eating is our busy schedules. Too often, we're eating on the run, dashing out the door, racing to the next thing, and arriving home late in the evening starving and impatient for dinner. We need food to be fast, portable, and convenient. So what do you do if you just don't have time to cook one night? What are your best options for food on the go?

The best choice is to plan ahead and have prepared meals in your fridge or freezer that you can simply reheat and enjoy. Every single recipe in *The Healing Kitchen* makes great leftovers for when you need an instant meal. But sometimes life gets in the way of our best efforts, and having a strategy for when that happens is the best way to guarantee success in those situations.

If you find yourself struggling to find time to prepare meals and/or constantly eating on the go—or worse, opting for old, unhealthy staples just because they're convenient—it may be time to critically evaluate the role that stress is playing in your health (see page 46). The solutions here are intended to make the occasional unusually busy day a little easier, not to help you sustain a stressful, frantic lifestyle that's not conducive to good health.

grab-and-go foods

These are great options if you need to run into your local grocery store and get something you can eat immediately:

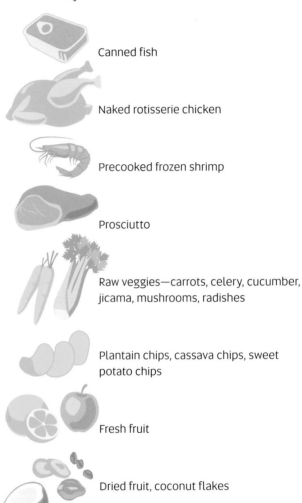

Canned fish

Naked rotisserie chicken

Precooked frozen shrimp

Prosciutto

Raw veggies—carrots, celery, cucumber, jicama, mushrooms, radishes

Plantain chips, cassava chips, sweet potato chips

Fresh fruit

Dried fruit, coconut flakes

Grab-and-go recipes
from *The Healing Kitchen*

If you need to eat on the run but can spare some time to prepare food ahead of time, these recipes are great options.

278
Cherry Balsamic Pâté served with Garlic & Thyme Crackers

279
Chewy Trail Mix Granola

268

280
Chicken Ranch Salad over Crackers

269
Crunchy Kale'nola

218
Honey-Garlic Drumsticks*

171
Honey-Lime Chicken & Strawberry Salad (cold)

110

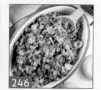
246
Lebanese Beef & Rice Stuffing**

224
Classic Roast Chicken* served with Orange & Olive Tapenade

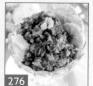
276

281
Lemon-Ginger Energy Balls

273
Lox & Everything Hors d'Oeuvre

217
Pesto Chicken Pasta (cold)

233
Seared Shrimp Pasta with White Sauce*

277
Smoked Salmon Spread served on cucumbers

270
Turkey Jerky

* Warm or cold.

**Can be a meal on its own served warm or cold.

Ultra-quick meals
from *The Healing Kitchen*

If you can spare twenty to thirty minutes to whip something together, these recipes are your best bets.

158
"Cheesy" Broccoli Soup

166
Antipasto Salad

200
Classic American Hamburgers

200
Greek Lamb Burgers

201
BBQ Chicken Burgers

141
Creamy Caesar Beef Skillet

144
Crispy Salmon Hash

142
Garlicky Greek Lamb Skillet

229
Lamb with Olive-Butternut Rice

194

194

226
Meatballs: Anti-Inflammatory, Mediterranean Lamb, Raisin & Spice

217
Pesto Chicken Pasta

233
Seared Shrimp Pasta with White Sauce

127
Pumpkin Spice Smoothie

126
Antioxidant Morning Smoothie

209
Speedy Shanghai Stir-Fry

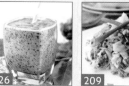
188
Taco Night

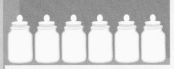
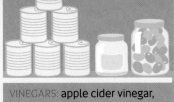

DRIED HERBS & SEASONINGS: basil, dill, marjoram, mint, oregano, rosemary, sage, thyme, garlic powder, onion powder, cinnamon, cloves, ginger, mace, sea salt, truffle salt

PICKLED STAPLES: artichoke hearts, olives, horseradish*

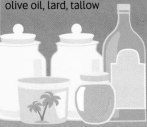

FATS: avocado oil, coconut oil, olive oil, lard, tallow

VINEGARS: apple cider vinegar, balsamic vinegar, pear cider vinegar, red wine vinegar

EMERGENCY PROTEINS: canned haddock, mackerel, oysters, salmon, sardines, shrimp, tuna

FLAVORINGS: anchovies, coconut aminos, fish sauce,* wasabi*

BAKING STAPLES: arrowroot starch, baking soda, blackstrap molasses, carob powder, coconut flour, cream of tartar, gelatin, honey, maple syrup, palm shortening, sweet potato flour, tapioca starch

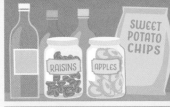

DRIED FRUIT: apples, bananas, coconut, dates, mangoes, raisins

EXTRAS: coconut wraps, nori wraps, apple chips, banana chips, cassava chips, plantain chips, sweet potato chips,* coconut flakes, coconut milk or cream

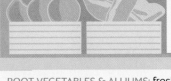

ROOT VEGETABLES & ALLIUMS: fresh garlic, ginger root, onions, sweet potatoes, winter squash

FRESH FRUIT: apples, avocados, bananas

Check ingredients for "no" foods.

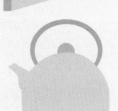

turning your kitchen into a healing kitchen

Now that you have the right information about how to eat healthy, the next big hurdle is actually doing it! It's time to turn your kitchen into a Healing Kitchen. This means throwing out (or donating to a food bank or composting) all of the foods in your home that you don't plan to eat anymore and restocking your freezer, fridge, and pantry with nutrient-dense choices.

If your family isn't going to join you on this health adventure, this is a good time to find strategies to make sure that you aren't exposed to things like gluten and figure out how you're going to handle the temptation of off-plan foods your family is eating. A strategy that works well for us is to have easy foods on hand that can be prepared quickly in a pinch, as well as comfort foods and treats for those times when food you shouldn't eat seems to be calling your name.

When it comes to restocking your pantry, you don't need to go out and buy everything in one enormous (and expensive!) shopping trip. Instead, add to your pantry a little each week, prioritizing those ingredients that you'll need for the meals you plan to make that week. Stocking a few emergency proteins and grab-and-go snacks also makes life easier!

How do you know what to put where? If you buy it refrigerated at the store, place it in your fridge at home. If you buy it frozen, put it in the freezer. And if you buy it off a shelf or out of a bin, put it in your pantry. Any pantry item that requires refrigeration upon opening will say so on the label. All fresh produce can be stored in the fridge to extend shelf life, and always refrigerate fresh produce after it's sliced.

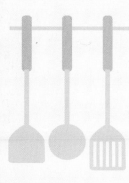

FROZEN INGREDIENTS

- Broth
- Meat: ground beef, chicken
- Fish and shellfish: salmon, tilapia, shrimp

- Vegetables: artichoke hearts, broccoli, carrots, cauliflower, celery, onions
- Fruit: bananas, berries, mangoes, pineapple

- Fresh herbs: basil, dill, mint, oregano, rosemary, tarragon, thyme (to best retain the flavors of fresh herbs, chop and mix with olive oil before freezing)

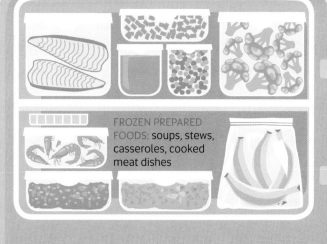

FROZEN PREPARED FOODS: soups, stews, casseroles, cooked meat dishes

Avoid freezing salads, delicate herbs, and hot foods that have not been cooled. The best containers for freezing are freezer-safe glass containers with tight-fitting lids, plastic freezer bags, and plastic lidded containers.

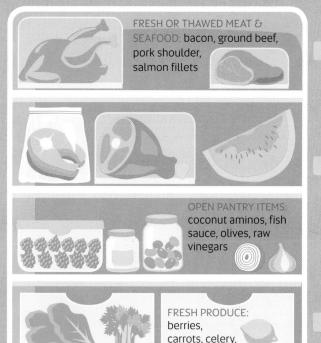

FRESH OR THAWED MEAT & SEAFOOD: bacon, ground beef, pork shoulder, salmon fillets

OPEN PANTRY ITEMS: coconut aminos, fish sauce, olives, raw vinegars

FRESH PRODUCE: berries, carrots, celery, cucumbers, kale, lemons, lettuce

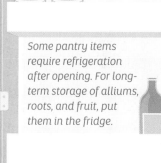

Some pantry items require refrigeration after opening. For long-term storage of alliums, roots, and fruit, put them in the fridge.

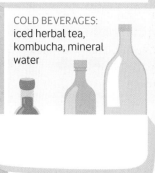

COLD BEVERAGES: iced herbal tea, kombucha, mineral water

ingredient swaps

standard american diet to autoimmune protocol swaps

Trying to figure out how to replace a component of a favorite meal?
These are some simple swaps for old favorites.

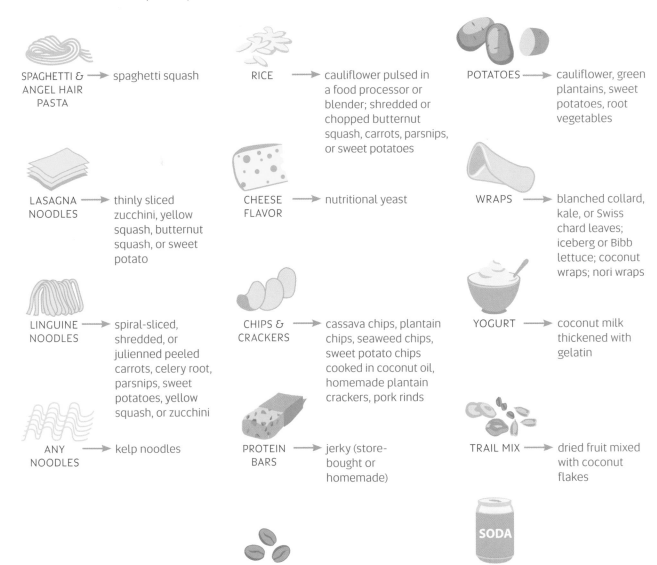

SPAGHETTI & ANGEL HAIR PASTA → spaghetti squash

LASAGNA NOODLES → thinly sliced zucchini, yellow squash, butternut squash, or sweet potato

LINGUINE NOODLES → spiral-sliced, shredded, or julienned peeled carrots, celery root, parsnips, sweet potatoes, yellow squash, or zucchini

ANY NOODLES → kelp noodles

RICE → cauliflower pulsed in a food processor or blender; shredded or chopped butternut squash, carrots, parsnips, or sweet potatoes

CHEESE FLAVOR → nutritional yeast

CHIPS & CRACKERS → cassava chips, plantain chips, seaweed chips, sweet potato chips cooked in coconut oil, homemade plantain crackers, pork rinds

PROTEIN BARS → jerky (store-bought or homemade)

COFFEE → dandelion, chicory, or carob tea

POTATOES → cauliflower, green plantains, sweet potatoes, root vegetables

WRAPS → blanched collard, kale, or Swiss chard leaves; iceberg or Bibb lettuce; coconut wraps; nori wraps

YOGURT → coconut milk thickened with gelatin

TRAIL MIX → dried fruit mixed with coconut flakes

SODA → sparkling water flavored with citrus slices or chopped fruit, kombucha

easy ingredient swaps

Looking at a recipe and don't have an ingredient on hand or can't find it at the store?
Here are some simple swaps for common ingredients.

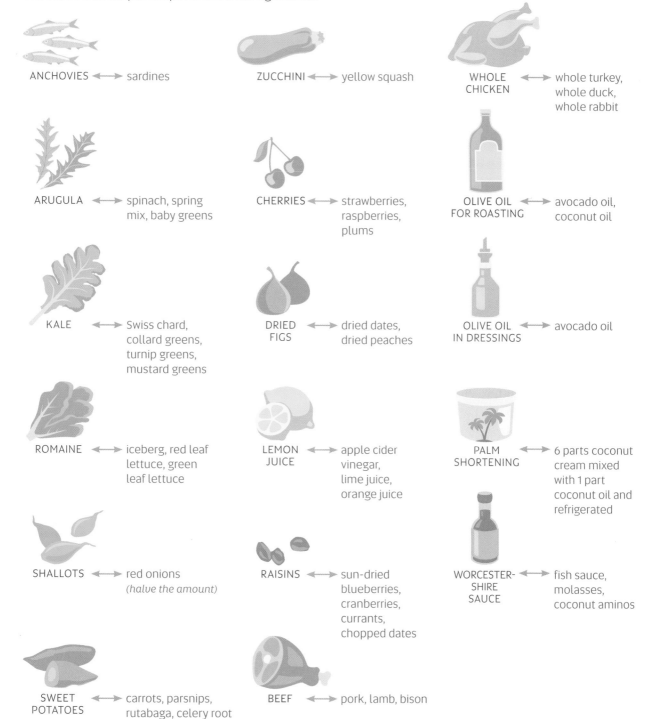

ANCHOVIES ←→ sardines

ZUCCHINI ←→ yellow squash

WHOLE CHICKEN ←→ whole turkey, whole duck, whole rabbit

ARUGULA ←→ spinach, spring mix, baby greens

CHERRIES ←→ strawberries, raspberries, plums

OLIVE OIL FOR ROASTING ←→ avocado oil, coconut oil

KALE ←→ Swiss chard, collard greens, turnip greens, mustard greens

DRIED FIGS ←→ dried dates, dried peaches

OLIVE OIL IN DRESSINGS ←→ avocado oil

ROMAINE ←→ iceberg, red leaf lettuce, green leaf lettuce

LEMON JUICE ←→ apple cider vinegar, lime juice, orange juice

PALM SHORTENING ←→ 6 parts coconut cream mixed with 1 part coconut oil and refrigerated

SHALLOTS ←→ red onions *(halve the amount)*

RAISINS ←→ sun-dried blueberries, cranberries, currants, chopped dates

WORCESTER-SHIRE SAUCE ←→ fish sauce, molasses, coconut aminos

SWEET POTATOES ←→ carrots, parsnips, rutabaga, celery root

BEEF ←→ pork, lamb, bison

herbs, spices, and flavor combos

Unfortunately, many seasonings end up on the "no" list because they're derived from nightshades, seeds, or other "no" foods. Here are the herbs, spices, and other flavorings that are on the "yes" list.

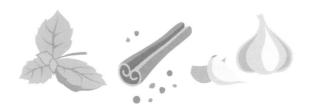

Herbs, spices, and other flavorings

basil (sweet, Thai, etc.)	cloves	lemongrass	rosemary	thyme
bay leaf	dill weed	mace	saffron	turmeric
chamomile	fennel leaf	marjoram	sage	truffle (whole truffles, truffle oil, or truffle salt)
chives	garlic	mint (peppermint, spearmint, etc.)	savory	
cilantro (coriander leaf)	ginger	oregano leaf	sea salt	vanilla extract
cinnamon	horseradish	parsley	tarragon	

Want to experiment with your own flavor combinations? Here are some great starting points.

ASIAN	Lemongrass, coconut aminos, fish sauce, garlic, ginger, lime
GREEK	Basil, oregano, lemon, olive oil, olives
ITALIAN	Balsamic vinegar, basil, garlic, marjoram, olive oil, oregano, rosemary, sage, thyme
MIDDLE EASTERN	Lemon, cinnamon, cloves, garlic, mace, mint, olive oil, olives, onion, turmeric

Here are some other ingredients that can help you achieve that perfect flavor and/or texture.

ACIDITY	Apple cider vinegar, balsamic vinegar, grapefruit, lemon, lime, orange
HEARTINESS	Butternut squash, carrot, celery root, plantain, rutabaga, sweet potato
SAVORY BOOST	Apple cider vinegar, balsamic vinegar, coconut aminos, fish sauce, molasses, mushrooms, truffle salt
SWEET ADDITIONS	Coconut milk, dried fruit, pureed fruit, fruit juice (in small quantities), ripe bananas and plantains, honey, maple syrup, molasses, sweet potatoes
TEXTURE	Apple chips, berries, coconut flakes, dried dates or figs, nori, raisins, roasted vegetables
THICKENERS	Arrowroot starch; tapioca starch; pureed plantain, sweet potato, or butternut squash

reinventing leftovers

Don't like leftovers? You're not alone. Plenty of people don't like the taste or texture of leftovers or find them boring. But just because you don't like leftovers doesn't mean that you have to give up the convenience of batch cooking and doom yourself to extra hours in the kitchen. There are lots of ways to turn leftovers into something new without a huge time commitment. And when in doubt, freeze leftovers for a quick meal down the road, once eating that particular food appeals to you again.

Here are some ideas for reinventing leftovers, either to create new meals or simply to be thrifty. You'll also find a meal plan based on reinventing leftovers on pages 96 and 97, and recipes that use leftovers are marked with an icon throughout the book.

- **Turn leftovers into soup:** Puree leftover roasted, steamed, or mashed root vegetables with broth to create a soup base. Bring to a low boil in a large pot and add leftover meat chopped into bite-sized pieces. Stir in a squeeze of lemon juice, large handfuls of chopped leafy green vegetables, and delicate herbs like parsley and cilantro. Continue cooking until the leafy greens have wilted and the meat is warmed through.

- **Use those broccoli stalks:** With a paring knife or vegetable peeler, remove the tough exterior of chopped broccoli stalks, toss with olive oil, sea salt, and lemon zest, and roast in a 400-degree oven until cooked through and golden.

- **Make easy bone broth:** Make the chicken broth on page 108 using the leftover carcass from a Classic Roast Chicken (page 224). You can even add the leftover herbs from the chicken to the pot for more flavor.

- **Save your veggie scraps:** Reserve vegetable scraps like broccoli stalks, carrot peels, carrot and celery ends, and cauliflower leaves to use in a vegetable- or meat-based broth for soups, stews, purees, and braising.

- **Reinvent the salad:** You can turn any leftover dish into a salad if you keep your refrigerator stocked with fresh heads of lettuce, arugula, spinach, or kale. Proteins such as Mojo Pulled Chicken (page 214), Beef or Pork Carnitas (page 186), and Classic Roast Chicken (page 224) are flavorful but won't overpower a salad. Add chopped nonstarchy vegetables like celery, cucumbers, radishes, and shallots, along with shredded vegetables like carrots and zucchini.

- **Make meat many ways:** Add leftover slow-cooked meats to soups, stews, salads, lettuce wraps, cauliflower rice bowls, or collard-wrapped burritos. If the meat dries out, heat it in a lidded pot with ½ cup bone broth or water until the moisture has been restored.

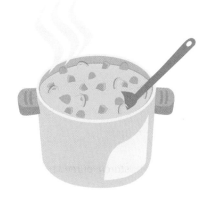

multitasking in the kitchen

If you aren't a seasoned cook, one of the hardest things to learn is how to multitask in the kitchen. It takes great skill to cook a meal with two or three components and have each dish ready to serve at the same time—let alone figure out how to cook another recipe at the same time in preparation for the following day! Yet figuring out how to multitask is one of the greatest strategies for minimizing the time you spend in the kitchen.

The best strategy for cooking multiple recipes at once is to think ahead. Read through each recipe that you want to prepare, noting how much hands-on time it requires, the total cook time, and how much chopping and other prep work you'll need to do ahead of time. One of the big secrets of successful multitasking is not taking on more than you can reasonably accomplish at once, and reading through each recipe is the best way to gauge this in advance. Make sure that you have all the ingredients and kitchen tools needed for all your recipes as well.

Most of the time, you'll want to do all the prep work for each recipe before you start cooking any of them. (There are exceptions, though, such as when one dish will simmer away for hours or bake for a long time.) Then figure out when to start each recipe by comparing their cook times. If one recipe takes forty minutes and another takes twenty minutes, start the one that takes forty minutes first. When that recipe is about halfway done, it's time to start the second one.

Multitasking in the kitchen is something that gets easier with experience—and it's definitely a skill worth mastering.

> *The best strategy for cooking multiple recipes at once is to think ahead.*

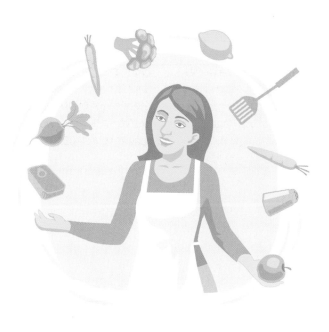

batch cooking

Batch cooking represents the height of kitchen multi-tasking and organization. It generally refers to cooking a large quantity of food—either a huge batch of a single dish or several dishes at once—in preparation for the days, week, or month ahead. You can approach batch cooking as "cooking for the freezer," "cooking for leftovers," or both simultaneously. Even though it may take a little longer to cook a double or triple batch of a recipe, the time you save over cooking that recipe on two or three occasions can be enormous.

Having a freezer full of already-cooked meals, ready to be reheated, can be a lifesaver. On busy weeknights when you arrive home starving, you can simply pull a meal out of the freezer and throw it directly into the microwave. Think of your freezer as your own fast food restaurant. And having a variety of ready-made meals in your freezer means that there's always more than one thing on the menu!

When freezing foods, let them cool prior to placing them in freezer-safe containers. If you're using a glass sealable container like a mason jar, place hot foods in the jar, leaving room at the top for expansion, and loosely secure the lid until the food cools, then tighten the lid before placing the jar in the freezer. This allows you to get a seal prior to freezing and extends the food's storage life in the freezer. Foods such as sausage patties and berries are best frozen on a baking sheet, separated so they aren't touching, and then placed in a freezer bag or other freezer-safe container once frozen; this prevents them from sticking to each other and makes it easier to grab what you need out of a large batch.

When choosing a freezer container, think about how many servings you want to freeze in each container. A large container is great for freezing a family meal's worth of food, whereas smaller containers are handy for individual portions or ingredients used in smaller quantities, like broth.

Thaw foods in the fridge prior to reheating. Before you go to bed, think about what you might want to pull out of the freezer for dinner tomorrow night and move it to the fridge; that way, your meal should be perfectly thawed and ready to heat up when you're ready to eat!

If you are cooking for leftovers, think about what will save you time when you reheat your meal. Will it help if you slice the entire roast tonight so that it's easy to serve tomorrow? Will it help if you refrigerate your leftovers as full dinner plates as opposed to putting the chicken in one container and the veggies in another?

Perhaps one of the most useful ways to approach a busy week is to spend a weekend afternoon batch cooking. In just three or four hours, you can cook all your meals for the entire week, meaning that you aren't spending any time preparing food during your hectic work/school week. To make this easy for you, we've included two batch cooking meal plans on pages 98 to 103.

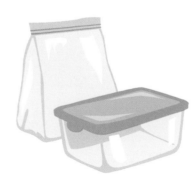

snack guide

It is generally healthier to eat large meals spaced about five to six hours apart and avoid snacking. But this isn't necessarily the best choice for everyone. For example, if you have a history of metabolic syndrome or adrenal insufficiency (adrenal fatigue), if you have difficulty managing chronic stress, or if your schedule forces you to go more than six hours between meals, you may find yourself in need of a snack.

Snack food options straight from the store

canned or pouched fish (salmon, tuna, sardines, herring, kippers)

canned shellfish (shrimp, crab, oysters, clams, mussels)

cassava chips

coconut flakes

dried fruit (dehydrated or freeze-dried; in moderation)

dried vegetables (dehydrated or freeze-dried; check ingredients for "no" foods)

fresh fruit

olives (check ingredients for "no" foods)

pickled herring and mackerel (check ingredients for "no" foods)

plantain chips

raw vegetables

sauerkraut (preferably raw; check ingredients for "no" foods)

seaweed snacks (check ingredients for "no" foods)

smoked fish (salmon, trout, kippers, etc.; can be hot-smoked or cold-smoked; check ingredients for "no" foods)

sweet potato chips

Snack recipes from *The Healing Kitchen*

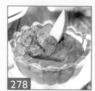
278
Cherry Balsamic Pâté

284
Cherry Lime Gummies

268
Chewy Trail Mix Granola

280
Chicken Ranch Salad over Crackers

269
Crunchy Kale'nola

279
Garlic & Thyme Crackers

281
Lemon-Ginger Energy Balls

273
Lox & Everything Hors d'Oeuvre

283
Mango Coconut Gummies

282
Monkey Bars

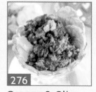
276
Orange & Olive Tapenade

284
Pomegranate Pear Gummies

271
Pulled Pork Sliders

274
Roasted Garlic & Pumpkin Hummus

277
Smoked Salmon Spread

275
Smoky Artichoke Baba Ghanoush

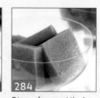
284
Strawberry Kiwi Gummies

270
Turkey Jerky

beverage guide

Trying to figure out what to drink? These options will keep you hydrated and have great flavor and added nutrients, and some even qualify as functional foods.

beet and other vegetable kvasses

carbonated or sparkling water

coconut milk (emulsifier-free)

coconut milk kefir

coconut water

homemade spa water

kombucha

lemon or lime juice

mineral water

soda water

tea, green or black

tea, herbal (including chamomile, chicory, cinnamon, citrus rind, clove, dandelion root, dried fruit, ginger, hibiscus, honeybush, lavender, lemon balm, marshmallow root, milk thistle, mint, rose hip, rooibos, turmeric, and yerba mate)

vegetable (green) juices and smoothies (in moderation)

water

water kefir

Beverage recipes from *The Healing Kitchen*

293
Citrus Fizz

294
Maple Mocha

292
Mint-ea Mojito

289
Moscow Mule

288
Red Sangria

291
Strawberry Lemonade Spritzer

290
Watermelon Lime Agua Fresca

let's get cooking (and healing)!

Now you know all the basics to get into your Healing Kitchen and create truly healthy and nourishing meals. This way of eating and living is founded in science, all of which is presented in detail in Sarah's book *The Paleo Approach*—that's where to go if you want to dive into the topic in more detail, understand more of the whys, learn where you can experiment individually, and troubleshoot challenges.

Healthy eating is really quite simple: choose a variety of high-quality meats, seafood, vegetables, and fruits, and choose foods based on their nutrient content with the goal of maximizing the nutritional merits of your diet. With the recipes in *The Healing Kitchen*, you'll be able to create amazing flavors, quickly and easily, with these health-promoting foods.

As you move forward, don't worry if you've tried "healthy eating" before and it hasn't worked. You've got this. Now that you know what healthy eating really is, you'll see how effective it can be. And that's the trick for sticking to something that's hard: it's not worth the effort if you don't see results, but once you do make gains, you'll stay motivated to keep working at it! And once you get past that initial learning curve, continuing becomes purely a matter of momentum.

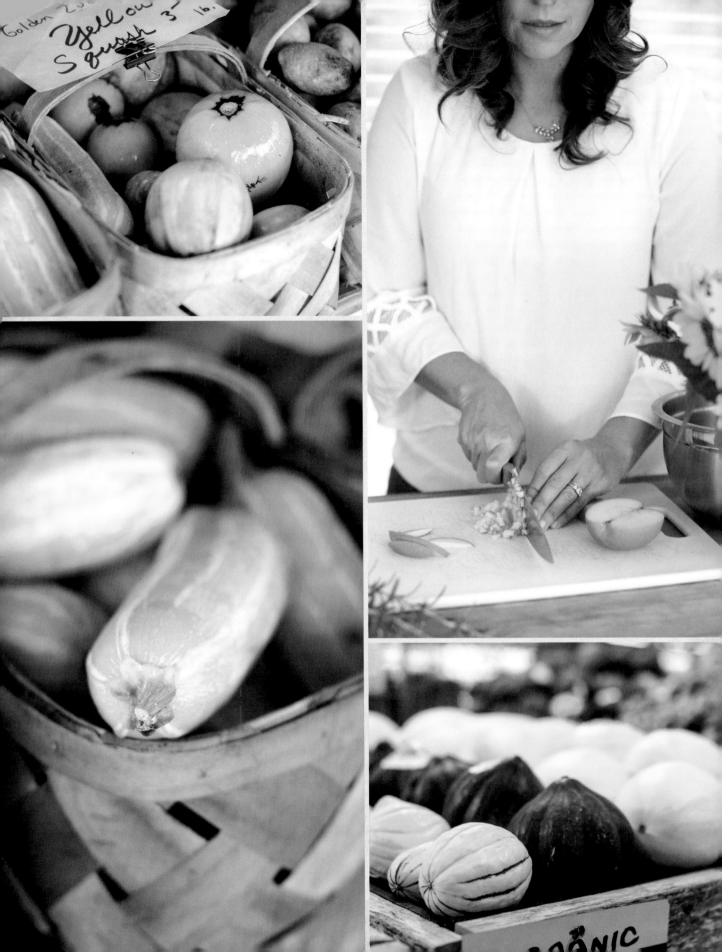

CHAPTER 4

meal plans and more!

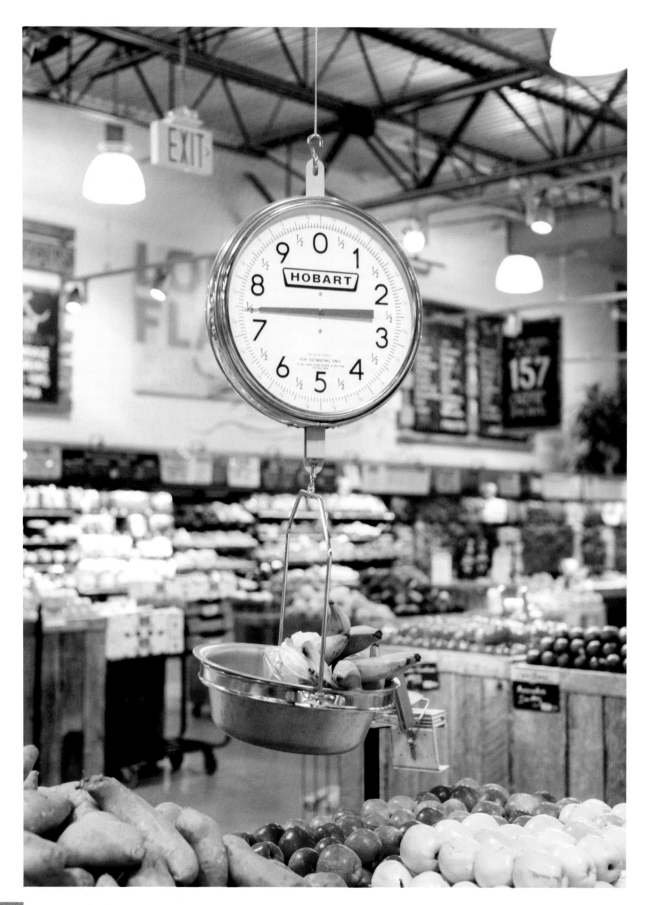

Meal plans are a great way to get organized for the week ahead and make sure that you aren't left wondering what to cook when you get home from work. We've included a whopping twelve meal plans in this book, four of them general and eight of them themed to cater to your specific needs.

These meal plans assume that you are feeding two people (or one very hungry person). If you're feeding just yourself, you may either halve the recipes or freeze the extra portions. If you're cooking for a family of more than two, you'll want to double or triple the amounts in the meal plans in order to have enough for the leftover meals that are built into each meal plan. (That may mean quadrupling or sextupling a recipe that is already doubled in the meal plan.) You can also round out your meals to feed a larger crew with additional simple sides, such as an extra salad, steamed vegetables, baked sweet potatoes or other root veggies, half an avocado, or a piece of fruit.

As you navigate each plan, first read through the recipes for the week. The weekend recipes tend to be more involved than the weekday ones, on the assumption that you have more time for food preparation on weekends than you do during the week. You'll also notice that in most of the meal plans, several meals are composed of leftovers.

Once you've read through the recipes for the week, have a look at the shopping list. If you strongly dislike or are sensitive to any food on the list, plan a substitute for either that ingredient or the entire dish and update your shopping list accordingly. If you'd rather have a can of salmon with some salad for lunch than a meal that requires preparation, that's fine, too. Don't like eating leftovers and don't mind spending more time in the kitchen? Cooking for a horde so big that even a triple batch is unlikely to provide leftovers? Go ahead and substitute new meals instead of leftovers in the plans. (Freeze leftovers if your goal is to

Most important, have fun. These meal plans are designed to make things easier for you. If they aren't achieving that goal, don't stick with them! Go ahead and devise your own meal plans.

enjoy a new flavor at every meal.) Remember to adjust the quantities of your recipes and shopping list accordingly.

Next, compare the items on your shopping list with what's actually in your pantry, fridge, and freezer. Strike off the list any foods that you already have on hand. Also figure out if you will need to order any items online. You'll want to order those items well in advance to make sure that they arrive in time. Finally, plan which items you are going to buy from which stores, farmstands, or farmers markets.

Now you're ready to go shopping. The shopping lists are designed for two weekly shopping trips: a big one over the weekend and a smaller one midweek, so that at the end of the week, you'll have fresher produce that's more nutrient dense. Items that you'll want to save for the midweek trip are marked with a star. Of course, if you prefer to make one big weekly shopping trip, the shopping lists work just as well.

If a dish uses a full recipe's worth or more of a dressing or condiment—for instance, Creamy Caesar Beef Skillet (page 141) uses a full recipe's worth of Caesar Dressing (page 110)—then the ingredients for that dressing or condiment are woven into the shopping list. If a dish uses less than that, though—for instance, Caesar Salad (page 165) uses only half a cup of Caesar Dressing—the dressing or condiment is listed separately, in case you already have enough on hand.

Most important, have fun. These meal plans are designed to make things easier for you. If they aren't achieving that goal, don't stick with them! Go ahead and devise your own meal plans. Or skip the meal plans altogether, buy whatever inspires you at the farmers market on Saturday morning, and then decide what to make from those ingredients when you get home. Figure out how to make this approach work for you—meal plans are just one tool in your toolbox.

general meal plan #1

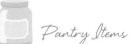

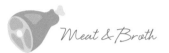

Meat & Broth

bacon, 4 slices thick-cut

☆ bacon, 9 slices regular

Beef Broth (page 109), 1½ cups

chicken breast, boneless, skinless, 1 pound, or ground chicken, 1 pound

chickens, 2 whole (4 pounds each)

Chicken or Pork Broth (pages 108–109), 3 cups

ground lamb, 2 pounds

ground pork, 5 pounds

ham, uncured, about ⅓ pound

prosciutto, 4 ounces

Seafood

clams, 3 (5- to 6-ounce) cans

☆ salmon, wild-caught, 4 (6-ounce) fillets

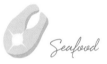

Fruit

avocados, 1½ medium

bananas, green, 3 medium (about 1⅓ pounds)

lemons, 2 medium

lime, ½ medium

peaches, 2 medium

plantain, green, 1 medium

☆ plantains, 1 pound green + 1 medium yellow

☆ red grapes, ¼ pound

☆ fruit of choice, 3 servings per person

☆ purchase midweek

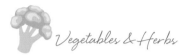

Vegetables & Herbs

arugula, 6 cups

basil leaves, 2¼ cups

carrots, 17 large (about 6 pounds)

celery, 4 or 5 stalks

cilantro, ¾ cup

curly kale, 1 large bunch

garlic, 2 heads

green cabbage, 1 head (about 1 pound)

green onions, 2

parsley, 3 tablespoons

parsnips, 4 large

red onions, 1 small + 2 large

romaine lettuce, 2 hearts + 1 head

rosemary, 4 sprigs

☆ rosemary, 1 tablespoon + 1 teaspoon minced

shallots, 5 large

spaghetti squash, 1 (4 pounds)

☆ spinach, 1 pound

thyme, 15 sprigs

☆ thyme leaves, 2 teaspoons chopped

turnip, 1 large

white sweet potatoes, 3 pounds (about 4 medium)

yellow onion, 1 medium

☆ mixed greens and veggies of choice for Simple Side Salad, 4 servings per person

☆ mixed spring salad greens or baby spinach, for serving

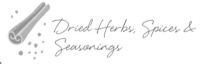

Dried Herbs, Spices & Seasonings

bay leaves, 2

dried oregano leaves, 2 tablespoons + 1 teaspoon

dried rubbed sage, 1½ tablespoons

dried thyme leaves, 1 teaspoon

garlic powder, 1½ teaspoons

ginger powder, 1 teaspoon

ground cinnamon, 2½ teaspoons

onion powder, 2¼ teaspoons

truffle salt, ¼ teaspoon

Pantry Items

albacore tuna, 1 (10-ounce) can

apple cider vinegar, 2½ teaspoons

arrowroot starch, 1¼ cups + 1½ teaspoons

artichoke hearts, ¼ cup sliced

bacon fat, 3 tablespoons

baking soda, 2 teaspoons

black olives, ¾ cup pitted + ½ cup chopped + ¼ cup sliced

coconut aminos, ¼ cup

coconut cream, 2 cups

coconut flour, ¾ cup

coconut milk, full-fat, 1 cup

coconut oil, ¼ cup + 1 tablespoon

cream of tartar, 1 teaspoon

dried apricots, ½ cup

extra-virgin olive oil, 1 cup + 1 teaspoon

fat of choice, ¼ cup

gelatin powder, unflavored, ½ teaspoon

hearts of palm, ⅔ cup chopped

honey, 2½ tablespoons + 1 teaspoon

honey or maple syrup, for serving

Medjool dates, 8

raisins, ½ cup, plus more for garnish if desired

vanilla extract, 1 teaspoon

Healing Kitchen Condiments & Spice Blends

Avocado Mayo (page 113) or Garlic-Dill Ranch Dressing (page 112), ½ cup

Caesar Dressing (page 110), ¾ cup

Country Herb Gravy (page 134), ½ to ¾ cup

Garlic & Herb Seasoning (page 123), ¼ cup

Garlic Sauce (page 106), 2½ tablespoons

Greek Dressing (page 110), ¼ cup

Honey Balsamic Dressing (page 110), ¼ cup + 3 tablespoons + 1 teaspoon

Smoky Artichoke Baba Ghanoush (page 275), ½ cup

Worcestershire Sauce (page 106), 1 teaspoon

	Breakfast	*Lunch*	*Dinner*
Sunday	130 ×2 Garlic & Herb Breakfast Sausage (freeze half) — 136 Oven-Baked Pancakes	194 Mediterranean Lamb Meatballs — 174 Peach & Kale Summer Salad	224 ×2 Classic Roast Chicken — 168 Roasted Root, Arugula & Balsamic Salad
Monday	LEFTOVER Garlic & Herb Breakfast Sausage — LEFTOVER Oven-Baked Pancakes	165 Make a Chicken Caesar Salad with leftover Classic Roast Chicken using the instructions on page 165	LEFTOVER Mediterranean Lamb Meatballs — LEFTOVER Peach & Kale Summer Salad — LEFTOVER Roasted Root, Arugula & Balsamic Salad
Tuesday	LEFTOVER Garlic & Herb Breakfast Sausage — 137 Cinnamon & Raisin Porridge	LEFTOVER Mediterranean Lamb Meatballs — 166 Antipasto Salad	209 Speedy Shanghai Stir-Fry
Wednesday	128 Chicken Hash Brown Patties — LEFTOVER Cinnamon & Raisin Porridge	162 New England Clam Chowder	227 Pesto Chicken Pizza made with leftover Classic Roast Chicken — LEFTOVER Antipasto Salad
Thursday	LEFTOVER Chicken Hash Brown Patties — Fruit	LEFTOVER New England Clam Chowder — Simple Side Salad (p. 112)	230 Bacon-Date Crusted Salmon — 258 Silky Potato Puree — 242 Spinach with Alliums & Lemon
Friday	135 Biscuits & Gravy (use frozen leftover Garlic & Herb Breakfast Sausage) — Fruit	172 Chunky Tuna Salad — 279 Garlic & Thyme Crackers	LEFTOVER Classic Roast Chicken — LEFTOVER Silky Potato Puree — Simple Side Salad (p. 112)
Saturday	LEFTOVER Biscuits & Gravy (use frozen leftover Garlic & Herb Breakfast Sausage) — Fruit	LEFTOVER New England Clam Chowder — Simple Side Salad (p. 112)	LEFTOVER Bacon-Date Crusted Salmon — LEFTOVER Spinach with Alliums and Lemon — Simple Side Salad (p. 112)

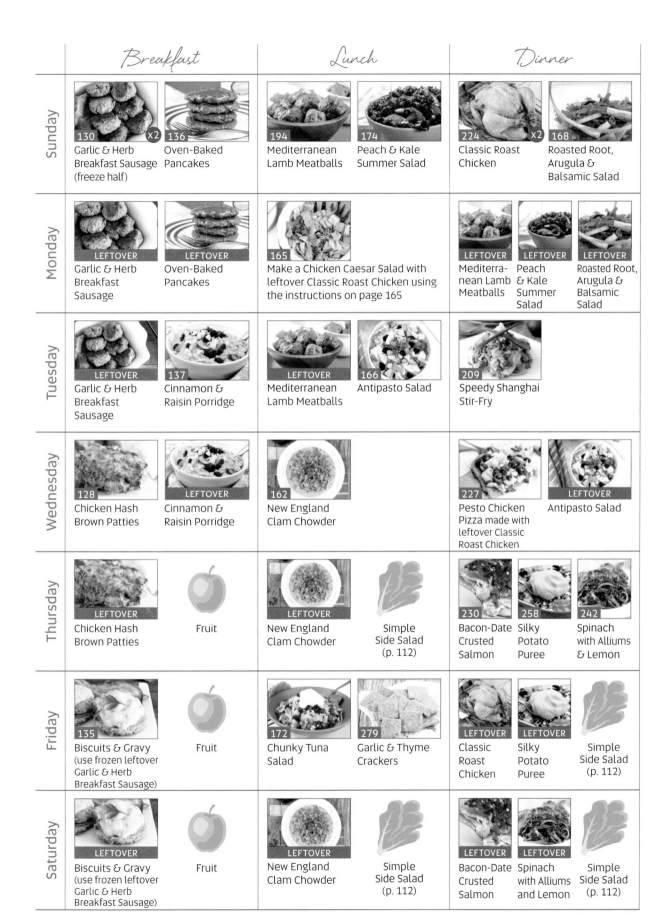

general meal plan #2

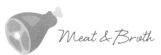

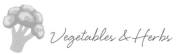

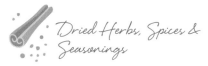

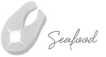

Meat & Broth

bacon, 22 slices

Beef Broth (page 109), 11 cups

chicken breast, boneless, skinless, 2 pounds

Chicken Broth (page 108) or water, ¼ cup

chicken thighs, boneless, skinless, 2 pounds

☆ ground beef, 2 pounds

ground lamb, 1½ pounds

ground pork, 2½ pounds

Pork Broth (page 109), ½ cup

☆ pork loin cutlets, boneless (about ½ inch thick), 2 pounds

pork shoulder, boneless, 3 pounds

Seafood

salmon fillets, wild-caught, skinless, 2 pounds

☆ shrimp, medium, precooked, 1½ pounds

Fruit

☆ apples, 2 Gala + 2 Golden Delicious

avocados, 2 large + 3½ medium

bananas, 3 medium-yellow medium

lemons, 3 medium

limes, 4 medium

☆ Mandarin oranges, 4

mango, 1 medium

pineapple, ⅓ whole (1 cup diced)

plantains, green, 2 large

☆ plantains, green, 2 medium

strawberries, ½ pint (about ⅓ pound)

fruit of choice, 2 servings per person

_____

☆ *purchase midweek*

Vegetables & Herbs

☆ basil leaves, ½ cup

broccoli, 1 medium head (about 1½ pounds) or 1 (12-ounce) bag florets

☆ broccoli, 1 large head (about 2 pounds)

carrots, 8 to 10 large (about 4 pounds) or 5 to 6 large + 2 (10-ounce) bags shredded

☆ carrots, 3 medium

☆ cauliflower, 1 large head (about 2 pounds)

celery, 6 stalks

☆ celery, 3 stalks

cilantro, ⅓ cup tightly packed + ¼ cup chopped

cucumber, ½ medium

☆ dill, ¼ cup chopped

English cucumber, ½ medium

☆ fennel bulb, 6 ounces

garlic, 2 heads

ginger, 1 (1-inch) piece

☆ green cabbage, 1 small head

☆ green onions, 1 bunch

leeks, 3 (about 1½ pounds)

lettuce, 10 to 12 leaves

mint, 2 tablespoons

☆ mushrooms, 8 ounces

orange sweet potatoes, 1½ pounds

radishes, ¼ pound

red cabbage, ¾ pound

red onion, 1 medium

romaine lettuce, 6 hearts

☆ rosemary, 1 sprig

☆ sage, 2 teaspoons minced

shallots, 2 large + 1 small

spaghetti squash, 1 (4 pounds)

☆ spinach, 3 ounces

☆ thyme, 5 sprigs

☆ white onion, 1 medium

white sweet potatoes, 3 pounds

yellow onion, 1 large

☆ zucchini, 2 medium

Dried Herbs, Spices & Seasonings

bay leaves, 5

cinnamon sticks, 2

dried mint, 1 teaspoon

dried rubbed sage, 2 teaspoons

dried thyme leaves, 1 tablespoon + ¾ teaspoon

garlic powder, 1½ teaspoons

ginger powder, ½ teaspoon

ground cinnamon, 1 tablespoon

ground mace, ¾ teaspoon

onion powder, 2¾ teaspoons

Pantry Items

apple cider vinegar, ¼ cup + 2 tablespoons + 1½ teaspoons

anchovies, about ½ (2-ounce) can

bacon fat or coconut oil, 2 tablespoons

baking soda, ½ teaspoon

coconut cream or full-fat coconut milk, ½ cup

coconut flour, ¼ cup

coconut milk, full-fat, 2 cups or 1 (13½-ounce) can + ¼ cup

coconut oil, 1 tablespoon

extra-virgin olive oil, 1 cup + 1 tablespoon

fish sauce, ½ teaspoon

honey, ¼ cup

plantain chips, salted, 4 cups (about 2 [3.25-ounce] bags)

raisins, 1 cup, plus more for garnish if desired

shredded coconut, unsweetened, ¾ cup, plus more for garnish if desired

Healing Kitchen Condiments & Spice Blends

Avocado Mayo (page 113), ½ cup

Garlic Sauce (page 106), ¼ cup

House Rub (page 122), 1 tablespoon

Strawberry Lime Dressing (page 110), ¾ cup

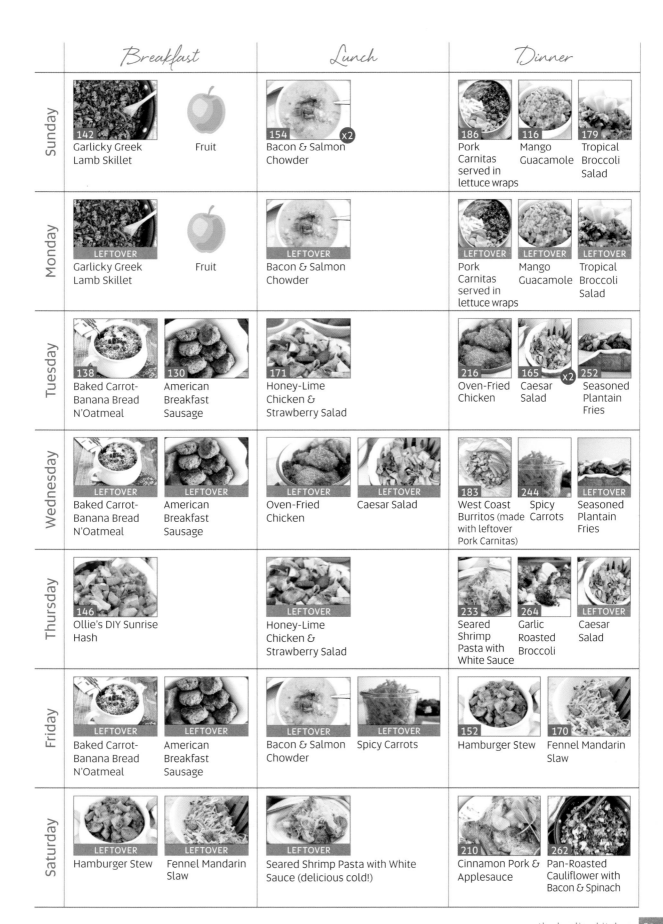

	Breakfast	Lunch	Dinner
Sunday	142 Garlicky Greek Lamb Skillet — Fruit	154 Bacon & Salmon Chowder (x2)	186 Pork Carnitas served in lettuce wraps — 116 Mango Guacamole — 179 Tropical Broccoli Salad
Monday	LEFTOVER Garlicky Greek Lamb Skillet — Fruit	LEFTOVER Bacon & Salmon Chowder	LEFTOVER Pork Carnitas served in lettuce wraps — LEFTOVER Mango Guacamole — LEFTOVER Tropical Broccoli Salad
Tuesday	138 Baked Carrot-Banana Bread N'Oatmeal — 130 American Breakfast Sausage	171 Honey-Lime Chicken & Strawberry Salad	216 Oven-Fried Chicken — 165 Caesar Salad (x2) — 252 Seasoned Plantain Fries
Wednesday	LEFTOVER Baked Carrot-Banana Bread N'Oatmeal — LEFTOVER American Breakfast Sausage	LEFTOVER Oven-Fried Chicken — LEFTOVER Caesar Salad	183 West Coast Burritos (made with leftover Pork Carnitas) — 244 Spicy Carrots — LEFTOVER Seasoned Plantain Fries
Thursday	146 Ollie's DIY Sunrise Hash	LEFTOVER Honey-Lime Chicken & Strawberry Salad	233 Seared Shrimp Pasta with White Sauce — 264 Garlic Roasted Broccoli — LEFTOVER Caesar Salad
Friday	LEFTOVER Baked Carrot-Banana Bread N'Oatmeal — LEFTOVER American Breakfast Sausage	LEFTOVER Bacon & Salmon Chowder — LEFTOVER Spicy Carrots	152 Hamburger Stew — 170 Fennel Mandarin Slaw
Saturday	LEFTOVER Hamburger Stew — LEFTOVER Fennel Mandarin Slaw	LEFTOVER Seared Shrimp Pasta with White Sauce (delicious cold!)	210 Cinnamon Pork & Applesauce — 262 Pan-Roasted Cauliflower with Bacon & Spinach

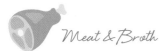

general meal plan #3

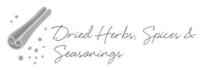

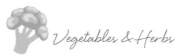

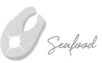

Meat & Broth

bacon, 18 slices

beef bottom round, 2 pounds

Beef Broth (page 109), 9½ cups

chickens, 2 whole (4 pounds each)

ground beef, 3 pounds

☆ ground chicken, thighs preferred, 2 pounds

ground pork, 2½ pounds

ham, uncured, about ⅓ pound

☆ pork loin roast, boneless, 2½ pounds

prosciutto, 7 ounces

Seafood

☆ salmon, wild-caught, 1 (8-ounce) fillet

☆ smoked salmon, 3 ounces

Fruit

apples, Gala, 2 medium

☆ bananas, green, 3 medium (about 1⅓ pounds)

lemons, 4 medium

orange, 1 medium

plantains, green, 2 large

red grapes, about ¼ pound

fruit of choice, 3 servings per person

☆ fruit of choice, 1 serving per person

Vegetables & Herbs

arugula, 5 ounces

basil leaves, ⅔ cup sliced + ¼ cup leaves

☆ broccoli, 1 large head (about 2 pounds)

carrots, 14 large (about 5 pounds)

cauliflower, 1 medium head (about 1½ pounds) or 1 (24-ounce) bag florets

☆ cauliflower, 1 medium head (about 1½ pounds) or 1 (24-ounce) bag florets

celery, 7 stalks

curly kale, 2 bunches

curly parsley, 3 cups chopped

English cucumber, 1 medium

garlic, 2 heads

ginger, 1 (2-inch) piece

green onions, 7

kale, 1 bunch

☆ kale, 1 bunch

mint, ¼ cup

orange sweet potatoes, 3 pounds (about 3 medium + 1 large)

☆ parsley, ⅓ cup chopped

red onion, ½ medium

romaine lettuce, 1 head

rosemary, 4 sprigs

☆ rosemary, 1 tablespoon chopped

thyme, 13 sprigs

white sweet potatoes, 3 pounds (about 3 medium + 1 large)

yellow onions, 4½ large

zucchini, 3 medium, OR spaghetti squash, 1 (4 pounds)

☆ mixed greens and veggies of choice for Simple Side Salad, 2 servings per person

Other

red wine, ½ cup

Dried Herbs, Spices & Seasonings

bay leaf, 1

cinnamon stick, 1

dried dill weed, ½ teaspoon

dried marjoram, 1 teaspoon

dried oregano leaves, 2 teaspoons

dried parsley, ¼ teaspoon

dried rubbed sage, 2 teaspoons

dried thyme leaves, 2¾ teaspoons

garlic powder, 1½ teaspoons

granulated garlic, ½ teaspoon

ginger powder, 1¼ teaspoons

ground cinnamon, 4¼ teaspoons

ground mace, 1½ teaspoons

Pantry Items

apple cider vinegar, 1½ teaspoons

arrowroot starch, ⅔ cup + 2 teaspoons

bacon fat or coconut oil, 1 tablespoon

baking soda, 1¼ teaspoons

black olives, pitted, ¾ cup

blackstrap molasses, 4 teaspoons

butternut squash puree, 1⅓ cups

coconut cream, ⅔ cup

coconut milk, full-fat, 1 cup

coconut flour, ¾ cup

coconut milk, full-fat, 1 cup

coconut oil, 3 tablespoons

cream of tartar, 1 teaspoon

dried Turkish figs, ½ cup chopped

hearts of palm, ⅔ cup chopped

honey, 3 tablespoons, plus more for serving

nutritional yeast, 1 tablespoon

raisins, 1 cup

sweet potato puree, 1 cup

vanilla extract, 1 teaspoon

Healing Kitchen Condiments & Spice Blends

Five-Spice Powder (page 123), ½ teaspoon

Greek Dressing (page 110), ¼ cup

☆ *purchase midweek*

	Breakfast	Lunch	Dinner
Sunday	130 American Breakfast Sausage — Fruit	161 Hearty Healing Beef Stew	224 x2 Classic Roast Chicken · 256 Spicy African Kale · 258 Silky Potato Puree
Monday	LEFTOVER American Breakfast Sausage — Fruit	LEFTOVER Hearty Healing Beef Stew	LEFTOVER Classic Roast Chicken · LEFTOVER Spicy African Kale · LEFTOVER Silky Potato Puree
Tuesday	140 Comforting Breakfast Casserole	LEFTOVER Classic Roast Chicken · 176 Grain-Free Tabbouleh	213 Prosciutto & Fig Bistro Pizza · 166 Antipasto Salad
Wednesday	LEFTOVER American Breakfast Sausage — Fruit	LEFTOVER Classic Roast Chicken · LEFTOVER Grain-Free Tabbouleh	196 Meat Sauce & Spaghetti · LEFTOVER Antipasto Salad
Thursday	LEFTOVER Comforting Breakfast Casserole	226 Raisin & Spice Meatballs · 244 Sweet Potato & Kale "Rice" Salad	LEFTOVER Meat Sauce & Spaghetti · Simple Side Salad (p. 112)
Friday	144 Crispy Salmon Hash — Fruit	LEFTOVER Raisin & Spice Meatballs · LEFTOVER Sweet Potato & Kale "Rice" Salad	208 Garlic & Rosemary Crusted Pork Loin · 250 Creamy Bacon Scalloped Sweet Potatoes · 264 Garlic Roasted Broccoli
Saturday	136 Oven-Baked Pancakes · 139 Spiced Candied Bacon	LEFTOVER Garlic & Rosemary Pork Loin · LEFTOVER Creamy Bacon Scalloped Sweet Potatoes	LEFTOVER Garlic & Rosemary Pork Loin · LEFTOVER Garlic Roasted Broccoli · Simple Side Salad (p. 112)

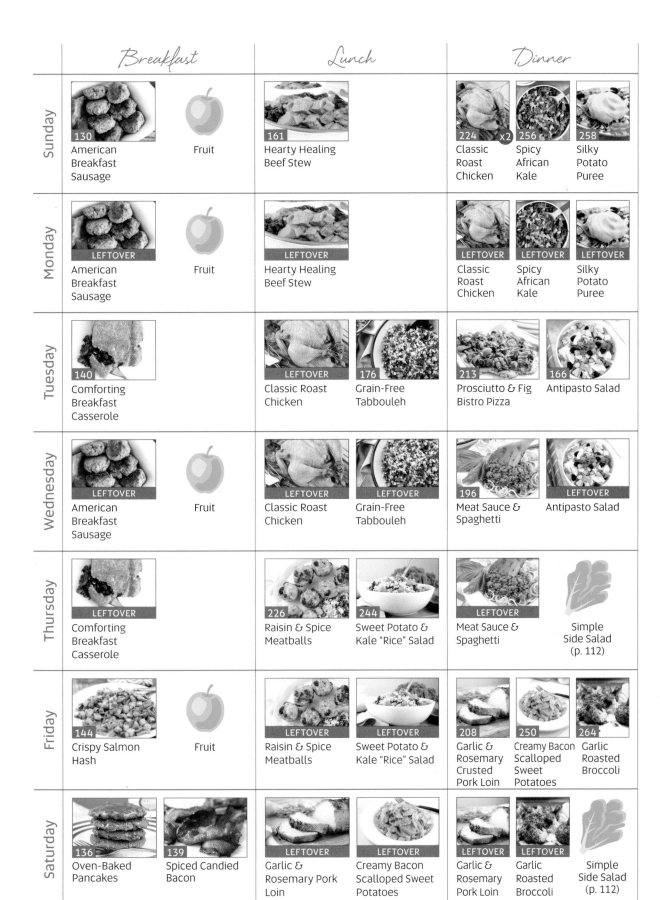

general meal plan #4

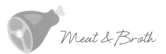

Meat & Broth

bacon, 18 slices + 1 serving per person

☆ chicken (rotisserie or breast), 3 cups shredded

Chicken Broth (page 108), 1 cup

☆ Chicken Broth (page 108), 1½ cups

chicken drumsticks, skin-on, 12

chicken tenders, 1 pound

ground beef, 2 pounds

☆ ground beef, 1 pound

☆ ground chicken, thighs preferred, 2 pounds

ground pork, 4 pounds

pork shoulder, boneless, 3 pounds

Seafood

smoked salmon, 4 ounces

Fruit

apple, Granny Smith, 1

avocados, 2 medium

☆ avocado, ⅓ medium

☆ bananas, green, 3 medium (about 1⅓ pounds)

☆ lemon, 1 medium

lime, 1 medium

mango, green, 1 medium

pineapple, ⅓ whole (1 cup diced)

fruit of choice, 3 servings per person

☆ fruit of choice, 1 serving per person

Vegetables & Herbs

asparagus, 1½ pounds

☆ basil leaves, 2 cups

broccoli, 1 medium head (about 1½ pounds) or 1 (12-ounce) bag florets

carrots, 5 or 6 large (about 2 pounds)

☆ carrots, 1⅓ pounds or 2 (10-ounce) bags shredded

celery, 2 stalks

cilantro, ⅓ cup finely chopped

☆ cilantro, ¾ cup loosely packed + ¼ cup chopped

cucumber, 1 medium

dill, ¼ cup chopped

garlic, 2 heads

ginger, 1 (1½-inch) piece

green onion, 1

lettuce, 6 to 8 leaves

orange sweet potatoes, 2 pounds (about 3 medium)

☆ parsley, ½ cup finely chopped

red onion, ½ medium

rosemary, ¼ cup finely chopped

☆ shallots, 4 large

spaghetti squash, 2 (4 pounds each)

☆ spaghetti squash, 1 (4 pounds)

white sweet potatoes, 2 pounds (about 3 medium)

yellow onions, 2 large

☆ yellow onion, 1 medium

mixed greens and veggies of choice for Simple Side Salad, 2 servings per person

☆ mixed greens and veggies of choice for Simple Side Salad, 1 serving per person

☆ desired toppings for BBQ Chicken Burgers

Healing Kitchen Condiments & Spice Blends

Avocado Mayo (page 113), ½ cup

Five-Spice Powder (page 123), 2 teaspoons

Garlic Sauce (page 106), ½ cup

Tangy Carolina BBQ Sauce (page 118), ⅓ cup

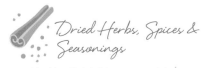

Dried Herbs, Spices & Seasonings

dried basil, 1 tablespoon + 1 teaspoon

dried oregano leaves, 2 teaspoons

dried rubbed sage, 1½ teaspoons

dried thyme leaves, ¾ teaspoon

garlic powder, ¼ teaspoon

ginger powder, 2¾ teaspoons

ground cinnamon, 1 tablespoon + 1 teaspoon

ground mace, 1¼ teaspoons

onion powder, ½ teaspoon

turmeric, ¼ teaspoon

Pantry Items

apple cider vinegar, ¾ cup + 1 teaspoon

arrowroot starch, 1 teaspoon

bacon fat, 2 tablespoons

baking soda, ¾ teaspoon

black olives, sliced, ⅓ cup

blackstrap molasses, 1 tablespoon

butternut squash puree, 2 (15-ounce) cans

canned sliced beets, 6 ounces (optional)

coconut aminos, ¼ cup

coconut flour, ¼ cup

coconut milk, full-fat, 2 cups

coconut oil, ¼ cup + 2 tablespoons

extra-virgin olive oil, 1¼ cups + 2 tablespoons

fish sauce, 2 tablespoons

honey, ½ cup + 1 tablespoon + 1 teaspoon, plus more for serving

maple syrup, for serving

pineapple chunks, 2 (14-ounce) cans

raisins, 1½ cups

shredded coconut, unsweetened, 1 cup

vanilla extract, 1 teaspoon

_____

☆ *purchase midweek*

	Breakfast	*Lunch*	*Dinner*
Sunday	**132** Bacon-Wrapped Apple & Cinnamon Sausage Fruit	**222** Coconut-Crusted Chicken Tenders with Pineapple Dipping Sauce **244** Spicy Carrots	**204** Hawaiian Pulled Pork **179** Tropical Broccoli Salad **LEFTOVER** Spicy Carrots
Monday	**LEFTOVER** Bacon-Wrapped Apple & Cinnamon Sausage Fruit	**LEFTOVER** Hawaiian Pulled Pork **LEFTOVER** Tropical Broccoli Salad **LEFTOVER** Spicy Carrots	**114** x2 **238** x2 Make It Bolognese! served over Spaghetti Squash Noodles Simple Side Salad (p. 112)
Tuesday	**137** x2 Cinnamon & Raisin Porridge **130** American Breakfast Sausage	 **218** Honey-Garlic Drumsticks **175** Smoked Salmon Potato Salad	**LEFTOVER** Hawaiian Pulled Pork **265** Gingered Asparagus **LEFTOVER** Spicy Carrots
Wednesday	**LEFTOVER** Bacon-Wrapped Apple & Cinnamon Sausage Fruit	**LEFTOVER** Hawaiian Pulled Pork **178** Thai Green Mango Salad	**LEFTOVER** Bolognese Sauce **LEFTOVER** Spaghetti Squash Noodles Simple Side Salad (p. 112)
Thursday	**LEFTOVER** Cinnamon & Raisin Porridge **LEFTOVER** American Breakfast Sausage	**LEFTOVER** Honey-Garlic Drumsticks **LEFTOVER** Smoked Salmon Potato Salad	**217** **LEFTOVER** Pesto Chicken Pasta using leftover Spaghetti Squash Noodles
Friday	**LEFTOVER** Cinnamon & Raisin Porridge **LEFTOVER** American Breakfast Sausage	 **194** Anti-Inflammatory Meatballs **242** x2 Carrot Pilaf with Lemon & Parsley **LEFTOVER** Gingered Asparagus	**201** BBQ Chicken Burgers wrapped in lettuce **252** Bacon Five-Spice Sweet Potato Fries
Saturday	**136** Oven-Baked Pancakes Bacon & fruit	**LEFTOVER** BBQ Chicken Burgers wrapped in lettuce **LEFTOVER** Bacon Five-Spice Sweet Potato Fries	**LEFTOVER** Anti-Inflammatory Meatballs **LEFTOVER** Carrot Pilaf with Lemon & Parsley Simple Side Salad (p. 112)

one-pot meal plan
for those who dislike doing dishes

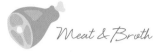

Meat & Broth

bacon, 13 slices

☆ beef bottom round, 2 pounds

Beef Broth (page 109), 4 cups

Bone Broth of choice (pages 108–109), 2 cups

chicken, 1 whole (4 pounds)

chicken breast, boneless, skinless, 2 pounds

Chicken Broth (page 108), 4 cups

Chicken or Beef Broth (pages 108–109), 6 cups

chicken thighs, boneless, skinless, 3 pounds

ground beef, 2 pounds

ground lamb, 1½ pounds

☆ ground lamb, 2 pounds

pork loin roast, boneless, 2½ pounds

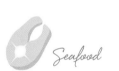

Seafood

shrimp, medium, 1 pound

Fruit

avocado, ½ medium

lemons, 2 medium

limes, 3 medium

oranges, 3 medium

plantains, green, 4 medium

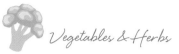

Vegetables & Herbs

basil leaves, ¼ cup chopped

broccoli, 1 large head (about 2 pounds)

☆ butternut squash, 3 pounds

carrots, 5 large (about 1½ pounds)

☆ carrots, 4 large (about 1¼ pounds)

cauliflower, 1 large head (about 2 pounds)

☆ celery, 4 stalks

cilantro, 1 cup finely chopped + ⅓ cup leaves

☆ cilantro, ¾ cup chopped

garlic, 3 heads

☆ green onions, 1 bunch

☆ kale, 1 bunch

lettuce, such as Boston or Bibb, 1 pound (about 2 large heads)

mushrooms, 1 pound

orange sweet potatoes, 4 medium (6 inches long)

☆ orange sweet potatoes, 1½ pounds

oregano leaves, ½ cup chopped

parsnips, 1½ pounds

red cabbage, about ¾ pound

red onion, 1 large

rosemary, 2 sprigs + 1 tablespoon finely chopped

shallots, 3 large

thyme, 5 sprigs

☆ thyme, 3 sprigs

yellow onions, 4 large

zucchini, 2 medium

mixed greens and veggies of choice for Simple Side Salad, 4 servings per person

☆ mixed greens and veggies of choice for Simple Side Salad, 2 servings per person

root vegetables, 1 serving per person

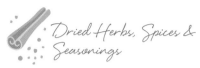

Dried Herbs, Spices & Seasonings

bay leaf, 1

cinnamon stick, 1

dried dill weed, 1 teaspoon

dried mint, 1 teaspoon

dried oregano leaves, 3 tablespoons

dried parsley, 1 teaspoon

dried rubbed sage, ½ teaspoon

dried thyme leaves, 1½ teaspoons

garlic powder, 1 teaspoon

ginger powder, 1¼ teaspoons

ground cinnamon, 2 teaspoons

onion powder, ¼ teaspoon

Pantry Items

anchovies, about ½ (2-ounce) can

coconut cream or full-fat coconut milk, ½ cup

coconut oil, 1 tablespoon

extra-virgin olive oil, 1 cup

extra-virgin olive oil or coconut oil, 3 tablespoons

fat, solid (such as duck fat, lard, or tallow), 2 tablespoons

fish sauce, 2½ teaspoons

Kalamata olives, pitted, 1½ cups

plantain chips, 4 ounces

raisins, 1 cup

sweet potato puree, 1 cup

Healing Kitchen Condiments & Spice Blends

Garlic Sauce (page 106), ¼ cup

Mango Guacamole (page 116), ⅔ cup

Other

red wine, ½ cup

☆ *purchase midweek*

*Roast the broccoli on a separate baking sheet for the last 20 minutes of cooking time for the pork loin.

**This meal is really two pots, but they are so delicious together, we had to include them both!

	Breakfast	*Lunch*	*Dinner*
Sunday	142 Garlicky Greek Lamb Skillet	224 Classic Roast Chicken with root vegetables on the side / Simple Side Salad (p. 112)	208 Garlic & Rosemary Crusted Pork Loin / 264 Garlic Roasted Broccoli* / 252 Garlic-Dill Parsnip Fries
Monday	LEFTOVER Garlicky Greek Lamb Skillet	LEFTOVER Classic Roast Chicken with root vegetables on the side / Simple Side Salad (p. 112)	LEFTOVER Garlic & Rosemary Crusted Pork Loin / LEFTOVER Garlic Roasted Broccoli / LEFTOVER Garlic-Dill Parsnip Fries
Tuesday	141 Creamy Caesar Beef Skillet	164 Lettuce Soup with cubed leftover / LEFTOVER Garlic & Rosemary Crusted Pork Loin	214 Mojo Pulled Chicken over shredded lettuce / 239 Caribbean Plantain Rice**
Wednesday	LEFTOVER Creamy Caesar Beef Skillet	219 Mojo-Mango Stuffed Sweet Potatoes using leftover Mojo Pulled Chicken / Simple Side Salad (p. 112)	232 Shrimp n' Cauli-Grits / Simple Side Salad (p. 112)
Thursday	LEFTOVER Mojo Pulled Chicken / LEFTOVER Caribbean Plantain Rice	158 Chicken "Tortilla" Soup using leftover Mojo Pulled Chicken	161 Hearty Healing Beef Stew
Friday	LEFTOVER Hearty Healing Beef Stew	229 Lamb with Olive-Butternut Rice x2	LEFTOVER Lamb with Olive-Butternut Rice / Simple Side Salad (p. 112)
Saturday	146 Ollie's DIY Sunrise Hash	LEFTOVER Chicken "Tortilla" Soup	LEFTOVER Lamb with Olive-Butternut Rice / Simple Side Salad (p. 112)

5 ingredients or less meal plan for those who like it simple

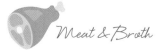

Meat & Broth

bacon, 6 or 7 slices + 1 serving per person

☆ bacon, 9 or 10 slices + 1 serving per person

Beef Broth (page 109), 1½ cups

chicken drumsticks, skin-on, 24

ground beef, 1 pound

☆ ground lamb, 2 pounds

ground pork, 3 pounds

pork loin roast, boneless, 2½ pounds

☆ pork shoulder, boneless, 3 pounds

prosciutto, 4 slices

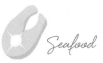

Seafood

salmon, wild-caught, 6 (6-ounce) fillets

Fruit

apples, any variety, 2 medium

☆ apples, any variety, 2 medium

avocado, 1 medium

bananas, 2 medium

blueberries, 2 cups

lemon, 1 medium

oranges, 2 medium

peaches, 2 medium

☆ plantains, green, 2 medium + 2 large

raspberries, 2 pints

fruit of choice, 2 servings per person

☆ fruit of choice, 1 serving per person

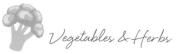

Vegetables & Herbs

broccoli, 1 large head (about 2 pounds)

carrots, 12 large (about 5 pounds)

☆ carrots, 5 or 6 large (about 2 pounds)

curly kale, 1 large bunch

garlic, 2 heads

ginger, 1 (3-inch) piece

green cabbage, 1 head (about 2 pounds)

parsnips, 8 large

rosemary, 1 tablespoon + 1 teaspoon finely chopped

shallots, 2 large

spaghetti squash, 2 (4 pounds each)

spinach, 2 handfuls

thyme leaves, 2 teaspoons chopped, or 1 teaspoon dried thyme leaves

Vidalia onions, 2 large

white sweet potatoes, 4 medium (about 2¾ pounds)

mixed greens and veggies of choice for Simple Side Salad, 4 servings per person

☆ mixed greens and veggies of choice for Simple Side Salad, 2 servings per person

☆ desired toppings for Greek Lamb Burgers

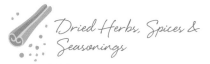

Dried Herbs, Spices & Seasonings

dried dill weed, 2½ teaspoons

dried rubbed sage, 1 tablespoon + ½ teaspoon

dried thyme leaves, 1 tablespoon

garlic powder, ½ teaspoon

ground cinnamon, 1 tablespoon + 2 teaspoons

onion powder, 1½ teaspoons

Pantry Items

apple cider vinegar, ¼ cup + 3 tablespoons

bacon or duck fat, 1 tablespoon

balsamic vinegar, ½ cup + 2 teaspoons

coconut milk, full-fat, 2½ cups

coconut oil, ¼ cup

extra-virgin olive oil, 1 cup + 2 tablespoons

fat of choice, 2 tablespoons

honey, ¾ cup

Kalamata olives, 2 tablespoons finely chopped

pineapple chunks, 1 (14-ounce) can

raisins, 1 cup, plus more for garnish if desired

tapioca starch, ½ cup

Healing Kitchen Condiments & Spice Blends

Garlic & Herb Seasoning (page 123), 2 tablespoons

Garlic Sauce (page 106), ¼ cup + 1 tablespoon (in addition to 1 full recipe, included in shopping list)

Honey Balsamic Dressing (page 110), 2 tablespoons

House Rub (page 122), 2 teaspoons

☆ *purchase midweek*

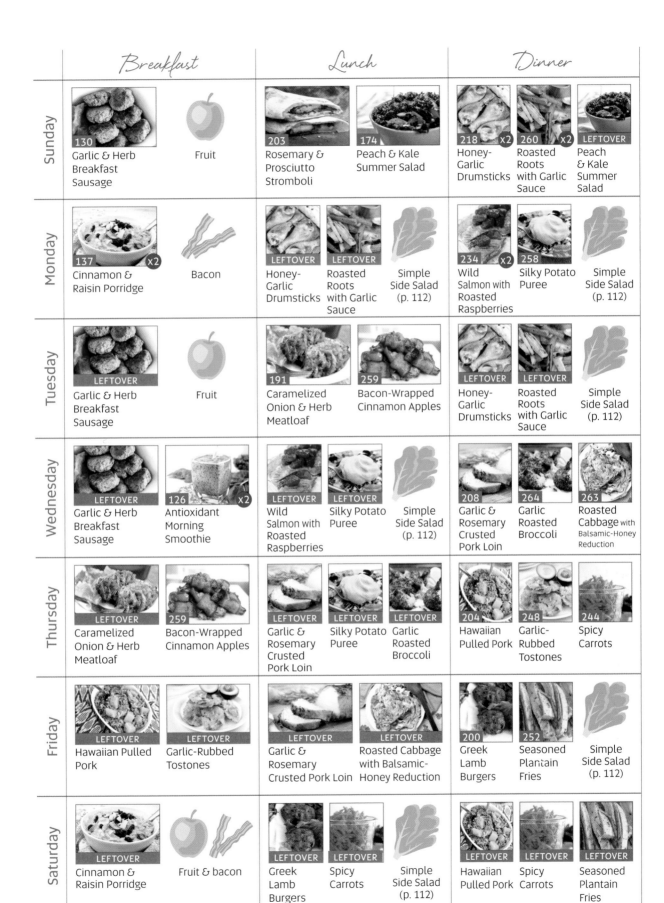

	Breakfast	Lunch	Dinner
Sunday	130 Garlic & Herb Breakfast Sausage / Fruit	203 Rosemary & Prosciutto Stromboli / 174 Peach & Kale Summer Salad	218 x2 Honey-Garlic Drumsticks / 260 x2 Roasted Roots with Garlic Sauce / LEFTOVER Peach & Kale Summer Salad
Monday	137 x2 Cinnamon & Raisin Porridge / Bacon	LEFTOVER Honey-Garlic Drumsticks / LEFTOVER Roasted Roots with Garlic Sauce / Simple Side Salad (p. 112)	234 x2 Wild Salmon with Roasted Raspberries / 258 Silky Potato Puree / Simple Side Salad (p. 112)
Tuesday	LEFTOVER Garlic & Herb Breakfast Sausage / Fruit	191 Caramelized Onion & Herb Meatloaf / 259 Bacon-Wrapped Cinnamon Apples	LEFTOVER Honey-Garlic Drumsticks / LEFTOVER Roasted Roots with Garlic Sauce / Simple Side Salad (p. 112)
Wednesday	LEFTOVER Garlic & Herb Breakfast Sausage / 126 x2 Antioxidant Morning Smoothie	LEFTOVER Wild Salmon with Roasted Raspberries / LEFTOVER Silky Potato Puree / Simple Side Salad (p. 112)	208 Garlic & Rosemary Crusted Pork Loin / 264 Garlic Roasted Broccoli / 263 Roasted Cabbage with Balsamic-Honey Reduction
Thursday	LEFTOVER Caramelized Onion & Herb Meatloaf / 259 Bacon-Wrapped Cinnamon Apples	LEFTOVER Garlic & Rosemary Crusted Pork Loin / LEFTOVER Silky Potato Puree / LEFTOVER Garlic Roasted Broccoli	204 Hawaiian Pulled Pork / 248 Garlic-Rubbed Tostones / 244 Spicy Carrots
Friday	LEFTOVER Hawaiian Pulled Pork / LEFTOVER Garlic-Rubbed Tostones	LEFTOVER Garlic & Rosemary Crusted Pork Loin / LEFTOVER Roasted Cabbage with Balsamic-Honey Reduction	200 Greek Lamb Burgers / 252 Seasoned Plantain Fries / Simple Side Salad (p. 112)
Saturday	LEFTOVER Cinnamon & Raisin Porridge / Fruit & bacon	LEFTOVER Greek Lamb Burgers / LEFTOVER Spicy Carrots / Simple Side Salad (p. 112)	LEFTOVER Hawaiian Pulled Pork / LEFTOVER Spicy Carrots / LEFTOVER Seasoned Plantain Fries

20 minutes or less meal plan
for those who aren't fans of the kitchen

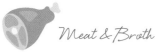
Meat & Broth

bacon, 2 servings per person

Beef Broth (page 109), 1½ cups

Bone Broth of choice (pages 108–109), 3 cups

Chicken Broth (page 108) or water, ¼ cup

ground beef, 2 pounds

ground lamb, 2 pounds

☆ ground lamb, 2 pounds

ground pork, 2 pounds

☆ ground pork, 1 pound

ham, uncured, about ⅓ pound

prosciutto, 4 ounces

rotisserie chicken, 1

☆ skirt steak, 1½ pounds

Seafood

salmon, wild-caught, 1 (8-ounce) fillet + 3 (6-ounce) fillets

☆ shrimp, medium, precooked, 1½ pounds

smoked salmon, 3 ounces

Fruit

avocados, 1⅓ medium

☆ avocado, 1 medium

☆ bananas, 2 medium

☆ blueberries, 2 cups

lemon, 1 large

lime, 1 medium

oranges, 2 medium

peaches, 2 medium

plantains, green, 2 medium

raspberries, 1 pint

red grapes, about ½ pound

fruit of choice, 3 servings per person

☆ fruit of choice, 2 servings per person

☆ purchase midweek

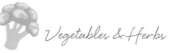
Vegetables & Herbs

☆ asparagus, 1½ pounds

basil leaves, 2¾ cups

☆ butternut squash, 3 pounds

☆ cauliflower, ½ head (about 1 pound)

celery, 3 stalks

cilantro, ¾ cup

☆ cucumbers, 2 servings per person

curly kale, 1 large bunch

☆ English cucumbers, 2 large

garlic, 1 large head

ginger, 1 (2-inch) piece

☆ green cabbage, 1 pound

green onions, 3 to 4 (2 ounces)

☆ mint, ½ cup sliced

☆ oregano leaves, ½ cup chopped

red onions, 3 large

romaine lettuce, 2 hearts + 1 head

☆ romaine lettuce, 2 hearts

shallots, 1¼ large

☆ shallots, 2 large

spaghetti squash, 2 (4 pounds each)

☆ spinach, 1 pound + 2 handfuls

thyme leaves, 2 tablespoons chopped

white sweet potatoes, 3 pounds (about 4 medium)

desired toppings for Classic American Hamburgers and Greek Lamb Burgers

mixed spring salad greens or baby spinach, for serving

Healing Kitchen Condiments & Spice Blends

Avocado Mayo (page 113) or Garlic-Dill Ranch Dressing (page 112), 1 cup

Caesar Dressing (page 110), ½ cup

Honey Balsamic Dressing (page 110), 2 tablespoons

Garlic & Herb Seasoning (page 123), 2 tablespoons

Greek Dressing (page 110), ¼ cup

Worcestershire Sauce (page 106), 1 tablespoon + 1 teaspoon

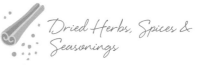
Dried Herbs, Spices & Seasonings

dried dill weed, 2½ teaspoons

dried parsley, ¼ teaspoon

dried rubbed sage, 2 teaspoons

garlic powder, 1½ teaspoons

ginger powder, 1 tablespoon

ground cinnamon, 1 tablespoon

ground mace, ½ teaspoon

onion powder, 2 teaspoons

truffle salt, ½ teaspoon

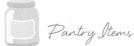
Pantry Items

albacore tuna, 2 (10-ounce) cans

apple cider vinegar, 1½ teaspoons

arrowroot starch, ½ teaspoon

balsamic vinegar, 1 teaspoon

black olives, ¾ cup pitted + ⅓ cup sliced

blackstrap molasses, 1 teaspoon

coconut aminos, ½ cup + 3 tablespoons

coconut milk, full-fat, 1¼ cups

coconut oil, ¼ cup + 3 tablespoons

dried apricots, 1 cup diced

extra-virgin olive oil, 1¼ cups

fat of choice, 2 tablespoons

fish sauce, 2½ teaspoons

hearts of palm, ⅔ cup chopped

honey, 1 tablespoon + 1 teaspoon

Kalamata olives, 1¼ cups pitted + 2 tablespoons finely chopped

nutritional yeast, ¼ cup

raisins, 1 cup

pumpkin or sweet potato puree, 2 cups

Other

frozen broccoli, 1 (16-ounce) bag

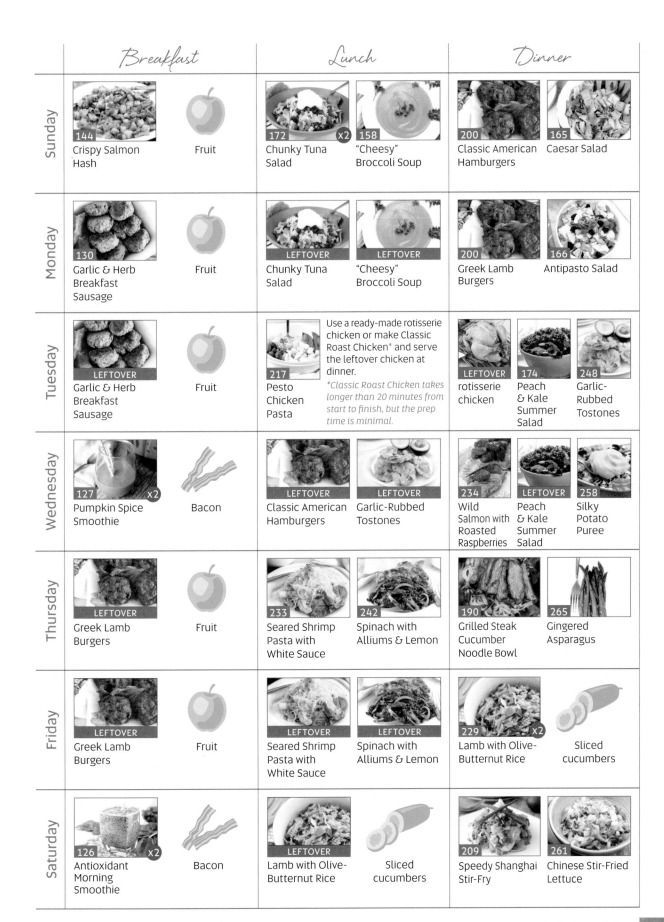

	Breakfast	Lunch	Dinner
Sunday	144 Crispy Salmon Hash · Fruit	172 (x2) Chunky Tuna Salad · 158 "Cheesy" Broccoli Soup	200 Classic American Hamburgers · 165 Caesar Salad
Monday	130 Garlic & Herb Breakfast Sausage · Fruit	LEFTOVER Chunky Tuna Salad · LEFTOVER "Cheesy" Broccoli Soup	200 Greek Lamb Burgers · 166 Antipasto Salad
Tuesday	LEFTOVER Garlic & Herb Breakfast Sausage · Fruit	217 Pesto Chicken Pasta · Use a ready-made rotisserie chicken or make Classic Roast Chicken* and serve the leftover chicken at dinner. *Classic Roast Chicken takes longer than 20 minutes from start to finish, but the prep time is minimal.	LEFTOVER rotisserie chicken · 174 Peach & Kale Summer Salad · 248 Garlic-Rubbed Tostones
Wednesday	127 (x2) Pumpkin Spice Smoothie · Bacon	LEFTOVER Classic American Hamburgers · LEFTOVER Garlic-Rubbed Tostones	234 Wild Salmon with Roasted Raspberries · LEFTOVER Peach & Kale Summer Salad · 258 Silky Potato Puree
Thursday	LEFTOVER Greek Lamb Burgers · Fruit	233 Seared Shrimp Pasta with White Sauce · 242 Spinach with Alliums & Lemon	190 Grilled Steak Cucumber Noodle Bowl · 265 Gingered Asparagus
Friday	LEFTOVER Greek Lamb Burgers · Fruit	LEFTOVER Seared Shrimp Pasta with White Sauce · LEFTOVER Spinach with Alliums & Lemon	229 (x2) Lamb with Olive-Butternut Rice · Sliced cucumbers
Saturday	126 (x2) Antioxidant Morning Smoothie · Bacon	LEFTOVER Lamb with Olive-Butternut Rice · Sliced cucumbers	209 Speedy Shanghai Stir-Fry · 261 Chinese Stir-Fried Lettuce

on-the-go meal plan for the busiest people

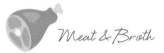

Meat & Broth

bacon, 40 slices

Beef Broth (page 109), 3 cups

Chicken Broth (page 108) or water, ½ cup

chickens, 2 whole (4 pounds each)

ground beef, 6 pounds

☆ ground beef, 2 pounds

ground pork, 3 pounds

☆ skirt steak, 1½ pounds

Seafood

shrimp, medium, precooked, 3 pounds

smoked salmon, 4 ounces

Fruit

apples, Granny Smith, 2

avocado, ½ medium

☆ avocados, 2 servings per person

lemons, 3 medium

limes, 3 medium

orange, ½ medium

☆ plantains, green, 2 medium

fruit of choice, 2 servings per person

☆ fruit of choice, 2 servings per person

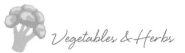

Vegetables & Herbs

basil leaves, 1 cup loosely packed

carrots, 10 large (about 4 pounds)

☆ carrots, 3 medium (about ½ pound)

cauliflower, 1 medium head

☆ celery, 3 stalks

cucumber slices, for serving

dill, 2 tablespoons chopped

☆ English cucumbers, 2 large

☆ ginger, 1 (1-inch) piece

mint, ½ cup sliced

mushrooms, 1 pound

☆ mushrooms, 8 ounces

orange sweet potatoes, 5½ pounds

rosemary, 5 sprigs + 2 tablespoons finely chopped

sage, 2 tablespoons minced, or dried rubbed sage, 2 teaspoons

shallots, 16 large

spaghetti squash, 2 (4 pounds each)

thyme, 10 sprigs + 1 teaspoon

☆ thyme, 5 sprigs

☆ white onion, 1 medium

yellow onions, 3 large

zucchini, 2 medium

☆ zucchini, 2 medium

mixed greens and veggies of choice for Simple Side Salad, 4 servings per person

☆ mixed greens and veggies of choice for Simple Side Salad, 1 serving per person

Other

frozen cherries, 1 (10-ounce) bag

sparkling water, ½ cup

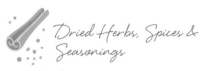

Dried Herbs, Spices & Seasonings

bay leaf, 1

dried rubbed sage, 1 teaspoon

garlic powder, 1¼ teaspoons

ginger powder, 1½ teaspoons

ground cinnamon, 2½ teaspoons

ground mace, ½ teaspoon

onion powder, ¼ teaspoon

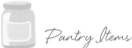

Pantry Items

anchovies, about ½ (2-ounce) can

apple chips, 6 ounces

balsamic vinegar, 1 teaspoon

black olives, pitted, 1 (6-ounce) can

capers, 2 tablespoons

coconut aminos, 1 tablespoon

coconut cream or full-fat coconut milk, ½ cup

coconut oil, ½ cup + 2 tablespoons

dried Turkish figs, 3 cups

extra-virgin olive oil, 1¼ cups + 1 tablespoon + 1 teaspoon

fish sauce, 2½ teaspoons

gelatin powder, unflavored, ¼ cup

Medjool dates, 4 large

wild-caught salmon, 1 (6-ounce) can

Healing Kitchen Condiments & Spice Blends

Cauli'fredo Sauce (page 119), 2 cups

Worcestershire Sauce (page 106), 2 tablespoons, or blackstrap molasses, 1 tablespoon

☆ *purchase midweek*

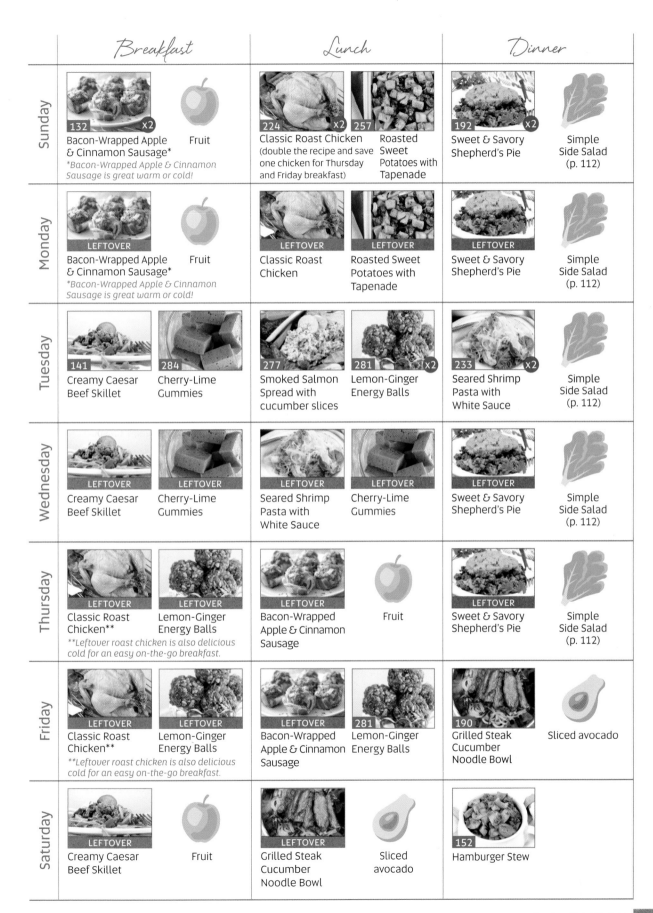

	Breakfast	Lunch	Dinner
Sunday	**132** x2 Bacon-Wrapped Apple & Cinnamon Sausage* / Fruit *Bacon-Wrapped Apple & Cinnamon Sausage is great warm or cold!*	**224** x2 Classic Roast Chicken (double the recipe and save one chicken for Thursday and Friday breakfast) / **257** Roasted Sweet Potatoes with Tapenade	**192** x2 Sweet & Savory Shepherd's Pie / Simple Side Salad (p. 112)
Monday	LEFTOVER Bacon-Wrapped Apple & Cinnamon Sausage* / Fruit *Bacon-Wrapped Apple & Cinnamon Sausage is great warm or cold!*	LEFTOVER Classic Roast Chicken / LEFTOVER Roasted Sweet Potatoes with Tapenade	LEFTOVER Sweet & Savory Shepherd's Pie / Simple Side Salad (p. 112)
Tuesday	**141** Creamy Caesar Beef Skillet / **284** Cherry-Lime Gummies	**277** Smoked Salmon Spread with cucumber slices / **281** x2 Lemon-Ginger Energy Balls	**233** x2 Seared Shrimp Pasta with White Sauce / Simple Side Salad (p. 112)
Wednesday	LEFTOVER Creamy Caesar Beef Skillet / LEFTOVER Cherry-Lime Gummies	LEFTOVER Seared Shrimp Pasta with White Sauce / LEFTOVER Cherry-Lime Gummies	LEFTOVER Sweet & Savory Shepherd's Pie / Simple Side Salad (p. 112)
Thursday	LEFTOVER Classic Roast Chicken** / LEFTOVER Lemon-Ginger Energy Balls **Leftover roast chicken is also delicious cold for an easy on-the-go breakfast.*	LEFTOVER Bacon-Wrapped Apple & Cinnamon Sausage / Fruit	LEFTOVER Sweet & Savory Shepherd's Pie / Simple Side Salad (p. 112)
Friday	LEFTOVER Classic Roast Chicken** / LEFTOVER Lemon-Ginger Energy Balls **Leftover roast chicken is also delicious cold for an easy on-the-go breakfast.*	LEFTOVER Bacon-Wrapped Apple & Cinnamon Sausage / **281** Lemon-Ginger Energy Balls	**190** Grilled Steak Cucumber Noodle Bowl / Sliced avocado
Saturday	LEFTOVER Creamy Caesar Beef Skillet / Fruit	LEFTOVER Grilled Steak Cucumber Noodle Bowl / Sliced avocado	**152** Hamburger Stew

family favorites
for those with kids to please

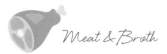

Meat & Broth

- bacon, 31 slices + 1 serving per person
- Beef Broth (page 109), 1½ cups
- Canadian bacon or ham, uncured, 6 ounces
- ☆ chicken, 1 whole (4 pounds)
- ☆ chicken, cooked and chopped, 1½ cups
- Chicken Broth (page 108), 1 cup
- chicken tenders, 1 pound
- chicken thighs, boneless, skinless, 2 pounds
- ground beef, 2 pounds
- ground chicken, thighs preferred, 2 pounds
- ground pork, 1½ pounds
- pork loin cutlets, boneless (about ½ inch thick), 4 pounds

Fruit

- apples, 4 Gala + 4 Golden Delicious + 1 Granny Smith
- ☆ avocado, 1 medium
- bananas, 3 medium
- ☆ bananas, 2 yellow medium + 3 green medium
- ☆ blueberries, 2 cups
- lemons, 2 medium
- lime, ½ medium
- ☆ oranges, 2 medium
- pineapple, 1
- plantains, green, 2 pounds + 2 large
- ☆ plantains, green, 1 pound
- fruit of choice, 1 serving per person
- ☆ fruit of choice, 3 servings per person

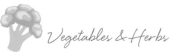

Vegetables & Herbs

- broccoli, 1 large head (about 2 pounds) + 1 medium head (about 1 pound) or 1 (12-ounce) bag florets
- ☆ Brussels sprouts, 1 pound
- carrots, 10 large (about 4 pounds) or 6 large (about 2½ pounds) + 2 (10-ounce) bags shredded
- ☆ carrots, 5 large (about 2 pounds)
- carrots, baby, 2 pounds
- chives, 2 tablespoons minced
- ☆ dill, 1 tablespoon
- garlic, 1 large head
- ☆ green onion, 1
- parsnips, 4 large
- ☆ red onions, 2 large + 1 small
- rosemary, 1 tablespoon finely chopped
- ☆ rosemary, 2 sprigs
- sage, 1 tablespoon + 1 teaspoon minced
- ☆ spinach, 1 pound + 2 handfuls
- thyme leaves, 2 tablespoons chopped
- ☆ thyme, 2½ teaspoons + 5 sprigs
- ☆ white sweet potatoes, 2 pounds (about 3 medium)
- ☆ yellow onion, 1 medium
- desired toppings for Classic American Hamburgers
- mixed greens and veggies of choice for Simple Side Salad, 1 serving per person

Healing Kitchen Condiments & Spice Blends

- Avocado Mayo (page 113), ½ cup
- Garlic Sauce (page 106), 2½ tablespoons
- House Rub (page 122), 2 teaspoons
- Garlic-Dill Ranch Dressing (page 112), ⅓ cup
- Worcestershire Sauce (page 106), 1 tablespoon

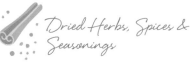

Dried Herbs, Spices & Seasonings

- cinnamon sticks, 4
- dried rubbed sage, ¼ teaspoon
- garlic powder, 2¼ teaspoons
- ginger powder, 1 teaspoon
- granulated garlic, ½ teaspoon
- ground cinnamon, 2½ tablespoons
- ground mace, 1¼ teaspoons
- onion powder, 2 teaspoons
- turmeric, ¼ teaspoon

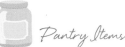

Pantry Items

- apple cider vinegar, 2 teaspoons
- arrowroot starch, ⅔ cup + 1 tablespoon
- bacon fat or coconut oil, ¼ cup
- baking soda, 1¾ teaspoons
- balsamic vinegar, 1 teaspoon
- blackstrap molasses, 1 tablespoon + 2 teaspoons
- coconut cream, 1 cup + 2 tablespoons
- coconut flour, 1 cup
- coconut milk, full-fat, 2 cups or 1 (13½-ounce) can + ¼ cup
- coconut oil, ½ cup + 2 tablespoons
- cream of tartar, 1 teaspoon
- extra-virgin olive oil, ½ cup + 3 tablespoons + 2 teaspoons
- fish sauce, 1 teaspoon
- honey, ¼ cup + 2 tablespoons
- honey or maple syrup, for serving
- pineapple chunks, 1 (14-ounce) can
- plantain chips, salted, 4 cups (about 2 {3.25-ounce] bags)
- raisins, 1¾ cups, plus more for garnish if desired
- shredded coconut, unsweetened, 1¾ cups, plus more for garnish if desired
- vanilla extract, 1 teaspoon

☆ *purchase midweek*

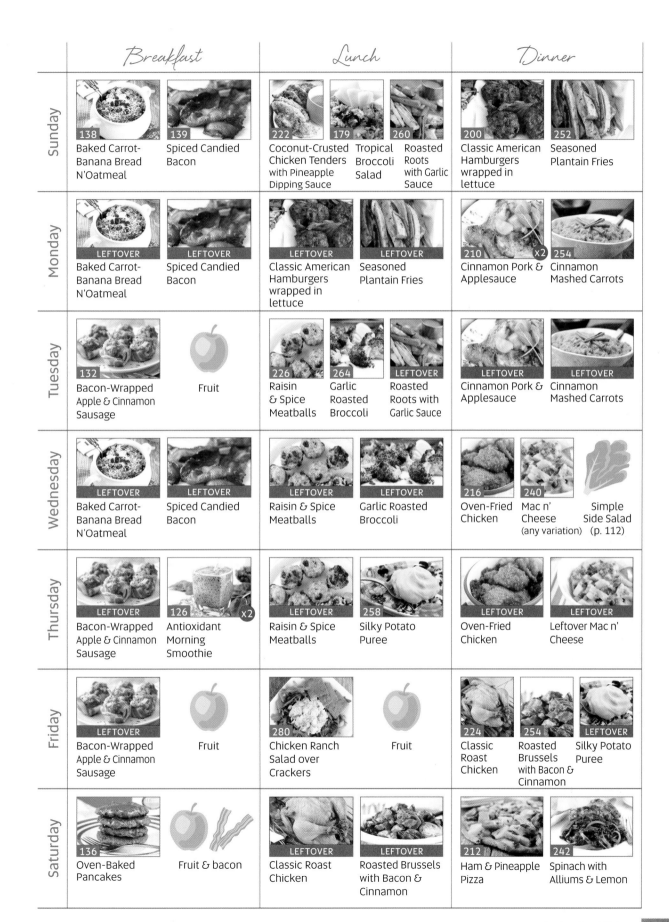

	Breakfast		Lunch			Dinner		
Sunday	**138** Baked Carrot-Banana Bread N'Oatmeal	**139** Spiced Candied Bacon	**222** Coconut-Crusted Chicken Tenders with Pineapple Dipping Sauce	**179** Tropical Broccoli Salad	**260** Roasted Roots with Garlic Sauce	**200** Classic American Hamburgers wrapped in lettuce	**252** Seasoned Plantain Fries	
Monday	LEFTOVER Baked Carrot-Banana Bread N'Oatmeal	LEFTOVER Spiced Candied Bacon	LEFTOVER Classic American Hamburgers wrapped in lettuce	LEFTOVER Seasoned Plantain Fries		**210** x2 Cinnamon Pork & Applesauce	**254** Cinnamon Mashed Carrots	
Tuesday	**132** Bacon-Wrapped Apple & Cinnamon Sausage	Fruit	**226** Raisin & Spice Meatballs	**264** Garlic Roasted Broccoli	LEFTOVER Roasted Roots with Garlic Sauce	LEFTOVER Cinnamon Pork & Applesauce	LEFTOVER Cinnamon Mashed Carrots	
Wednesday	LEFTOVER Baked Carrot-Banana Bread N'Oatmeal	LEFTOVER Spiced Candied Bacon	LEFTOVER Raisin & Spice Meatballs	LEFTOVER Garlic Roasted Broccoli		**216** Oven-Fried Chicken	**240** Mac n' Cheese (any variation)	Simple Side Salad (p. 112)
Thursday	LEFTOVER Bacon-Wrapped Apple & Cinnamon Sausage	**126** x2 Antioxidant Morning Smoothie	LEFTOVER Raisin & Spice Meatballs	**258** Silky Potato Puree		LEFTOVER Oven-Fried Chicken	LEFTOVER Leftover Mac n' Cheese	
Friday	LEFTOVER Bacon-Wrapped Apple & Cinnamon Sausage	Fruit	**280** Chicken Ranch Salad over Crackers	Fruit		**224** Classic Roast Chicken	**254** Roasted Brussels with Bacon & Cinnamon	LEFTOVER Silky Potato Puree
Saturday	**136** Oven-Baked Pancakes	Fruit & bacon	LEFTOVER Classic Roast Chicken	LEFTOVER Roasted Brussels with Bacon & Cinnamon		**212** Ham & Pineapple Pizza	**242** Spinach with Alliums & Lemon	

leftovers reinvented
for those who like to mix it up

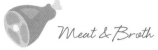

Meat & Broth

☆ baby back ribs, 3 pounds

bacon, 9 slices

Bone Broth of choice (pages 108–109), 1 cup

chicken breast, boneless, skinless, 2 pounds

☆ chicken breast, boneless, skinless, 2 pounds

☆ chicken breast, boneless, skinless, 2 pounds, or ground chicken breast, 2 pounds

Chicken Broth (page 108) or water, ⅔ cup

Chicken or Beef Broth (pages 108–109), 6 cups

chicken thighs, boneless, skinless, 3 pounds

chickens, 2 whole (4 pounds each)

ground beef, 2 pounds

ground pork, 2½ pounds

pork shoulder, boneless, 3 pounds

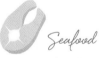

Seafood

☆ salmon, wild-caught, 2 (8-ounce) fillets

☆ smoked salmon, 6 ounces

Fruit

apples, 1 per person

avocados, 2 large + 3 medium + 3 servings per person

☆ avocado, 1 medium + 1 small + 1 serving per person

lemons, 7 medium

limes, 6 medium

☆ Mandarin oranges, 4

mango, 1 ripe + 1 green

oranges, 4 medium

plantains, 2 green-yellow + 4 green

☆ plantains, 2 green-yellow

☆ *purchase midweek*

Vegetables & Herbs

☆ arugula, 1 serving per person

carrots, 10 large (about 4 pounds)

cauliflower, 1 medium head (about 1½ pounds) or 1 (24-ounce) bag florets

cilantro, 2½ cups finely chopped

☆ cucumbers, 2 medium

☆ dill, ½ cup chopped

☆ fennel bulb, 6 ounces

garlic, 3 heads

☆ green cabbage, 1 small head

☆ green onion, 1

iceberg lettuce, shredded, 2 servings per person

☆ iceberg lettuce, 1 large head

mushrooms, 1 pound

orange sweet potatoes, 4 medium (6 inches long)

red onions, 2 large

romaine lettuce, 2 hearts

rosemary, 4 sprigs

shallots, 2 large

spinach, 1 pound

thyme, 10 sprigs + 1 teaspoon

white sweet potatoes, 2 pounds

☆ white sweet potatoes, 1 medium + 2 pounds

yellow onions, 1 large + 1 medium

zucchini, 2 medium

mixed greens and veggies of choice for Simple Side Salad, 1 serving per person

☆ mixed greens and veggies of choice for Simple Side Salad, 1 serving per person

Healing Kitchen Condiments & Spice Blends

House Rub (page 122), 2 tablespoons

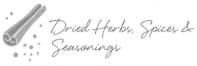

Dried Herbs, Spices & Seasonings

dried dill weed, 1 teaspoon

dried oregano leaves, 2 tablespoons + 2 teaspoons

dried parsley, ½ teaspoon

dried rubbed sage, 1½ teaspoons

dried thyme leaves, 1 tablespoon + 1¼ teaspoons

garlic powder, 2¾ teaspoons

ginger powder, 1 tablespoon + ¾ teaspoon

ground cinnamon, 1 teaspoon

ground mace, ¾ teaspoon

onion powder, 1½ teaspoons1

Pantry Items

anchovies, about ½ (2-ounce) can

apple cider vinegar, 1 cup + 2 tablespoons

bacon fat, ½ cup + 1 tablespoons

bacon or duck fat, 1 tablespoon

baking soda, 1 teaspoon

balsamic vinegar, 1 teaspoon

black olives, pitted, 1 (6-ounce) can

blackstrap molasses, 2 tablespoons

coconut cream, 1 cup

coconut cream or full-fat coconut milk, 1 cup

coconut oil, ½ cup + 1 tablespoon

coconut sugar or maple sugar, 1 tablespoon

cream of tartar, 2 teaspoons

extra-virgin olive oil, 2¼ cups + 1 tablespoon + 1 teaspoon

fat of choice, 2 teaspoons

fish sauce, 1 tablespoon + 1¾ teaspoon

honey, 1 teaspoon

Medjool dates, 4 large

plantain chips, 4 ounces

sweet potato puree, 1 cup

tapioca starch, ½ cup

	Breakfast	*Lunch*	*Dinner*
Sunday	128 (x2) Chicken Hash Brown Patties — 130 American Breakfast Sausage	214 116 121 Mojo Pulled Chicken topped with Mango Guacamole in Plantain Wraps — Simple Side Salad (p. 112)	224 (x2) 276 Classic Roast Chicken (reserve 3 cups shredded chicken for Saturday lunch) topped with Orange-Olive Tapenade — 242 Spinach with Alliums & Lemon
Monday	LEFTOVER LEFTOVER Chicken Hash Brown Patties stacked with leftover American Breakfast Sausage & sliced avocado	LEFTOVER LEFTOVER Leftover Mojo Pulled Chicken on top of shredded lettuce with leftover Mango Guacamole	165 Leftover Classic Roast Chicken made into Chicken Caesar Salad topped with diced avocado (double the Caesar Dressing, page 110)
Tuesday	141 Creamy Caesar Beef Skillet using leftover Caesar Dressing	219 Mojo-Mango Stuffed Sweet Potatoes — (reserve 2 baked sweet potatoes for Thursday breakfast)	158 Chicken "Tortilla" Soup using leftover Mojo Pulled Chicken — 188 Toasted Lime Cilantro Cauli-Rice
Wednesday	LEFTOVER LEFTOVER Chicken Hash Brown Patties stacked with leftover American Breakfast Sausage and thinly sliced apples	LEFTOVER Chicken "Tortilla" Soup topped with diced avocado	206 BBQ Pulled Pork (reserve extra Tangy Carolina BBQ Sauce for Friday dinner) — 248 (x2) Garlic-Rubbed Tostones — 178 Thai Green Mango Salad
Thursday	LEFTOVER Creamy Caesar Beef Skillet served over a baked 6-inch sweet potato	271 Pulled Pork Sliders using leftover BBQ Pulled Pork and Garlic-Rubbed Tostones topped with shredded lettuce	168 Grilled Chicken Souvlaki Salad
Friday	144 (x2) Crispy Salmon Hash	168 Greek Gyro Wraps using leftover Grilled Chicken Souvlaki — LEFTOVER Thai Green Mango Salad	118 Oven-Baked BBQ Ribs using leftover Tangy BBQ Sauce — 170 Fennel Mandarin Slaw
Saturday	LEFTOVER Crispy Salmon Hash served cold over arugula salad with diced avocado and Greek Dressing (page 110)	LEFTOVER LEFTOVER Shredded Chicken & Fennel Mandarin Slaw using leftover Classic Roast Chicken and leftover Fennel Mandarin Slaw	206 BBQ Pulled Pork Stromboli using leftover BBQ Pulled Pork — Simple Side Salad (p. 112)

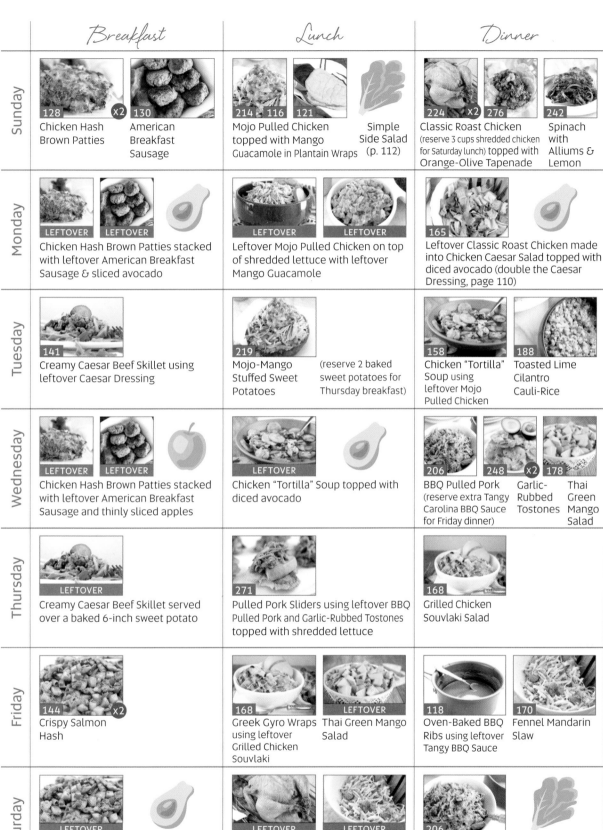

batch cooking meal plan #1 with cooking video

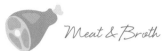

Meat & Broth

bacon, 33 slices regular + 8 slices thick-cut

Beef Broth (page 109) or water, ½ cup

Bone Broth of choice (pages 108–109), 1 cup

Chicken Broth (page 108), 2 cups

Chicken or Pork Broth (pages 108–109), 6 cups

chickens, 2 whole (4 pounds each)

ground beef, 1 pound + 1 pound lean

ground pork, 3 pounds

pork shoulder, boneless, 3 pounds

Fruit

apples, 2 Gala + 2 Granny Smith

lemons, 2½ medium

plantains, green, 4 pounds + 2 medium + 2 large

fruit of choice, 4 servings per person

☆ fruit of choice, 3 servings per person

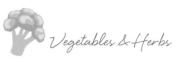

Vegetables & Herbs

basil leaves, 4 cups loosely packed

carrots, 12 large (about 5 pounds)

celery, 4 to 6 stalks

chives, ¼ cup minced

cilantro, 1½ cups loosely packed

garlic, 1 head

parsley, ¼ cup + 2 tablespoons chopped

parsnips, 1½ pounds

rosemary, 4 sprigs + 2 tablespoons chopped

spaghetti squash, 2 (4 pounds each)

thyme, 18 to 20 sprigs

turnips, 2 large

yellow onions, 5 medium

mixed greens and veggies for Simple Side Salad, 2 servings per person

☆ mixed greens and veggies for Simple Side Salad, 4 servings per person

root vegetables of choice, 3 pounds

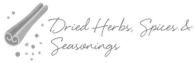

Dried Herbs, Spices & Seasonings

bay leaves, 4

dried mint, 2 tablespoons

garlic powder, 1 teaspoon

ginger powder, 1 teaspoon

granulated garlic, ¼ teaspoon

ground cinnamon, 1 tablespoon + 1 teaspoon

ground cloves, ⅛ teaspoon

ground mace, ½ teaspoon

onion powder, 1 teaspoon

turmeric, ½ teaspoon

Pantry Items

apple cider vinegar, 2 teaspoons

arrowroot starch, 1 tablespoon + 1 teaspoon

bacon fat or coconut oil, 1 tablespoon

black olives, ⅔ cup sliced

blackstrap molasses, 2 teaspoons

clams, 6 (5- to 6-ounce) cans

coconut cream, 6¼ cups

coconut sugar or maple sugar, 1 tablespoon

extra-virgin olive oil, 1 cup + 1 tablespoon + 1 teaspoon

extra-virgin olive oil or avocado oil, 2 tablespoons

Healing Kitchen Condiments & Spice Blends

Tangy Carolina BBQ Sauce (page 118), ¾ cup

☆ *purchase midweek*

how to organize your batch cooking session

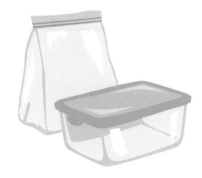

1. Prepare the BBQ Pulled Pork in a slow cooker or pressure cooker.

2. Meanwhile, bake the Bacon-Wrapped Apple & Cinnamon Sausage and the Comforting Breakfast Casserole in a 350-degree oven at the same time, according to their individual cooking times.

3. While the sausage and casserole are in the oven, cook the New England Clam Chowder on the stovetop.

4. Once the sausage and casserole are out of the oven, increase the temperature to 400 degrees and bake the Classic Roast Chicken and Spaghetti Squash Noodles (for the Pesto Chicken Pasta).

5. Once the clam chowder is off the stove, make the Lebanese Beef & Rice Stuffing and Mac n' Cheese.

6. While the Lebanese Beef & Rice Stuffing and Mac n' Cheese are cooking, make the Pronto Pesto for the Pesto Chicken Pasta in a blender.

7. Make the Pesto Chicken Pasta using the prepared Classic Roast Chicken and Spaghetti Squash Noodles.

8. Prepare your salad dressing of choice to serve with the Simple Side Salads throughout the week. Simple Side Salads can also be prepared and stored in the fridge separately from the dressing.

9. Freeze meals (other than salads) for Thursday, Friday, and Saturday. Thaw in the refrigerator overnight before reheating.

 Want to see how we organize our time for batch cooking? Check out our how-to video for this meal plan here: thepaleomom. com/thehealingkitchenvideos

	Breakfast	*Lunch*	*Dinner*
Sunday	132 x2 Bacon-Wrapped Apple & Cinnamon Sausage / Fruit	162 x2 New England Clam Chowder	224 x2 Classic Roast Chicken (double the recipe and add 3 pounds root vegetables around the chicken) / 246 Lebanese Beef & Rice Stuffing
Monday	LEFTOVER Bacon-Wrapped Cinnamon & Apple Sausage / Fruit	LEFTOVER Classic Roast Chicken and root vegetables / LEFTOVER Beef & Rice Stuffing	206 BBQ Pulled Pork / 240 x2 Mac n' Cheese / Simple Side Salad (p. 112)
Tuesday	140 Comforting Breakfast Casserole / Fruit	LEFTOVER New England Clam Chowder	LEFTOVER BBQ Pulled Pork / LEFTOVER Mac n' Cheese / Simple Side Salad (p. 112)
Wednesday	LEFTOVER Bacon-Wrapped Apple & Cinnamon Sausage / Fruit	217 x2 Pesto Chicken Pasta using leftover Classic Roast Chicken	LEFTOVER New England Clam Chowder
Thursday	LEFTOVER Comforting Breakfast Casserole / Fruit	LEFTOVER Pesto Chicken Pasta	LEFTOVER New England Clam Chowder / Simple Side Salad (p. 112)
Friday	LEFTOVER Bacon-Wrapped Apple & Cinnamon Sausage / Fruit	LEFTOVER BBQ Pulled Pork / LEFTOVER Mac n' Cheese / Simple Side Salad (p. 112)	LEFTOVER New England Clam Chowder / Simple Side Salad (p. 112)
Saturday	LEFTOVER Bacon-Wrapped Apple & Cinnamon Sausage / Fruit	LEFTOVER New England Clam Chowder / Simple Side Salad (p. 112)	Leftover meal of choice from earlier in the week

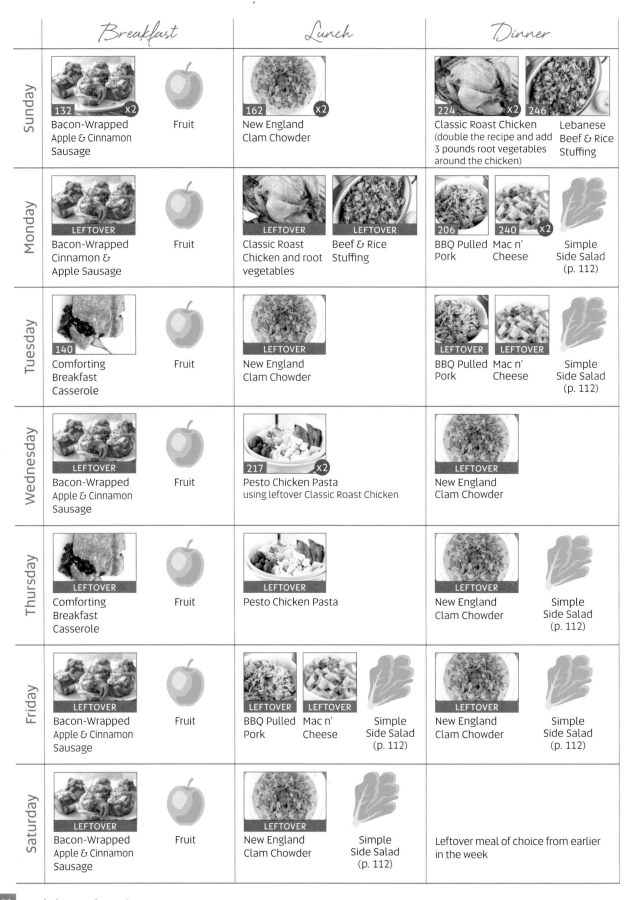

batch cooking meal plan #2 with cooking video

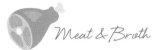

Meat & Broth

bacon, 10 slices

☆ bacon, 6 slices

beef bottom round, 4 pounds

Beef Broth (page 109), 8 cups

Bone Broth of choice (pages 108–109), 2 cups

chicken breast, boneless, skinless, 2 pounds

Chicken Broth (page 108) or water, 1⅓ cups

Chicken or Beef Broth (pages 108–109), 6 cups

chicken thighs, boneless, skinless, 3 pounds

ground beef, 4 pounds

☆ pork shoulder, boneless, 6 pounds

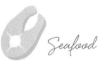

Seafood

shrimp, medium, 2 pounds

Fruit

avocado, 1 medium

☆ avocado, 1 serving per person

lemons, 2 large

limes, 4 medium

oranges, 3 medium

☆ peaches, 2 medium

☆ plantains, green, 2 large

fruit of choice, 3 servings per person

☆ fruit of choice, 2 servings per person

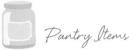

Vegetables & Herbs

basil leaves, ½ cup chopped

broccoli, 2 large heads (about 4 pounds)

carrots, 8 large (about 3½ pounds)

cauliflower, 2 large + 2 medium heads (about 7 pounds total), or 2 large heads (about 4 pounds) + 2 (12-ounce) bags florets

celery, 8 stalks

cilantro, 2 cups chopped

☆ curly kale, 1 large bunch

garlic, 3 heads

green onion, 1

kale, 2 bunches

mushrooms, 2 pounds

orange sweet potatoes, 4 medium (6 inches long)

red onion, 1 medium

☆ shallot, 1 small

thyme, 6 sprigs

yellow onions, 8 large

zucchini, 4 medium

mixed greens and veggies of choice for Simple Side Salad, 2 servings per person

Other

red wine, 1 cup

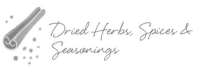

Dried Herbs, Spices & Seasonings

bay leaves, 2

cinnamon sticks, 2

dried oregano leaves, 2 tablespoons + 2 teaspoons

dried parsley, 2 teaspoons

dried thyme leaves, 1½ teaspoons

garlic powder, 1½ teaspoons

ginger powder, 1½ teaspoons

ground cinnamon, ½ teaspoon

onion powder, ½ teaspoon

Pantry Items

anchovies, about 1 (2-ounce) can

apple cider vinegar, ¼ cup + 2 tablespoons

coconut cream or full-fat coconut milk, 1 cup

coconut oil, 1 tablespoon

extra-virgin olive oil, 1½ cups + 1 tablespoon

fat of choice, 1 tablespoon + 1 teaspoon

fat, solid (such as duck fat, lard, or tallow), ¼ cup

fish sauce, 1 tablespoon + 2 teaspoons

pineapple chunks, 2 (14-ounce) cans

plantain chips, 4 ounces

sweet potato puree, 2 cups

Healing Kitchen Condiments & Spice Blends

Honey Balsamic Dressing (page 110), 2 tablespoons

House Rub (page 122), 2 teaspoons

Mango Guacamole (page 116), ⅔ cup

☆ *purchase midweek*

how to organize your batch cooking session

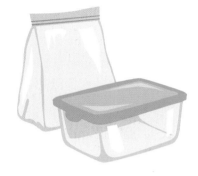

1. Prepare the Mojo Pulled Chicken and cook in your slow cooker or pressure cooker.

2. Once the chicken is done, clean out the cooking vessel, then prepare the Hawaiian Pulled Pork. If using a slow cooker, you may not be able to cook both in the same day. If this is the case, you may cook the pork overnight the night before and shred it the following morning.

3. In a 425-degree oven, bake the Seasoned Plantain Fries and Garlic Roasted Broccoli according to their individual cooking times, and at the same time bake the sweet potatoes for the Mojo-Mango Stuffed Sweet Potatoes for 45 minutes to 1 hour, until tender.

4. Meanwhile, make a triple batch of Caesar Dressing in a blender.

5. Prepare the Creamy Caesar Beef Skillet on the stovetop on one burner and the Hearty Healing Beef Stew on another burner.

6. Once the stovetop is available, prepare the Shrimp n' Cauli-Grits and Toasted Lime Cilantro Cauli-Rice.

7. Meanwhile, prepare the Mango Guacamole for the stuffed sweet potatoes in a blender or food processor. Assemble the Mojo-Mango Stuffed Sweet Potatoes using shredded Mojo Pulled Chicken, but store the Mango Guacamole separately until serving.

8. The Peach & Kale Summer Salad should be prepared less than 24 hours in advance. You can make the Honey Balsamic Dressing (and double the recipe so you have extra dressing for Simple Side Salads throughout the week) today as well as chop the shallots and kale and store them in the refrigerator to quickly throw together in the middle of the week. Then on Thursday night, prepare the salad in 10 minutes while you reheat the pork and plantain fries. You may assemble the Chicken "Tortilla" Soup during your batch cook session or you may prepare it the night you want to serve it. Either way, don't add the plantain chips until just before serving.

9. Freeze meals (other than salads) for Thursday, Friday, and Saturday. Thaw in the refrigerator overnight before reheating.

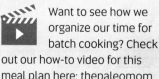

Want to see how we organize our time for batch cooking? Check out our how-to video for this meal plan here: thepaleomom.com/thehealingkitchenvideos

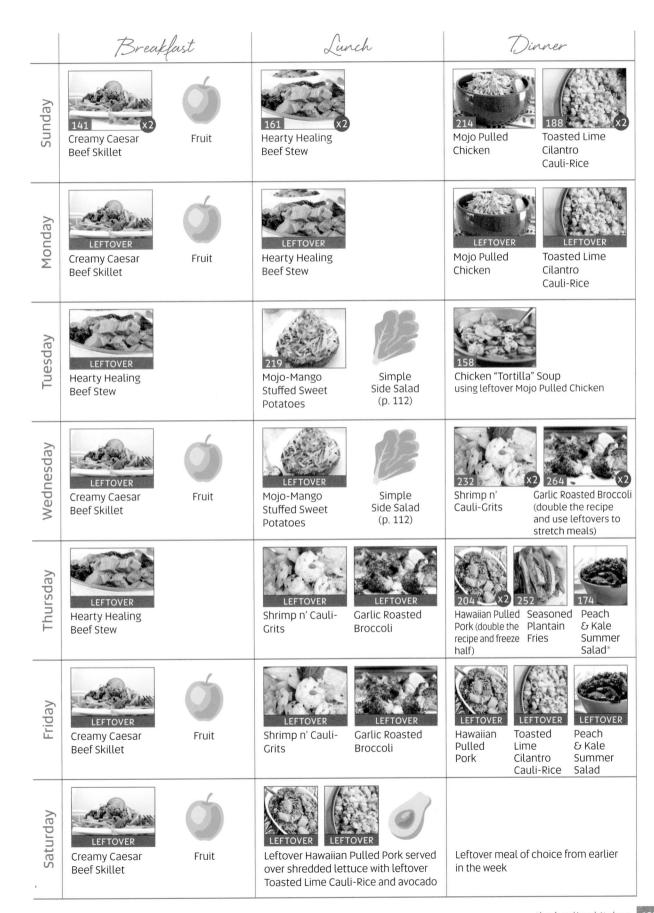

	Breakfast	*Lunch*	*Dinner*
Sunday	141 x2 Creamy Caesar Beef Skillet / Fruit	161 x2 Hearty Healing Beef Stew	214 Mojo Pulled Chicken / 188 x2 Toasted Lime Cilantro Cauli-Rice
Monday	LEFTOVER Creamy Caesar Beef Skillet / Fruit	LEFTOVER Hearty Healing Beef Stew	LEFTOVER Mojo Pulled Chicken / LEFTOVER Toasted Lime Cilantro Cauli-Rice
Tuesday	LEFTOVER Hearty Healing Beef Stew	219 Mojo-Mango Stuffed Sweet Potatoes / Simple Side Salad (p. 112)	158 Chicken "Tortilla" Soup using leftover Mojo Pulled Chicken
Wednesday	LEFTOVER Creamy Caesar Beef Skillet / Fruit	LEFTOVER Mojo-Mango Stuffed Sweet Potatoes / Simple Side Salad (p. 112)	232 x2 Shrimp n' Cauli-Grits / 264 x2 Garlic Roasted Broccoli (double the recipe and use leftovers to stretch meals)
Thursday	LEFTOVER Hearty Healing Beef Stew	LEFTOVER Shrimp n' Cauli-Grits / LEFTOVER Garlic Roasted Broccoli	204 x2 Hawaiian Pulled Pork (double the recipe and freeze half) / 252 Seasoned Plantain Fries / 174 Peach & Kale Summer Salad*
Friday	LEFTOVER Creamy Caesar Beef Skillet / Fruit	LEFTOVER Shrimp n' Cauli-Grits / LEFTOVER Garlic Roasted Broccoli	LEFTOVER Hawaiian Pulled Pork / LEFTOVER Toasted Lime Cilantro Cauli-Rice / LEFTOVER Peach & Kale Summer Salad
Saturday	LEFTOVER Creamy Caesar Beef Skillet / Fruit	LEFTOVER LEFTOVER Leftover Hawaiian Pulled Pork served over shredded lettuce with leftover Toasted Lime Cauli-Rice and avocado	Leftover meal of choice from earlier in the week

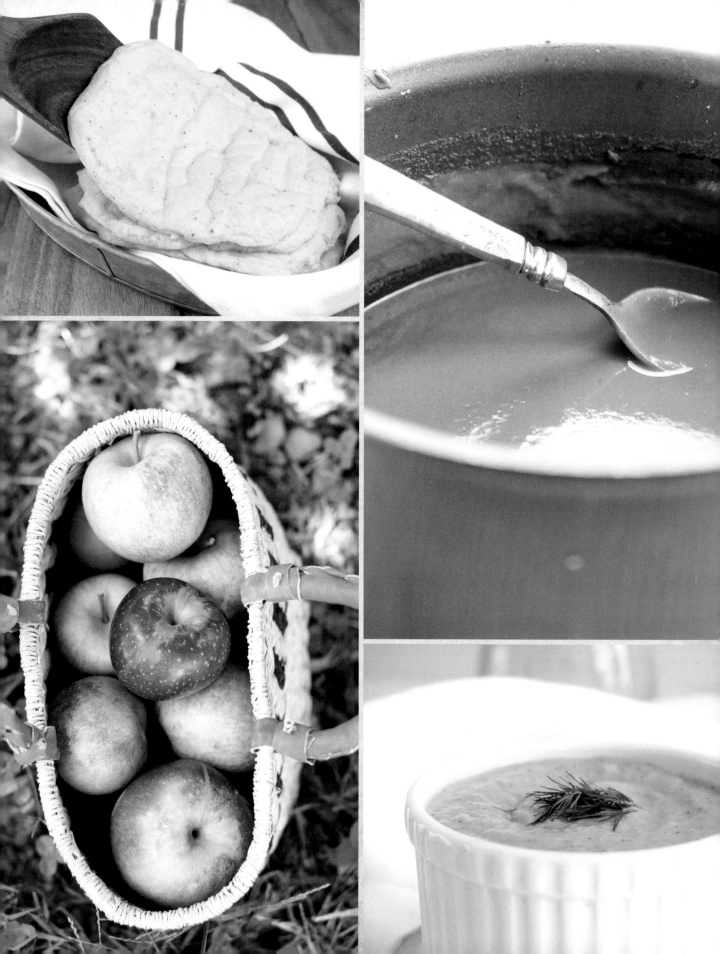

kitchen basics

worcestershire sauce

Makes ⅓ cup | Prep Time: 5 minutes | Cook Time: 10 minutes | Total Time: 15 minutes

⅔ cup apple cider vinegar

2 tablespoons honey

1½ tablespoons blackstrap molasses

2 teaspoons fish sauce

½ teaspoon ginger powder

½ teaspoon garlic powder

½ teaspoon onion powder

½ teaspoon fine sea salt

¼ teaspoon ground cinnamon

1. Whisk all the ingredients together in a small saucepan. Bring to a boil over medium-high heat.

2. Reduce to a simmer over medium-low heat and cook uncovered for 5 to 8 minutes, until the liquid has reduced to the thickness of runny honey. Be careful not to over-reduce the liquid or it will caramelize and thicken too much. Remove from the heat and transfer to a glass container to cool.

Serving Suggestions
Use as you would store-bought Worcestershire sauce to add a savory flavor to beef, pork, and lamb dishes, such as Classic American Hamburgers (page 200).

Storage
Store in a sealed glass container at room temperature for up to 2 weeks or in the refrigerator for up to 1 month.

garlic sauce

Makes 1 cup | Prep Time: 5 minutes | Total Time: 5 minutes + 30 minutes to rest

½ cup extra-virgin olive oil

½ cup full-fat coconut milk

¼ cup peeled garlic cloves, chopped

1 tablespoon fresh lemon juice

½ teaspoon fine sea salt

Place all the ingredients in a blender and puree on high speed until emulsified and smooth, about 1 minute. Allow the garlic flavor to mellow for at least 30 minutes before serving.

Serving Suggestions
Use as a marinade in Honey-Garlic Drumsticks (page 218) or when roasting root vegetables in Roasted Roots with Garlic Sauce (page 260), which is transformed into a light salad in Roasted Root, Arugula & Balsamic Salad (page 168).

Storage
Store in a sealed glass container in the refrigerator for up to 1 week.

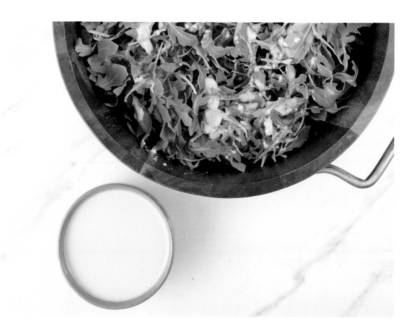

caramelized onions

Makes 2½ cups | Prep Time: 5 minutes | Cook Time: 20 minutes | Total Time: 25 minutes

1 tablespoon extra-virgin olive oil

2 large Vidalia onions, thinly sliced

Make Ahead

Thinly slice the onions, wrap in paper towels, and store in a plastic bag in the refrigerator for up to 3 days.

Serving Suggestions

Use in Caramelized Onion & Herb Meatloaf (page 191) or on top of Classic American Hamburgers (page 200).

Storage

Once cool, store in a sealed glass container in the refrigerator for up to 1 week or in the freezer for up to 6 months.

1. Heat the olive oil in a medium saucepan over medium heat. Add the onions and toss to coat in the oil. Cover the pan with a lid.

2. Cook for about 20 minutes, stirring the onions and scraping up the browned bits on the bottom of the pan with a wooden spoon every 5 minutes, until the onions are golden brown and tender.

roasted garlic

Makes 1 cup | Prep Time: 5 minutes | Cook Time: 35 minutes | Total Time: 40 minutes

1 cup peeled garlic cloves (see Tip)

1 tablespoon extra-virgin olive oil

½ teaspoon fine sea salt

Tip

Buy prepeeled garlic to save yourself the hassle of peeling all those cloves by hand.

Serving Suggestions

Use in Roasted Garlic & Pumpkin Hummus (page 274), blend ¼ cup roasted garlic with 2 ripe avocados for a roasted garlic and avocado dip, or mash roasted garlic and use to top grilled steak.

Storage

Once cool, store in a sealed glass container in the refrigerator for up to 1 week.

1. Preheat the oven to 375 degrees. Line a rimmed baking sheet with parchment paper.

2. Toss the garlic cloves with the olive oil and salt on the prepared baking sheet and spread into a single layer. Roast for 35 minutes, tossing halfway through cooking, until the garlic is lightly golden brown and has taken on a sweet flavor.

bone broth

Bone broth can be made from the bones of well-raised chickens, pigs, cattle, and fish. Also known as stock in the restaurant industry, it adds flavor and nutrition to a variety of dishes, such as soups, stews, purees, braises, and sauces. Quantity will depend on the amount of water that your cooking vessel holds. The amount of bones called for should fit in a 6-quart slow cooker or pressure cooker or a large stockpot.

chicken broth

Makes 4 to 5 quarts | Prep Time: 10 minutes | Cook Time: 2 to 48 hours, depending on cooking method |
Total Time: 2 hours 10 minutes to 48 hours 10 minutes, depending on cooking method

2 whole roasted chicken carcasses

1 tablespoon apple cider vinegar

5 cloves garlic, peeled

2 teaspoons fine sea salt

3 cups chopped vegetables such as carrots, onions, and celery (optional)

2 sprigs fresh rosemary or thyme

Filtered water

Tip

All of the recipes in this book that include the option to use a pressure cooker were made using an electric model with a digital controller. This third-generation pressure cooker is very different from the stovetop model that your grandmother or great-grandmother would have used. Today's pressure cookers are incredibly safe and easy to use, and some are even available with smart programming. The brand I use is Instant Pot.

Storage

Once cool, store in a sealed glass container in the refrigerator for up to 1 week or in the freezer for up to 3 months.

Pressure cooker instructions (see Tip): Put all the ingredients (including the vegetables, if using) in the pressure cooker insert and fill with water to the maximum fill line. Seal the lid and set the pressure cooker's manual timer to 120 minutes. Release the pressure when the timer goes off.

Slow cooker instructions: Put all the ingredients except the vegetables (if using) in the slow cooker insert. Add enough water to cover the carcasses and no higher than the fill line recommended by the manufacturer. Cook on low for 48 hours, adding the vegetables to the slow cooker when 6 to 8 hours of cooking time remains.

Stovetop instructions: Put all the ingredients except the vegetables (if using) in a large stockpot. Add enough water to cover the carcasses, leaving at least 1 inch of space at the top of the pot. Bring to a boil, cover with a lid, and reduce to a low simmer for 24 hours, adding the vegetables to the pot when 6 to 8 hours of cooking time remains.

To strain broth: Set a colander or mesh strainer over a large heat-safe bowl in the sink. Slowly and carefully pour the contents of the pot into the colander, allowing the broth to drain into the bowl. Discard the bones and vegetables, if used, or let the bones cool completely, then store them a plastic bag in the freezer to be used again to make one more pot of broth within 3 months of freezing.

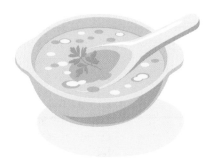

pork broth

Makes 4 to 5 quarts | Prep Time: 5 minutes | Cook Time: 2 hours 45 minutes to 48 hours 45 minutes, depending on cooking method | Total Time: 2 hours 50 minutes to 48 hours 50 minutes, depending on cooking method

2 to 3 pounds pork bones

1 tablespoon apple cider vinegar

2 teaspoons fine sea salt

Filtered water

Storage
Once cool, store in a sealed glass container in the refrigerator for up to 1 week or in the freezer for up to 3 months.

For all methods: Before adding the bones, roast the bones on a large parchment-lined rimmed baking sheet in a 350-degree oven for 45 minutes or until browned.

Pressure cooker instructions (see Tip, opposite): Put all the ingredients in the pressure cooker insert and fill with water to the maximum fill line. Seal the lid and set the pressure cooker's manual timer to 120 minutes. Release the pressure when the timer goes off.

Slow cooker instructions: Put all the ingredients in the slow cooker insert and fill with enough water to cover the bones, not exceeding the fill line recommended by the manufacturer. Cook on low for 48 hours.

Stovetop instructions: Put all the ingredients in a large stockpot. Add enough water to cover the bones, leaving at least 1 inch of space at the top of the pot. Bring to a boil, cover with a lid, and reduce to a low simmer for 24 to 36 hours.

To strain broth: Set a colander or mesh strainer over a large heat-safe bowl in the sink. Slowly and carefully pour the contents of the pot into the colander, allowing the broth to drain into the bowl. Discard the bones or let cool completely, then store in a plastic bag in the freezer to be used again to make one more pot of broth within 3 months of freezing.

beef broth

Makes 4 to 5 quarts | Prep Time: 5 minutes | Cook Time: 2 hours 45 minutes to 48 hours 45 minutes, depending on cooking method | Total Time: 2 hours 50 minutes to 48 hours 50 minutes, depending on cooking method

2 to 3 pounds beef bones, such as marrow bones

1 tablespoon apple cider vinegar

2 teaspoons fine sea salt

Filtered water

Storage
Once cool, store in a sealed glass container in the refrigerator for up to 1 week or in the freezer for up to 3 months.

For all methods: Before adding the bones, roast the bones on a large parchment-lined rimmed baking sheet in a 350-degree oven for 45 minutes or until browned.

Pressure cooker instructions (see Tip, opposite): Put all the ingredients in the pressure cooker insert and fill with water to the maximum fill line. Seal the lid and set the pressure cooker's manual timer to 120 minutes. Release the pressure when the timer goes off.

Slow cooker instructions: Put all the ingredients in the slow cooker insert and fill with enough water to cover the bones, not exceeding the fill line recommended by the manufacturer. Cook on low for 48 hours.

Stovetop instructions: Put all the ingredients in a large stockpot. Add enough water to cover the bones, leaving at least 1 inch of space at the top of the pot. Bring to a boil, cover with a lid, and reduce to a low simmer for 24 hours.

To strain broth: Set a colander or mesh strainer over a large heat-safe bowl in the sink. Slowly and carefully pour the contents of the pot into the colander, allowing the broth to drain into the bowl. Discard the bones or let cool completely, then store in a plastic bag in the freezer to be used again to make one more pot of broth within 3 months of freezing.

greek dressing

Makes about 1 cup | Prep Time: 5 minutes |
Total Time: 5 minutes

½ cup extra-virgin olive oil

¼ cup apple cider vinegar

2 tablespoons fresh lemon juice

2 cloves garlic, pressed

2 teaspoons dried oregano leaves

½ teaspoon fine sea salt

Whisk all the ingredients together until combined.
Stir before serving.

Serving Suggestions
*Use in Antipasto Salad (page 166) or Grilled Chicken
Souvlaki Salad (page 168).*

Storage
*Store in a sealed glass container in the refrigerator for up
to 1 month. The oil and vinegar will separate. Allow the
dressing to come to room temperature before stirring or
shaking vigorously to re-emulsify it.*

honey balsamic dressing

Makes about ¾ cup | Prep Time: 5 minutes |
Total Time: 5 minutes

½ cup extra-virgin olive oil

¼ cup balsamic vinegar

2 tablespoons honey

½ teaspoon fine sea salt

Whisk together all the ingredients until combined.
Stir before serving.

Serving Suggestions
*Use in Peach & Kale Summer Salad (page 174) or Sweet &
Smoky Spa Salad (page 166).*

Storage
*Store in a sealed glass container in the refrigerator for up
to 2 weeks. The oil and vinegar will separate. Allow the
dressing to come to room temperature before stirring or
shaking vigorously to re-emulsify it.*

strawberry lime dressing

Makes about 1 cup | Prep Time: 8 minutes |
Total Time: 8 minutes

½ cup strawberries

¼ cup extra-virgin olive oil

1 tablespoon fresh lime juice

1 tablespoon coconut aminos (optional)

½ teaspoon fine sea salt

¼ teaspoon ginger powder

Remove the green tops from the strawberries. Place
all the ingredients in a blender and blend on high
speed until very smooth.

Serving Suggestions
*Use in Honey-Lime Chicken & Strawberry Salad (page 171)
or as a marinade for chicken breasts or drumsticks before
roasting in the oven.*

Storage
*Store in a sealed glass container in the refrigerator for up
to 1 week.*

caesar dressing

Makes about 1 cup | Prep Time: 8 minutes |
Total Time: 8 minutes

½ cup coconut cream or full-fat coconut milk

½ cup mashed avocado

¼ cup extra-virgin olive oil

2 cloves garlic, pressed

1 tablespoon fresh lemon juice

2 teaspoons mashed anchovies

½ teaspoon fish sauce

½ teaspoon fine sea salt

¼ teaspoon garlic powder

¼ teaspoon onion powder

Place all the ingredients in a blender and blend on
high speed until smooth.

Serving Suggestion
Use in Caesar Salad (page 165).

Storage
*Store in a sealed glass container in the refrigerator for up
to 1 week.*

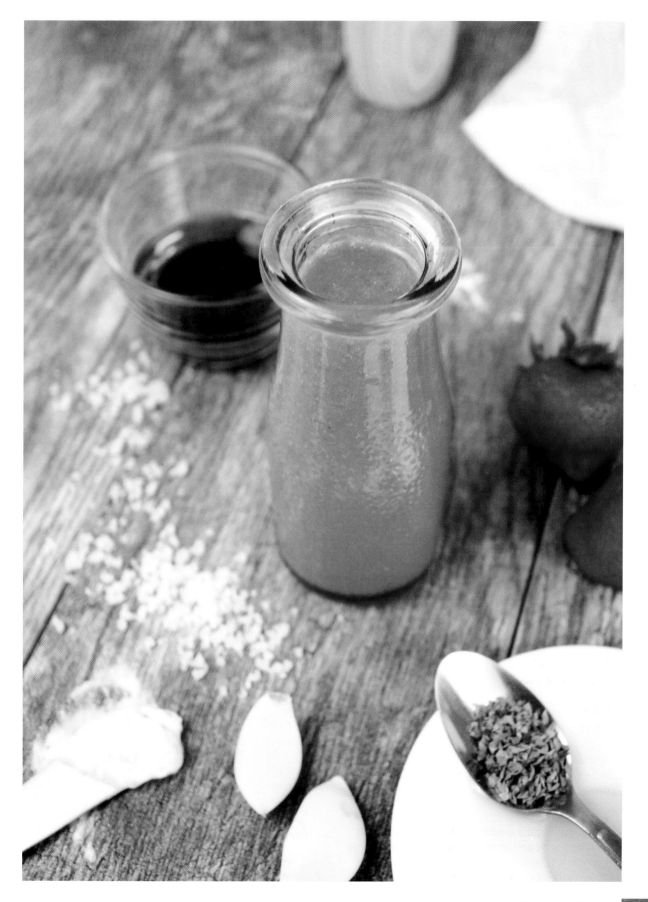

garlic-dill ranch dressing

Makes 1¼ cups | Prep Time: 10 minutes | Total Time: 10 minutes

¾ cup coconut cream, chilled

⅓ cup palm shortening

¼ cup plus 2 tablespoons extra-virgin olive oil

2 teaspoons apple cider vinegar

1 teaspoon lemon juice

1 tablespoon minced yellow onion

1½ teaspoons dried chives

1 teaspoon minced garlic

1 teaspoon minced fresh dill

½ teaspoon dried dill weed

½ teaspoon dried parsley

¼ teaspoon garlic powder

¼ teaspoon onion powder

1. In a mixing bowl, combine the coconut cream, palm shortening, olive oil, vinegar, and lemon juice.

2. Beat with a hand mixer on medium speed until smooth and creamy. At this point, you have a basic mayonnaise that can be used in cold sauces, dressings, and salads.

3. Add the remaining ingredients and mix with a spoon until well combined.

Storage

Store in a sealed glass container in the refrigerator for up to 1 week.

simple side salad

A simple side salad is a fantastic way to round out any meal that is lacking in greens. Build your own by mixing and matching some of the easy-to-source ingredients below. Make a double batch of one of our dressings for quick salads throughout the week!

Arugula

Lettuce

Spinach

Carrots (shredded or matchstick)

Cucumbers

Mushrooms

Onions

Radishes

Beets (raw, roasted, or steamed)

Avocados

Olives

Basil

Cilantro

Dill

Parsley

avocado mayo

Makes 1 cup | Prep Time: 5 minutes | Total Time: 5 minutes

2 large ripe avocados, peeled and pitted

¼ cup plus 2 tablespoons extra-virgin olive oil

1½ tablespoons fresh lemon juice

1 teaspoon apple cider vinegar

½ teaspoon fine sea salt

¼ teaspoon garlic powder

Place the pitted and peeled avocados in a blender. With the blender running, slowly drizzle in the olive oil to combine the avocados with the oil. Add the remaining ingredients and puree until smooth.

Serving Suggestions

Use as you would regular mayo in any mayo-based salad, such as Chunky Tuna Salad (page 172), or use warm or cold as a creamy and tangy dressing. You can also use it to top Plantain Wraps (page 121) or leftover cooked chicken, cilantro, and red onion for a tasty meal on the go.

Storage

Store in a sealed glass container in the refrigerator for up to 2 days. To prevent the avocado from browning, pour a thin layer of lukewarm water on top of the mayo and seal with a lid. When ready to serve, gently pour out the water and give the mayo a good stir.

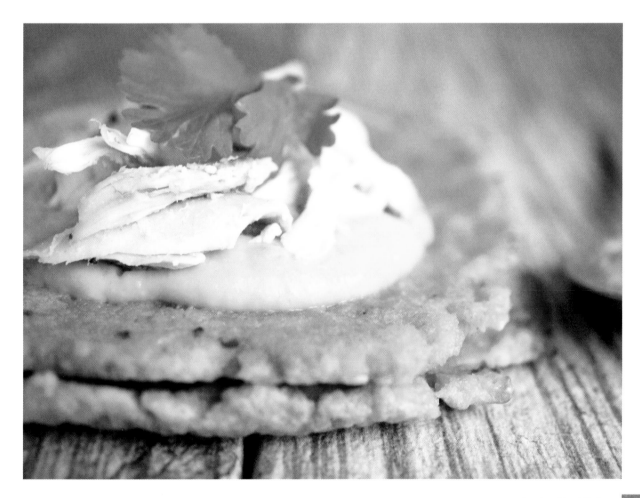

sweet marinara sauce

Makes 3 cups | Prep Time: 5 minutes | Cook Time: 25 minutes | Total Time: 30 minutes

2 cups chopped yellow onions

3 cloves garlic, minced

1 tablespoon extra-virgin olive oil

1 (15-ounce) can butternut squash puree (see Tip) or 2 scant cups homemade butternut squash puree

½ cup Chicken Broth (page 108)

3 ounces canned sliced beets, drained (optional, for color)

1 teaspoon dried basil

1 teaspoon dried oregano leaves

2 teaspoons apple cider vinegar

1 teaspoon fish sauce

½ teaspoon fine sea salt

1. In a large saucepan over medium heat, sauté the onions and garlic in the olive oil for 10 minutes, until the onions are softened and caramelized.

2. Add the butternut squash puree, chicken broth, beets (if using), basil, and oregano to the pan and bring to a low boil. Cover and simmer over medium-low heat for 15 minutes, scraping the bottom of the pan a few times to ensure that the sauce does not stick.

3. Transfer to a blender, add the vinegar, fish sauce, and salt, and puree until smooth.

Tip
Buy canned butternut squash puree for quick preparation. Canned sweet potato puree can be used as a replacement for butternut squash puree.

Store & Reheat
Once cool, store in a sealed glass container in the refrigerator for up to 1 week or in the freezer for up to 6 months. Reheat in a saucepan over medium-low heat until warm.

make it bolognese!

Makes 2 cups | Prep Time: 5 minutes | Cook Time: 7 minutes | Total Time: 12 minutes

1 pound ground beef, crumbled

2 cups Sweet Marinara Sauce (above)

1 tablespoon plus 1 teaspoon chopped fresh rosemary

1 teaspoon dried basil

⅛ teaspoon ground mace

Place all the ingredients in a large saucepan over medium heat. Bring to a simmer and maintain a simmer for 5 to 7 minutes, until the ground beef is cooked through. Stir well before serving.

Serving Suggestions
Serve over Spaghetti Squash Noodles (page 238) for a healthy updated take on a traditional weeknight meal. You may also use julienned or spiral-sliced zucchini or yellow squash, which can be served raw or lightly sautéed in olive oil and salt, in place of spaghetti squash.

Store & Reheat
Once cool, store in a sealed glass container in the refrigerator for up to 4 days or in the freezer for up to 3 months. Reheat in a saucepan over medium-low heat until warm.

tzatziki sauce

Makes 1 cup | Prep Time: 10 minutes | Total Time: 10 minutes

1½ cups peeled, seeded, and chopped cucumber (see Tip)

½ cup coconut cream, chilled

½ cup mashed avocado

2 tablespoons fresh lemon juice

2 tablespoons chopped fresh dill

1 clove garlic, chopped

½ teaspoon fine sea salt

Place all the ingredients in a food processor or blender and blend on high speed until smooth.

Tip

To quickly seed a cucumber, slice it in half lengthwise and draw the tip of a spoon along the seeded portion to scoop out the seeds in one go.

Serving Suggestions

Use as a dressing in Grilled Chicken Souvlaki Salad (page 168) or as a dip with sliced cucumbers, baby carrots, radishes, and celery sticks.

Storage

Store in a sealed glass container in the refrigerator for up to 2 days.

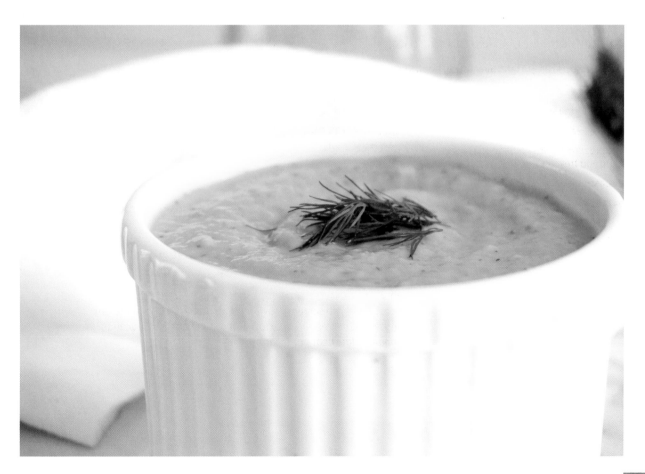

pronto pesto

Makes about ⅔ cup | Prep Time: 8 minutes | Total Time: 8 minutes

2 cups loosely packed fresh basil leaves

¾ cup loosely packed fresh cilantro leaves

⅓ cup mashed avocado

1 tablespoon chopped garlic

1 teaspoon apple cider vinegar

½ teaspoon fine sea salt

½ cup extra-virgin olive oil

Place all the ingredients except the olive oil in a food processor and blend until the herbs are finely chopped. While the food processor is running, slowly pour in the olive oil to make a smooth pesto sauce. Pesto is best served after the flavors are allowed to marry for at least 1 hour.

Serving Suggestions
Use in Pesto Chicken Pasta (page 217), on Pesto Chicken Pizza (page 227), or as a dip for Mediterranean Lamb Meatballs (page 194) or Roasted Roots with Garlic Sauce (page 260).

Storage
Store in a sealed glass container in the refrigerator for up to 2 days.

mango guacamole

Makes 2 cups | Prep Time: 8 minutes | Total Time: 8 minutes

2 large ripe avocados, peeled and pitted

1 cup chopped mango

⅓ tightly packed cup chopped fresh cilantro leaves

2 tablespoons diced shallot

2 tablespoons fresh lime juice

½ teaspoon fine sea salt or truffle salt (see Tip, page 122)

Place all the ingredients in a food processor and pulse until chopped to the desired consistency.

Serving Suggestions
Use in Mojo-Mango Stuffed Sweet Potatoes (page 219), as a replacement for Easy Guacamole on Taco Night (page 188), or as a dip for sliced and toasted Plantain Wraps (page 121), plantain chips, or cucumber slices.

Storage
Store in a sealed glass container in the refrigerator for up to 2 days. To prevent the avocado from browning, pour a thin layer of lukewarm water on top of the guacamole and seal with a lid. When ready to serve, gently pour out the water and give the guacamole a good stir.

cilantro chimichurri

Makes 1½ cups | Prep Time: 10 minutes | Total Time: 10 minutes

2 cups packed fresh cilantro leaves

1 cup chopped unpeeled zucchini

2 tablespoons apple cider vinegar

1 tablespoon chopped garlic

½ teaspoon fine sea salt

½ cup extra-virgin olive oil

Place all the ingredients except the olive oil in a food processor and blend until finely chopped. While the food processor is running, slowly pour in the olive oil and continue processing until well combined.

Serving Suggestions
Use on Garlic-Rubbed Tostones (page 248) or as a salad dressing over Beef Carnitas (page 186), chopped romaine lettuce, and sliced avocado.

Storage
Store in a sealed glass container in the refrigerator for up to 2 days. The flavor deepens nicely when the chimichurri is refrigerated overnight.

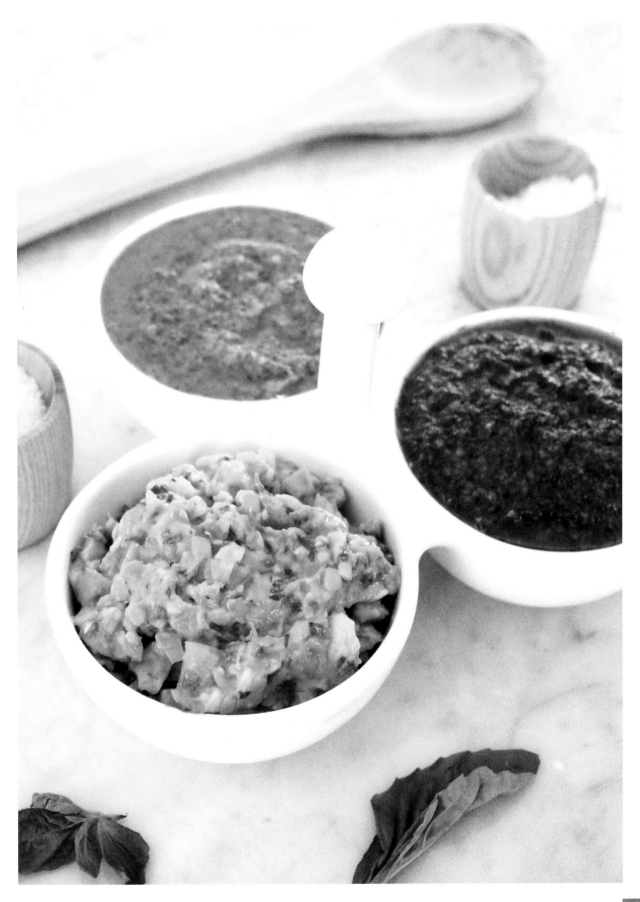

tangy carolina bbq sauce

Makes 2 cups | Prep Time: 5 minutes | Cook Time: 12 minutes | Total Time: 17 minutes

1 cup sweet potato puree (see Tip)

¾ cup apple cider vinegar

3 tablespoons bacon fat

2 tablespoons blackstrap molasses

1 teaspoon fish sauce

1 teaspoon fine sea salt

1 teaspoon ginger powder

½ teaspoon onion powder

¼ teaspoon garlic powder

Tip

Buy canned sweet potato puree for quick preparation.

Serving Suggestions

Use in BBQ Pulled Pork (page 206) or BBQ Chicken Burgers (page 201).

Storage

Once cool, store in a sealed glass container in the refrigerator for up to 2 weeks.

Whisk together all the ingredients in a small saucepan over medium heat. Bring to a low boil and whisk continuously while maintaining a low boil for 2 to 3 minutes, until slightly thickened. This sauce is thinner than traditional BBQ sauce.

Oven-Baked BBQ Ribs. Rub 2 tablespoons of House Rub (page 122) on 3 pounds of baby back ribs. Wrap tightly in foil and place in the refrigerator overnight. Preheat the oven to 250 degrees, unwrap the foil, and brush ½ cup of Tangy Carolina BBQ Sauce on the ribs. Tightly wrap in foil again and place on a rimmed baking sheet. Bake for 3½ to 4 hours, until the ribs are fall-off-the-bone tender. Remove from the foil, brush lightly with more BBQ sauce, and broil on high for 3 to 4 minutes, until the top is browned. Serve with additional warmed BBQ sauce for dipping, with Mac n' Cheese (page 240) or Smoked Salmon Potato Salad (page 175) on the side.

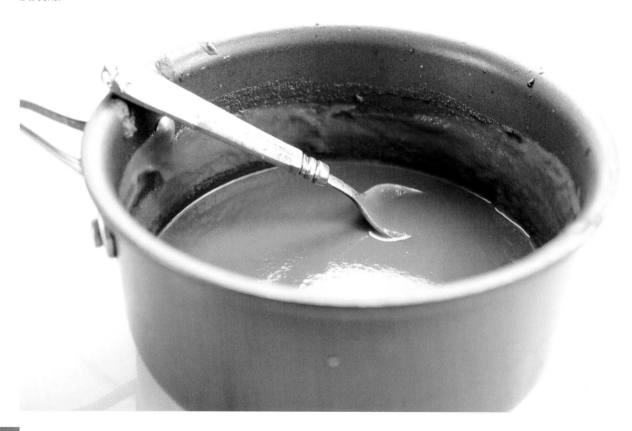

cauli'fredo sauce

Makes 1 cup | Prep Time: 5 minutes | Cook Time: 8 minutes | Total Time: 13 minutes

2 cups cauliflower florets (about ½ head)

1 tablespoon minced garlic

1 tablespoon extra-virgin olive oil

1 teaspoon fine sea salt

¼ cup Chicken Broth (page 108) or water

Serving Suggestions

Use in Seared Shrimp Pasta (page 233) or toss with steamed broccoli for a creamy side dish.

Storage

Once cool, store in a sealed glass container in the refrigerator for up to 4 days or in the freezer for up to 6 months.

1. Steam the cauliflower in a lidded steamer basket set over a pot of boiling water for 4 to 5 minutes, until tender. Drain and transfer to a blender.

2. Meanwhile, in a small skillet over medium heat, cook the garlic in the olive oil for 2 to 3 minutes, until fragrant, making sure that the garlic does not burn.

3. Spoon the garlic into the blender, add the salt and chicken broth, and puree on high speed until smooth. For a thinner sauce, add more broth or water 2 tablespoons at a time until the desired thickness is reached.

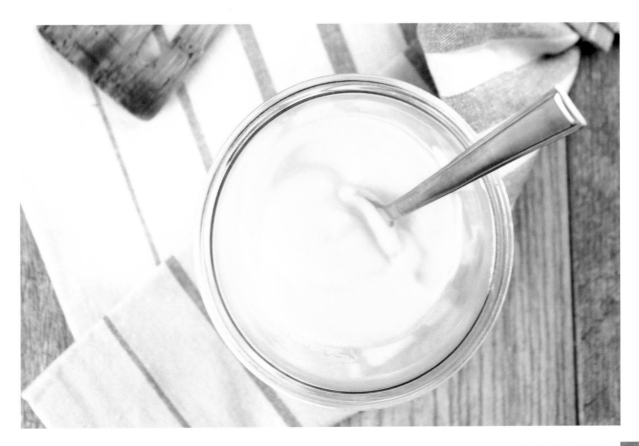

thin pizza crust

Makes one 10-inch crust | Prep Time: 5 minutes | Cook Time: 13 minutes | Total Time: 18 minutes

⅔ cup arrowroot starch

¼ cup plus 2 tablespoons coconut flour

1 teaspoon cream of tartar

½ teaspoon baking soda

¼ teaspoon fine sea salt or truffle salt (see Tip, page 122)

2 tablespoons extra-virgin olive oil

½ cup warm water

Serving Suggestions
Use this crust for Prosciutto & Fig Bistro Pizza (page 213), Ham & Pineapple Pizza (page 212), Pesto Chicken Pizza (page 227), or Spinach & Garlic Lover's Pizza (page 228).

Storage
Once cool, store wrapped in plastic wrap in the refrigerator for up to 24 hours or in the freezer for up to 3 months.

1. Preheat the oven to 425 degrees. Line a cookie sheet or pizza pan with parchment paper.

2. In a mixing bowl, whisk together the dry ingredients. Slowly pour in the olive oil, continuously stirring the mixture as you pour. Mix in the warm water thoroughly. The dough will be slightly crumbly, but once you roll it out in Step 3, it will bind together well.

3. Place the dough on the prepared cookie sheet or pizza pan. Lay another sheet of parchment paper on top of the dough and use your hands or a rolling pin to smooth the dough into a crust about ¼ inch thick. You may roll it into the desired shape, such as a circle, oval, or rectangle.

4. Bake for 12 to 13 minutes, until light golden brown and crisp. Use immediately in one of our pizza recipes, or let cool and store as directed.

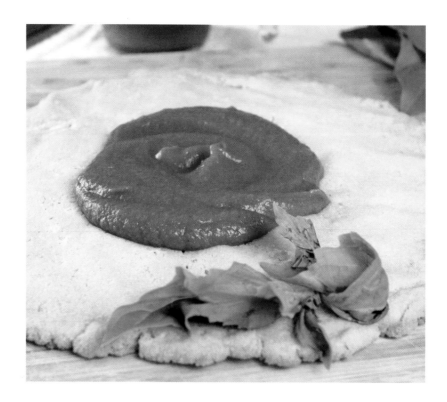

plantain wraps

Makes 6 wraps | Prep Time: 7 minutes | Cook Time: 10 minutes | Total Time: 17 minutes

2 green-yellow plantains (see Tip)

¼ cup extra-virgin olive oil

2 tablespoons water

1 teaspoon cream of tartar

½ teaspoon baking soda

½ teaspoon fine sea salt

Tip

For best results, the plantains should be mostly green with some hints of yellow. They may be slightly spotted. If using green plantains, you may need to add an extra tablespoon of water if the plantains don't puree easily.

Serving Suggestions

Use as wraps for Chunky Tuna Salad (page 172) or Beef or Pork Carnitas (page 186) with Mango Guacamole (page 116).

Store & Reheat

Once cool, store in a sealed glass container at room temperature for up to 1 day or in the refrigerator for up to 3 days. Reheat in a 300-degree oven for a few minutes until warm. Plantain wraps are most pliable when warm; they stiffen up considerably at room temperature or when refrigerated.

1. Preheat the oven to 425 degrees. Line a cookie sheet with parchment paper.

2. Prepare the plantains by slicing them lengthwise from tip to tip and using your fingers to peel off the skins. Roughly chop the plantains and place in a high-powered blender or food processor with the rest of the ingredients. Blend on low speed for several minutes, until smooth, scraping down the sides as needed. A few small chunks remaining will not affect the recipe.

3. Scoop six ⅓-cup mounds of batter onto the prepared cookie sheet, leaving at least 3 inches of space between them. Using your hands or the back of a silicone spatula, spread the dough into even 6-inch rounds about ¼ inch thick.

4. Bake for 10 minutes, until the wraps are golden brown and firm to the touch and have risen slightly.

5. Let cool for a few minutes before using as soft pita wrap replacements or slicing into triangles and serving with salad.

Venezuelan "Arepas." Stuff warmed Plantain Wraps with warmed Beef Carnitas (page 186), diced avocado, and Cilantro Chimichurri (page 116). Serve with Garlic-Rubbed Tostones (page 248) on the side, if desired.

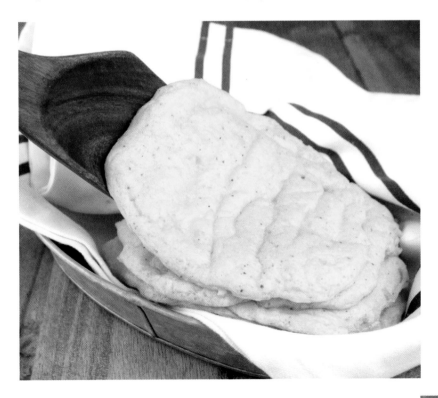

seasoning mixes

house rub

Makes ¼ cup | Prep Time: 5 minutes |
Total Time: 5 minutes

1 tablespoon plus 1 teaspoon fine sea salt

2 teaspoons dried oregano leaves

2 teaspoons dried thyme leaves

2 teaspoons garlic powder

2 teaspoons onion powder

2 teaspoons ginger powder

½ teaspoon turmeric powder

Whisk all the ingredients together in a small bowl until well combined.

Serving Suggestions
Use as a dry rub for all cuts of meat, including chicken, beef, pork, lamb, and turkey.

Storage
Store in a sealed glass or wooden container at room temperature for up to 3 months.

umami dust

Makes ¼ cup | Prep Time: 7 minutes |
Total Time: 7 minutes

1 ounce dried shiitake mushrooms

1 tablespoon truffle salt (see Tip)

1 teaspoon fine sea salt

In a high-powered blender or spice grinder, finely grind the dried mushrooms into a powder. Transfer to a small bowl and whisk in the salts until well combined.

Tip
Truffle salt is a specialty seasoning that can often be found in the spice aisle of larger grocery stores, online, or at specialty spice shops. Look for pure truffle salt that contains just two ingredients: sea salt and truffles. Truffle salt adds a savory flavor to meat, poultry, and vegetable dishes and can be used for both finishing and cooking.

Serving Suggestions
Use to flavor steamed or roasted vegetables or savory dishes like burgers, steaks, roasted chicken thighs, and grilled pork chops.

Storage
Store in a sealed glass or wooden container at room temperature for up to 6 months.

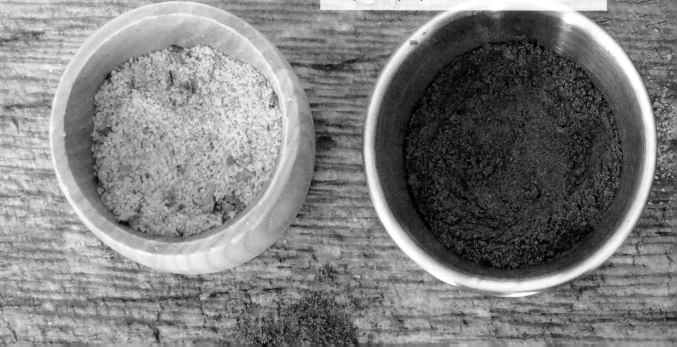

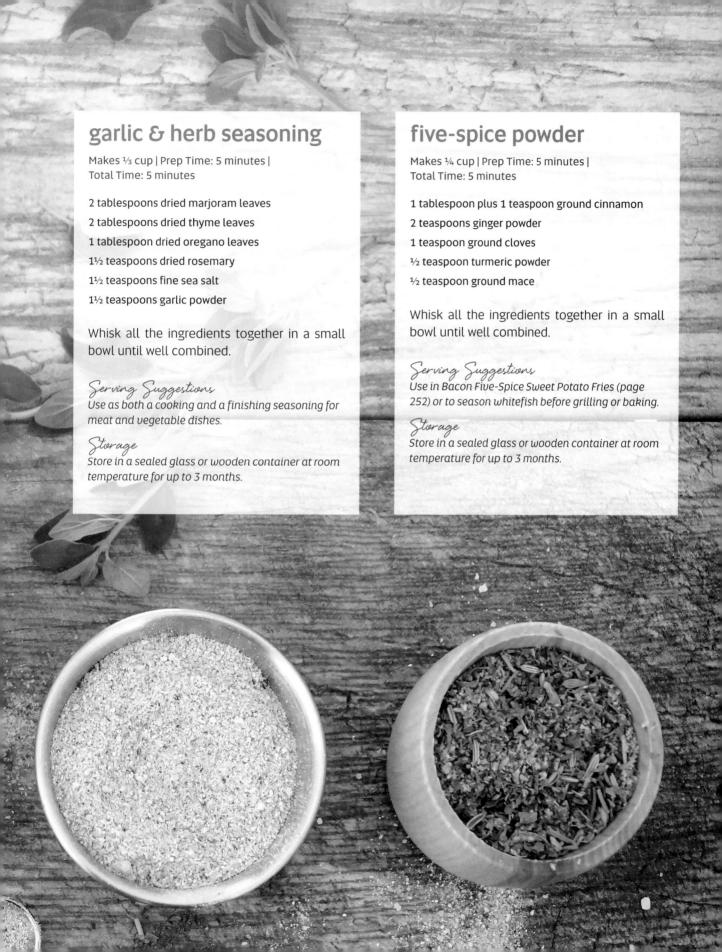

garlic & herb seasoning

Makes ⅓ cup | Prep Time: 5 minutes |
Total Time: 5 minutes

2 tablespoons dried marjoram leaves

2 tablespoons dried thyme leaves

1 tablespoon dried oregano leaves

1½ teaspoons dried rosemary

1½ teaspoons fine sea salt

1½ teaspoons garlic powder

Whisk all the ingredients together in a small bowl until well combined.

Serving Suggestions
Use as both a cooking and a finishing seasoning for meat and vegetable dishes.

Storage
Store in a sealed glass or wooden container at room temperature for up to 3 months.

five-spice powder

Makes ¼ cup | Prep Time: 5 minutes |
Total Time: 5 minutes

1 tablespoon plus 1 teaspoon ground cinnamon

2 teaspoons ginger powder

1 teaspoon ground cloves

½ teaspoon turmeric powder

½ teaspoon ground mace

Whisk all the ingredients together in a small bowl until well combined.

Serving Suggestions
Use in Bacon Five-Spice Sweet Potato Fries (page 252) or to season whitefish before grilling or baking.

Storage
Store in a sealed glass or wooden container at room temperature for up to 3 months.

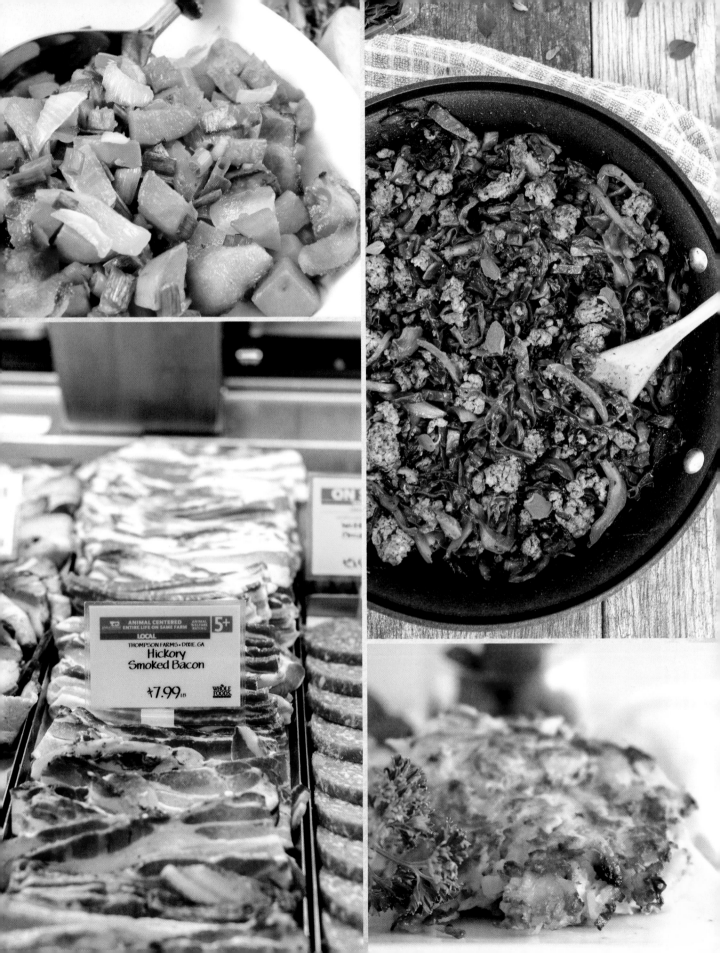

ANIMAL CENTERED
ENTIRE LIFE ON SAME FARM

5+

LOCAL

THOMPSON FARMS • DIXIE, GA

Hickory
Smoked Bacon

$7.99 LB

WHOLE FOODS

antioxidant morning smoothie

Serves 1 | Prep Time: 5 minutes | Total Time: 5 minutes

1 banana, chilled

Handful of spinach leaves

1 cup blueberries, chilled

½ cup mashed avocado

⅓ cup fresh orange juice

⅛ teaspoon fine sea salt

Place all the ingredients in a blender and blend until pureed. Serve immediately or chill for up to 12 hours until ready to serve.

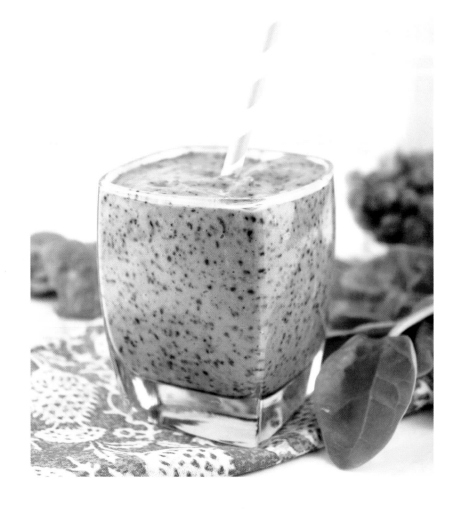

pumpkin spice smoothie

Serves 1 | Prep Time: 5 minutes | Total Time: 5 minutes

1 cup canned pumpkin or sweet potato puree, chilled

¾ cup full-fat coconut milk, chilled

1½ teaspoons honey

½ teaspoon blackstrap molasses

1 teaspoon ground cinnamon

¼ teaspoon ground mace

¼ teaspoon fine sea salt

Place all the ingredients in a blender and blend on high speed until pureed. For a thinner smoothie, add ¼ cup additional coconut milk or water.

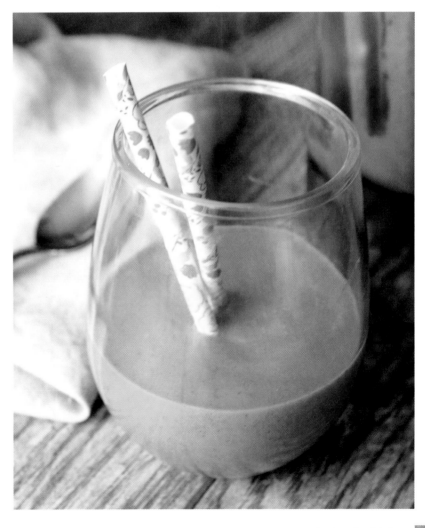

chicken hash brown patties 🍲

Makes 12 patties, serves 4 | Prep Time: 10 minutes | Cook Time: 18 minutes | Total Time: 28 minutes

1 pound white sweet potatoes

1 pound boneless, skinless chicken breast, chopped, or 1 pound ground chicken breast

1 teaspoon garlic powder

1 teaspoon dried thyme leaves

¾ teaspoon fine sea salt

¼ teaspoon onion powder

3 tablespoons bacon fat, divided

½ teaspoon Garlic & Herb Seasoning (page 123; optional)

1. Peel the sweet potatoes, then shred them using your food processor's shredder attachment. If you're using chopped chicken breast, put the chicken breast through the shredder as well to finely grind it.

2. Transfer the shredded sweet potatoes and chicken to a large mixing bowl. Using your hands, mix in the garlic powder, thyme, salt, and onion powder until evenly incorporated.

3. Heat 1 tablespoon of the bacon fat in a large, deep skillet over medium heat. Scoop ⅓ cup of the chicken mixture into the pan and flatten it with a spatula until it's about ½ inch thick. Working quickly, repeat this step until you fill the pan with patties, without overcrowding the pan. Cook the patties for 2 to 3 minutes per side until golden brown and cooked through. Sprinkle the patties immediately with Garlic & Herb Seasoning, if desired.

4. Repeat Step 3 until all of the hash brown mixture is used up.

Make Ahead
Prepare the recipe through Step 2 and store the mixture in the refrigerator for up to 24 hours prior to cooking.

Serving Suggestion
Make breakfast protein stacks by layering a Chicken Hash Brown Patty with Garlic & Herb Breakfast Sausage (page 130) and sliced avocado.

Store & Reheat
Once cool, store in a sealed glass container in the refrigerator for up to 4 days or in the freezer for up to 3 months. Reheat in a skillet greased with bacon fat on medium heat until warmed through.

Change It Up
Replace the white sweet potatoes with an equal amount of another starchy root, such as regular sweet potato, parsnip, or celery root.

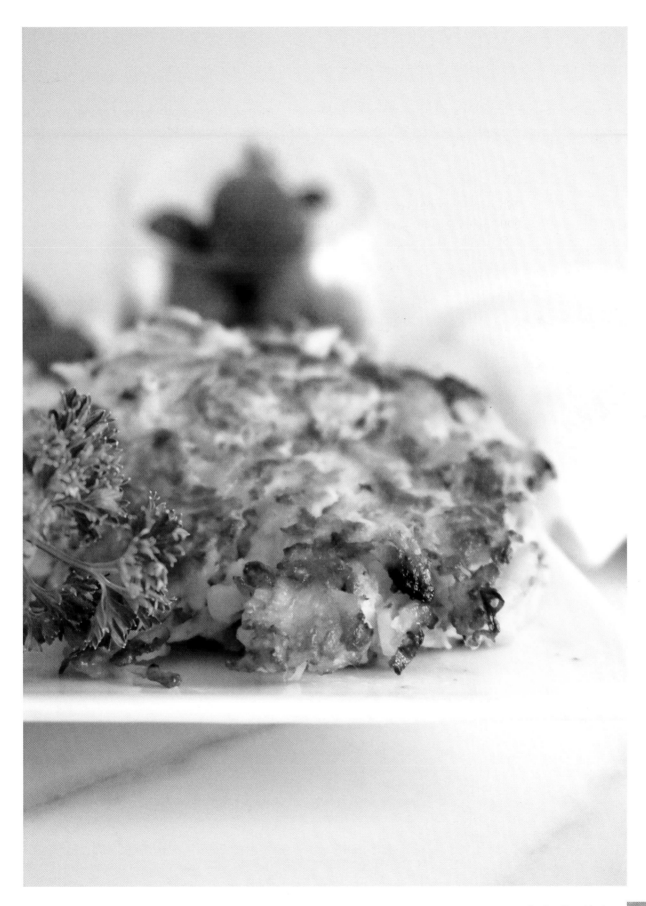

garlic & herb breakfast sausage

Serves 6 | Prep Time: 8 minutes | Cook Time: 12 minutes | Total Time: 20 minutes

2 pounds ground pork

2 tablespoons Garlic & Herb Seasoning (page 123)

2 teaspoons dried rubbed sage

1 teaspoon onion powder

½ teaspoon fine sea salt

2 tablespoons fat of choice

1. In a large bowl, mix together all the ingredients except the fat. Form the mixture into 15 patties that are 2 inches wide and about ¾ inch thick.

2. Heat the fat in a large, deep skillet over medium-high heat. Brown the patties on both sides for a total of 10 to 12 minutes, until the center is no longer pink and the outside is a crispy golden brown. Cook them in two batches if needed to avoid overcrowding the pan. You may need to lower the temperature slightly toward the end of the cooking time if the pan gets too hot and the outsides of the patties begin to burn.

Make Ahead
Prepare the sausage mixture as directed in Step 1. Store in the refrigerator overnight before cooking the following morning.

Serving Suggestions
Use in Biscuits & Gravy (page 135) or stack on top of Chicken Hash Brown Patties (page 128) for an on-the-go breakfast.

Store & Reheat
Transfer the cooked patties to a glass container lined with a layer of paper towels. Once cool, cover with a lid and store in the refrigerator for up to 3 days or in the freezer for up to 3 months. Reheat in a skillet over medium heat until warm.

american breakfast sausage

Serves 6 to 10 | Prep Time: 10 minutes | Cook Time: 25 minutes | Total Time: 35 minutes + at least 8 hours to chill

1½ teaspoons dried rubbed sage

¼ teaspoon ginger powder

¾ teaspoon ground mace

¾ teaspoon dried thyme leaves

2½ pounds ground pork

1½ teaspoons fine sea salt

Store & Reheat
Once cool, store in a sealed glass container in the refrigerator for up to 3 days. If freezing, freeze on a baking sheet and then transfer to a resealable freezer bag or container. Reheat frozen patties in the microwave or by frying in a skillet.

1. Combine the dried spices in a spice grinder and grind into a fine powder. You can also do this using a mortar and pestle, clean coffee grinder, mini blender, or mini food processor.

2. Place the ground herbs, pork, and salt in a large bowl. Use your hands to fully incorporate the spices into the meat. Alternatively, mix in the bowl of a stand mixer on low speed for 3 to 4 minutes. Cover with plastic wrap and refrigerate overnight or for up to 24 hours.

3. Preheat the oven to 400 degrees.

4. Form 4- to 8-ounce patties with your hands, just as you would make hamburger patties. (How big you make the patties will depend on how big a serving size you are aiming for.) Place the patties on a rimmed baking sheet, spaced about 1 inch apart. You may need two baking sheets, depending on how thick you make the patties.

5. Bake for 15 to 25 minutes, depending on thickness, until the internal temperature reaches a minimum of 160 degrees. Alternatively, you can fry the patties in a skillet or on a griddle over medium-high heat.

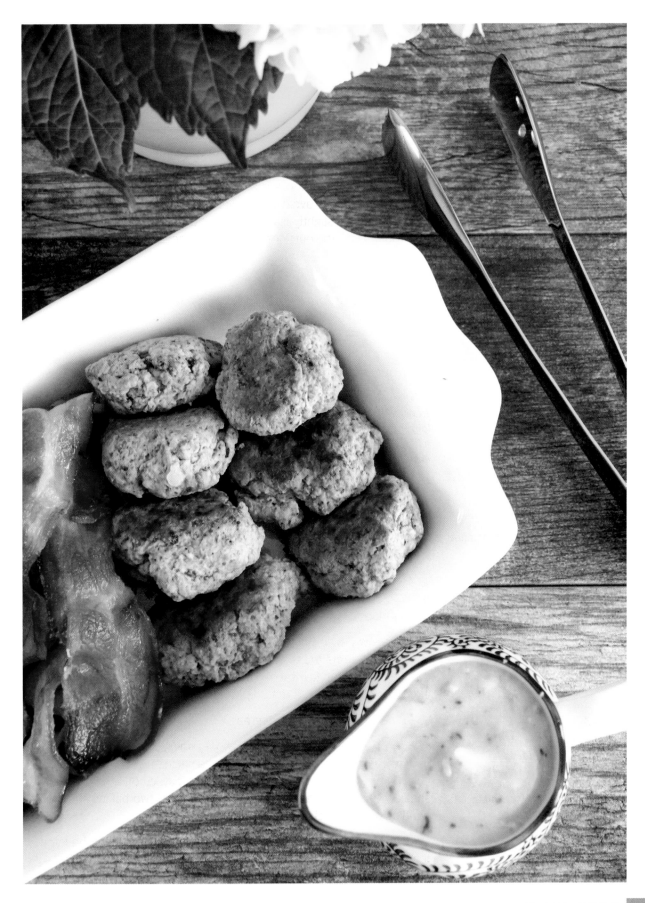

bacon-wrapped apple & cinnamon sausage

Makes 15 pieces | Prep Time: 10 minutes | Cook Time: 25 minutes | Total Time: 35 minutes

15 slices bacon (not thick-cut)

1½ pounds ground pork

1 Granny Smith apple, finely diced

1 tablespoon finely chopped fresh rosemary

½ teaspoon ground cinnamon

½ teaspoon fine sea salt

¼ teaspoon ground mace

Make Ahead

Prepare the sausage mixture up to 1 day in advance and store covered in the refrigerator until ready to assemble the cups.

Serving Suggestion

Serve with Pumpkin Spice Smoothie (page 127) for a fall-themed morning meal.

Store & Reheat

Once cool, store in a sealed glass container in the refrigerator for up to 4 days or in the freezer for up to 3 months. To reheat, place in a muffin pan or on a rimmed baking sheet and reheat in a 350-degree oven until warm in the center.

Change It Up

In place of the ground pork mixture, use either American Breakfast Sausage (page 130) or Garlic & Herb Breakfast Sausage (page 130), scaling down the recipe to use the recommended 1½ pounds of meat.

1. Preheat the oven to 350 degrees. Have on a hand two 12-cup muffin pans.

2. Cut the bacon slices in half widthwise. Do not use thick-cut bacon, as it will be difficult to mold into the muffin cups and will not cook properly. Lay 2 half-slices in an X shape inside a muffin cup. Fold any overhang into the inside rim of the cup. Repeat with the rest of the bacon to make a total of 15 cups. If you prefer your bacon crispier, we highly suggest prebaking the bacon cups for 7 to 10 minutes, carefully draining rendered fat, then proceeding with step 3.

3. Place the rest of the ingredients in a medium bowl and combine with your hands. Form fifteen ¼ cup–size balls of sausage with your hands and press them into the prepared bacon cups.

4. Bake for 20 to 25 minutes, until the sausage is cooked through and the edges of the bacon are crispy. Immediately use a spoon to remove the cups to a paper towel–lined plate so that they are not sitting in all the juices. Let cool slightly and serve either warm or cold for an on-the-go breakfast.

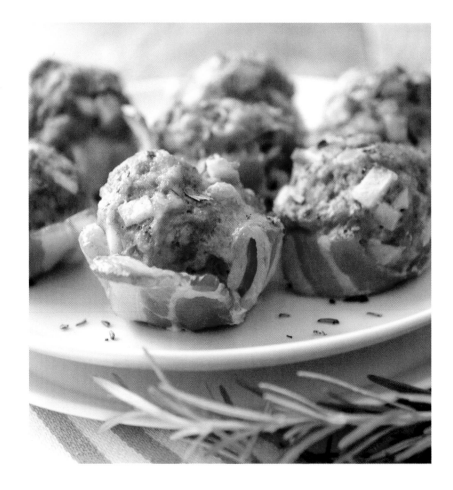

bacon-herb biscuits

Makes 5 biscuits | Prep Time: 15 minutes | Cook Time: 29 minutes | Total Time: 44 minutes

3 slices bacon, chopped into ½-inch pieces

1 tablespoon minced garlic

1 teaspoon chopped fresh thyme

8 ounces peeled and chopped yellow plantain (about 1 medium; see Tip)

2 tablespoons bacon fat (from above)

½ cup arrowroot starch

2 tablespoons coconut flour

1 teaspoon dried oregano leaves

½ teaspoon unflavored gelatin powder

1 teaspoon apple cider vinegar

¾ teaspoon baking soda

½ teaspoon fine sea salt

2 tablespoons warm water

Honey, for drizzling (optional)

1. Preheat the oven to 375 degrees. Line a cookie sheet with parchment paper.

2. In a large skillet over medium heat, cook the bacon until crispy. Stir in the garlic and thyme and cook until the garlic is fragrant, about 1 minute.

3. Spoon the bacon-herb mixture into a small bowl, reserving the bacon fat for use in Step 4. Set aside.

4. Place the plantain in a food processor or high-powered blender and pulse until broken up into small pieces. Add the remaining ingredients, except the bacon-herb mixture, and blend until a smooth, wet dough has formed.

5. Spoon the mixture into a mixing bowl. Stir in the bacon-herb mixture.

6. Scoop ¼ cup of the dough at a time onto the prepared cookie sheet and use your hands to form 5 round biscuits, spacing them at least 1 inch apart. Bake for 20 minutes, until golden brown with crusted tops. Remove from the oven and let cool slightly on the cookie sheet before removing to a serving plate. Slice in half and drizzle with honey, if desired.

Tip

When selecting a yellow plantain for this recipe, make sure that it does not have any brown or black spots. Spots indicate that the starch has started to convert to sugar, which will affect the texture of this recipe. For the most accurate measurement, use a kitchen scale to measure 8 ounces of peeled and chopped plantain.

Store & Reheat

Once cool, store in a sealed glass container or tightly wrapped in plastic wrap in the refrigerator for up to 2 days or in the freezer for up to 3 months. To reheat, wrap in a damp paper towel and microwave in 10-second increments, or wrap in foil and warm in a 300-degree oven.

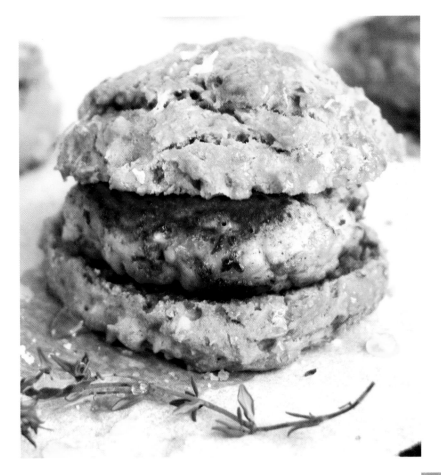

country herb gravy

Makes 1 cup | Prep Time: 7 minutes | Cook Time: 10 minutes | Total Time: 17 minutes

2 tablespoons bacon fat or 4 slices bacon

1 large white sweet potato (about 1 pound), peeled and cubed

1½ cups Beef or Chicken Broth (pages 108–109), divided, plus more if needed

2 teaspoons chopped fresh sage

1 teaspoon chopped fresh rosemary

½ teaspoon dried thyme leaves

½ teaspoon fine sea salt

Make Ahead
Chop the sweet potato up to 2 days in advance. Store wrapped in paper towels in a plastic bag in the refrigerator until ready to use.

Serving Suggestions
Use in Biscuits & Gravy (opposite) or Beef Pot Pie (page 182), or serve with Oven-Fried Chicken (page 216).

Store & Reheat
Once cool, store in a sealed glass container in the refrigerator for up to 10 days or in the freezer for up to 3 months. Reheat in the microwave or in a small saucepan over low heat until warm.

1. Place the bacon fat in a blender. If you do not have bacon fat on hand, cook the bacon in a medium saucepan over medium heat until the fat has rendered. Drain the fat (about 2 tablespoons) into a blender and reserve the cooked bacon for another use.

2. Bring the sweet potatoes and 1 cup of the broth to a boil in a medium saucepan (or the pan you used to render the bacon fat) over medium-high heat. Maintain a low boil until the potatoes are fork-tender, 8 to 10 minutes.

3. Transfer the potatoes and broth from the pan to the blender and puree with the remaining ½ cup of broth, herbs, and salt. Add additional broth if needed to thin out the gravy, keeping in mind that the gravy tends to thicken up once refrigerated.

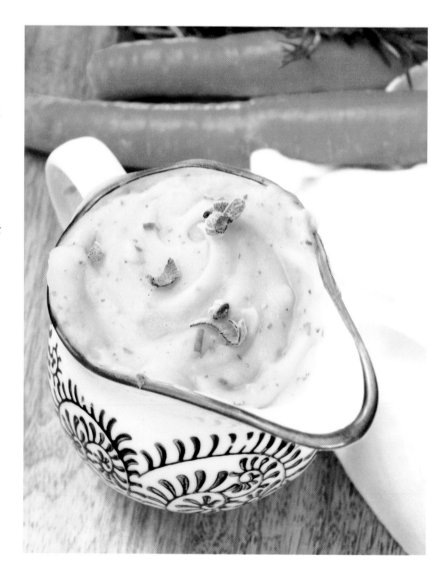

biscuits & gravy

Makes 5 sandwiches | Prep Time: 5 minutes | Total Time: 5 minutes

1 recipe Bacon-Herb Biscuits (page 133), sliced in half

½ to ¾ cup Country Herb Gravy (opposite), as desired

5 patties breakfast sausage of choice (page 130)

Tip
Do not assemble until ready to serve.

Store & Reheat
The biscuits, gravy, and sausage should be stored separately in the refrigerator or freezer according to their individual storage instructions.

When ready to assemble the sandwiches, warm all the ingredients. Place a sausage patty on the bottom half of each sliced biscuit and place on individual serving plates. Pour the warm gravy over the sausage, then cap each patty with a biscuit top. If eating with a knife and fork, you may assemble the sandwiches and pour the gravy over the top. Serve immediately. You may also assemble the sandwiches cold, pour the gravy over them, and then place them in a baking dish in a 350-degree oven for 10 minutes or until warm.

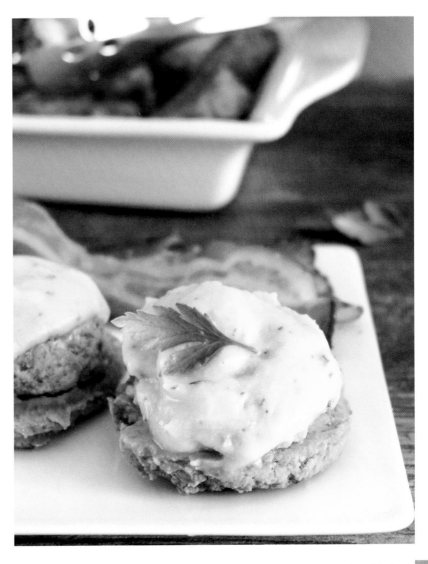

oven-baked pancakes

Makes seven 3-inch pancakes | Prep Time: 7 minutes | Cook Time: 25 minutes | Total Time: 32 minutes

3 green bananas (about 1⅓ pounds)

¼ cup coconut flour

2 tablespoons coconut oil, melted

1 tablespoon honey

1 teaspoon arrowroot starch

1 teaspoon ground cinnamon

1 teaspoon vanilla extract

¾ teaspoon baking soda

½ teaspoon apple cider vinegar

¼ teaspoon fine sea salt

Honey or maple syrup, for serving

1. Preheat the oven to 350 degrees. Line a cookie sheet with parchment paper.

2. Place all the ingredients in a blender and puree until smooth.

3. Scoop a scant ¼ cup of the batter onto the prepared cookie sheet. Repeat to make 7 pancakes, leaving about 2 inches between them. Using the back of a spoon in a circular motion, smooth each pancake into a circle about 3 inches wide and ⅓ inch high.

4. Bake for 23 to 25 minutes, until lightly browned and cooked through. Let rest for 5 minutes before serving. Serve drizzled with honey or maple syrup.

Store & Reheat

Once cool, store in a sealed glass container or plastic bag in the refrigerator for up to 5 days or in the freezer for up to 6 months. Reheat in a 300-degree oven until warm.

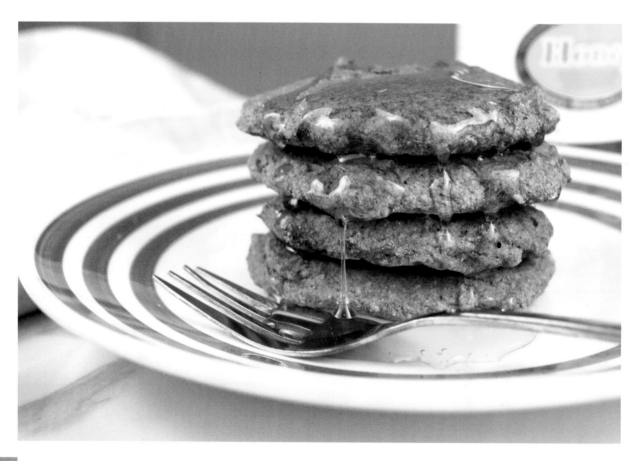

cinnamon & raisin porridge

Serves 3 to 4 | Prep Time: 5 minutes | Cook Time: 15 minutes | Total Time: 20 minutes

1 recipe Spaghetti Squash Noodles (page 238), precooked

1 cup full-fat coconut milk

½ cup raisins, plus more for garnish if desired

1½ tablespoons honey

1½ teaspoons ground cinnamon

Toasted coconut flakes, for garnish (optional)

1. Combine all the ingredients in a medium saucepan and bring to a boil over medium-high heat. Reduce the heat to maintain a simmer, cover with the lid ajar to allow moisture to escape, and cook for 12 to 15 minutes, stirring once or twice to ensure that the squash does not stick to the pan.

2. Serve the porridge as is or briefly use an immersion blender to break up the spaghetti squash noodles into smaller pieces to more closely resemble a traditional porridge.

3. Garnish with additional raisins and toasted coconut flakes, if desired.

Store & Reheat
Once cool, store in a sealed glass container in the refrigerator for up to 5 days or in the freezer for up to 3 months. To reheat, bring to a low boil in a small saucepan over medium heat.

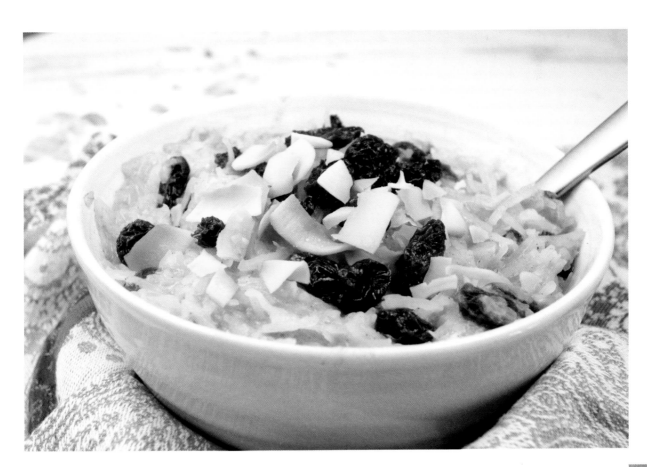

baked carrot-banana bread n'oatmeal

Serves 5 to 7 | Prep Time: 8 minutes | Cook Time: 55 minutes | Total Time: 1 hour 3 minutes

2 (10-ounce) bags shredded carrots or 1⅓ pounds carrots, peeled and shredded

1 (13½-ounce) can full-fat coconut milk

1 cup mashed medium-yellow bananas (about 3 medium)

¾ cup unsweetened shredded coconut, plus more for garnish if desired

½ cup raisins, plus more for garnish if desired

¼ cup coconut flour

2 tablespoons honey, liquid

2 teaspoons ground cinnamon

1 teaspoon fine sea salt

½ teaspoon baking soda

Store & Reheat

Once cool, store in a sealed glass container in the refrigerator for up to 10 days or in the freezer for up to 1 year. Reheat covered in a 300-degree oven until warm.

1. Preheat the oven to 350 degrees.

2. In a large mixing bowl, combine all the ingredients until the shredded carrots are well coated and the ingredients evenly mixed.

3. Spoon the mixture into a 9 by 13-inch glass casserole dish and press down firmly with a spatula.

4. Bake, covered tightly in foil, for 55 minutes or until the carrots are tender and the n'oatmeal is still moist. Let cool for 5 minutes before serving. Garnish with additional shredded coconut and raisins, if desired.

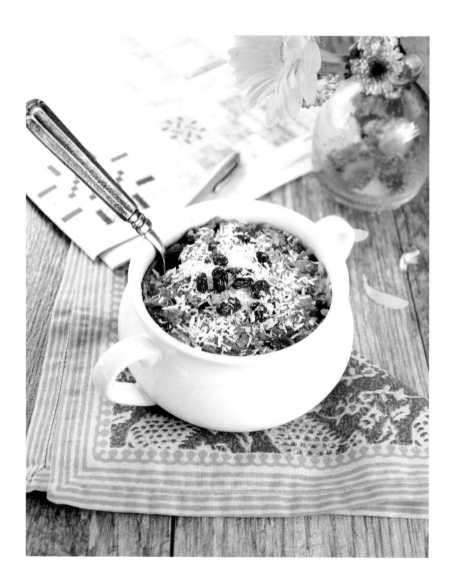

spiced candied bacon

Serves 4 to 6 | Prep Time: 5 minutes | Cook Time: 25 minutes | Total Time: 30 minutes

12 slices bacon

2 tablespoons honey

2 teaspoons blackstrap molasses

½ teaspoon ground cinnamon

½ teaspoon granulated garlic

¼ teaspoon ground mace

Make Ahead

Complete Steps 1 and 2. Cover the baking sheet with plastic wrap and place in the refrigerator for up to 24 hours, until ready to cook.

Store & Reheat

Once cool, store in a sealed glass container in the refrigerator for up to 3 days. Reheat by briefly searing in a skillet over medium-high heat.

1. Preheat the oven to 350 degrees. Line a large rimmed baking sheet with parchment paper. Place the bacon on the baking sheet, leaving space between the slices.

2. Whisk together the remaining ingredients. Using a pastry brush or basting brush, brush the mixture onto both sides of the bacon slices.

3. Bake for 20 to 25 minutes, until caramelized and crispy, flipping the bacon halfway through cooking. Drain on paper towels and serve warm.

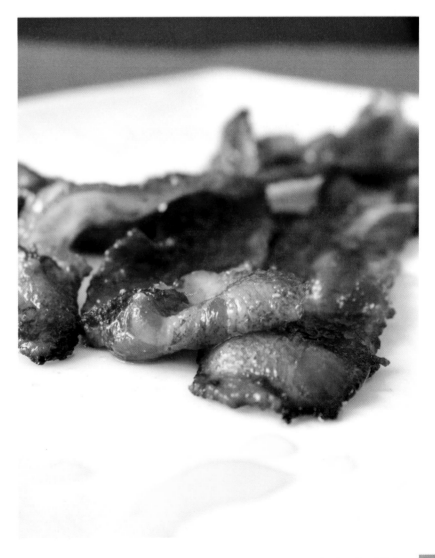

comforting breakfast casserole

Serves 4 | Prep Time: 7 minutes | Cook Time: 48 minutes | Total Time: 55 minutes

1 tablespoon bacon fat or coconut oil

2 Gala apples, diced

1 yellow onion, diced

1½ teaspoons ground cinnamon, divided

1 pound ground beef

1 teaspoon fine sea salt, divided

2 teaspoons blackstrap molasses

2 large green plantains, peeled and chopped

2 tablespoons extra-virgin olive oil or avocado oil

Make Ahead

Prepare the casserole through Step 4. Once cool, cover and refrigerate for up to 2 days before baking.

Store & Reheat

Once cool, cover the casserole dish and store in the refrigerator for up to 3 days or in the freezer for up to 3 months. Reheat in a 350-degree oven until warm.

1. Preheat the oven to 350 degrees.

2. Heat the bacon fat in a large skillet over medium-high heat. Add the apples and onion and sauté until tender and lightly browned, 8 to 10 minutes. Stir in 1 teaspoon of the cinnamon.

3. Add the ground beef and ¾ teaspoon of the salt to the skillet and cook until the beef is browned and no longer pink. Stir in the molasses. Transfer the mixture to an 8 by 8-inch glass baking dish.

4. Place the plantains, olive oil, remaining ½ teaspoon of cinnamon, and remaining ¼ teaspoon of salt in a blender and puree until smooth. Spread evenly on top of the ground beef mixture using either a silicone spatula or your hands.

5. Bake for 25 to 30 minutes, until the plantain crust has the texture of thick cornbread all the way through, then broil on high for 2 to 3 minutes until the top is golden brown.

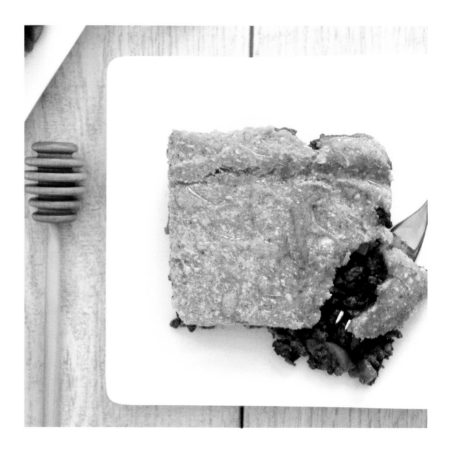

creamy caesar beef skillet

Serves 6 | Prep Time: 10 minutes | Cook Time: 17 minutes | Total Time: 27 minutes

2 tablespoons extra-virgin olive oil

1½ cups chopped yellow onions

2 zucchini, halved lengthwise and cut into semicircles (leave peel on)

1 pound sliced mushrooms

1 teaspoon fine sea salt, divided

2 pounds ground beef

1 recipe Caesar Dressing (page 110)

2 teaspoons fish sauce

Arugula, for serving (optional)

Store & Reheat

Once cool, store in a sealed glass container in the refrigerator for up to 4 days or in the freezer for up to 3 months. Reheat in a skillet over medium heat until warm.

1. Heat the olive oil in a large, deep skillet over medium-high heat. Add the onion and sauté for 2 minutes until fragrant and beginning to soften.

2. Add the zucchini, mushrooms, and ½ teaspoon of the salt to the skillet and toss the vegetables together. Cook for 8 to 10 minutes, stirring frequently, until the vegetables are tender but not mushy; the mushrooms should still have a medium bite to them. Transfer to a strainer set over the sink and drain the liquid from the vegetables. Set the vegetables aside.

3. Crumble the ground beef into the same skillet and season with the remaining ½ teaspoon of salt. Cook over medium-high heat for 4 to 5 minutes, until browned and no longer pink.

4. Add the vegetables back to the skillet along with the Caesar Dressing and fish sauce and turn off the heat. Toss the meat and vegetables in the dressing until thoroughly coated and creamy. Serve on a bed of arugula, if desired.

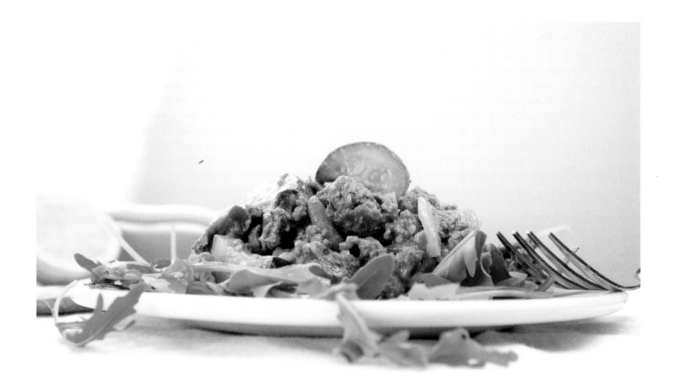

garlicky greek lamb skillet

Serves 4 | Prep Time: 8 minutes | Cook Time: 12 minutes | Total Time: 20 minutes

1½ pounds ground lamb, crumbled

1 teaspoon dried mint

½ teaspoon dried rubbed sage

½ teaspoon ground cinnamon

½ teaspoon fine sea salt

4 cups thinly sliced red cabbage (about ¾ pound)

1 cup thinly sliced yellow onions

¼ cup water

¼ cup Garlic Sauce (page 106)

2 teaspoons fresh lime or lemon juice

Make Ahead

Slice the cabbage and onions up to 2 days in advance and store wrapped in paper towels in a sealed plastic bag in the refrigerator until ready to use.

Store & Reheat

Once cool, store in a sealed glass container in the refrigerator for up to 3 days or in the freezer for up to 3 months. Reheat in a skillet over medium heat until warm.

1. In a large, deep skillet over medium-high heat, cook the lamb until browned on the outside and lightly pink on the inside. Stir in the mint, sage, cinnamon, and salt. Use a slotted spoon to transfer the seasoned lamb to a bowl, leaving the fat in the skillet.

2. Reduce the heat to medium. Add the cabbage and onions to the skillet and sauté in the rendered lamb fat for 4 to 5 minutes, until softened and lightly browned. Pour in the water, cover the skillet tightly, and steam-cook the vegetables until tender, 2 to 3 minutes.

3. Remove the lid and stir in the seasoned lamb, Garlic Sauce, and lime juice. Serve warm.

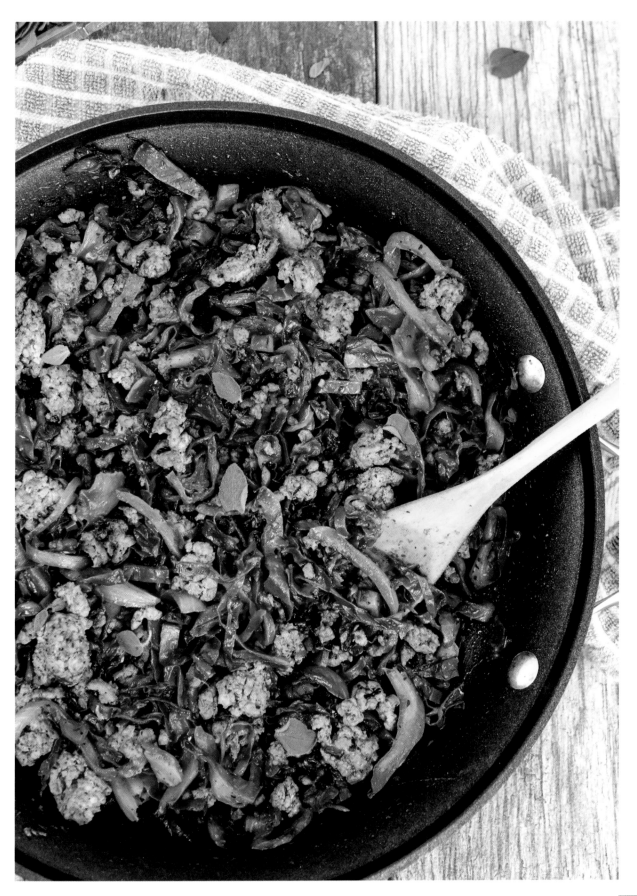

crispy salmon hash

Serves 2 | Prep Time: 8 minutes | Cook Time: 12 minutes | Total Time: 20 minutes

3 tablespoons extra-virgin olive oil, divided

1 pound white sweet potatoes, peeled and cut into ⅓-inch dice

½ teaspoon truffle salt (see Tip, page 122) or fine sea salt, divided

½ teaspoon dried dill weed

¼ teaspoon dried parsley

1½ teaspoons grated lemon zest

1 tablespoon fresh lemon juice

1 (8-ounce) wild-caught salmon fillet, pin bones removed (see Tip, page 230), chopped

3 ounces smoked salmon, chopped

1. Heat 2 tablespoons of the olive oil in a large skillet over medium-high heat. Add the potatoes and allow them to brown for several minutes without disturbing them. Add ¼ teaspoon of the salt, dill, and parsley to the skillet. Stir the potatoes and continue cooking for 3 to 4 more minutes, until crisp-tender.

2. While the potatoes are cooking, whisk together the remaining 1 tablespoon of olive oil, lemon zest, lemon juice, and remaining ¼ teaspoon of salt. Set aside.

3. Add the salmon to the skillet and cook until opaque, about 2 minutes.

4. Remove the hash from the heat and toss with the lemon oil. Serve warm.

Store & Reheat
Once cool, store in a sealed glass container in the refrigerator for up to 2 days. Reheat in a small greased skillet over medium heat.

Change It Up
Replace the white sweet potatoes with diced parsnips. Replace the dried parsley with 2 tablespoons of finely chopped fresh parsley.

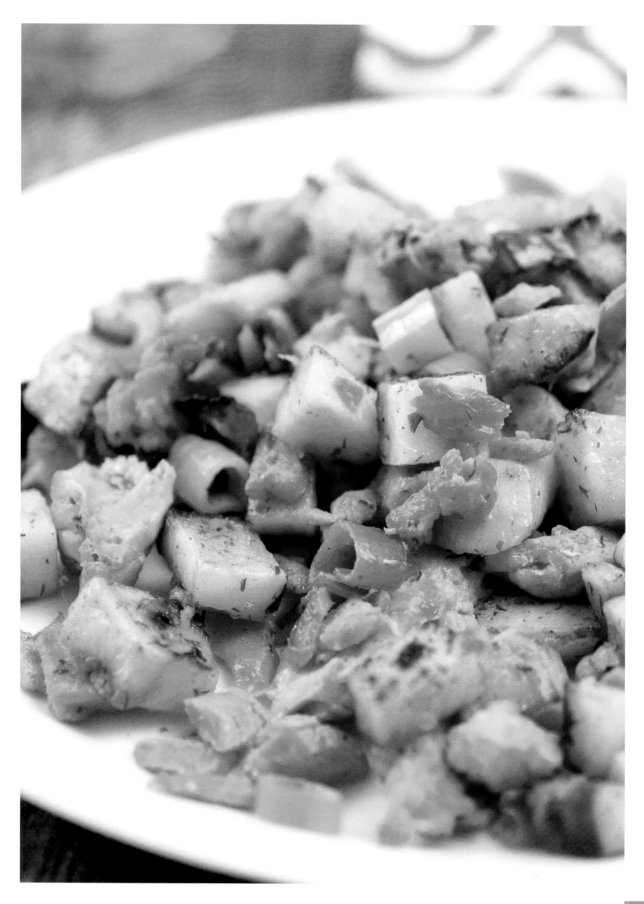

ollie's diy sunrise hash 🍲

Serves 4 | Prep Time: 10 minutes | Cook Time: 18 minutes | Total Time: 28 minutes

8 slices bacon, chopped (see Tip)

1 cup chopped yellow onion

1½ pounds orange sweet potatoes, peeled and chopped into ½-inch pieces

3 cloves garlic, minced

1 bunch green onions, sliced

¼ teaspoon fine sea salt or truffle salt (see Tip, page 122)

1. In a large, deep skillet over medium heat, cook the bacon with the onion until the fat has rendered and the bacon has begun to crisp up, 3 to 5 minutes.

2. Add the sweet potatoes and garlic to the pan and increase the heat to medium-high. Cook without disturbing for 4 to 5 minutes, until the bottoms of the sweet potatoes are lightly browned. Toss and continue to cook in the same manner, tossing only every few minutes, until the potatoes are crispy and cooked through.

3. Remove from the heat and stir in the green onions and salt.

Tip
Use sharp kitchen shears to cut the bacon quickly.

Make Ahead
Peel and chop the sweet potatoes and store wrapped in paper towels in a sealed plastic bag in the refrigerator for up to 5 days until ready to use.

Store & Reheat
Once cool, store in a sealed glass container in the refrigerator for up to 3 days or in the freezer for up to 3 months. Reheat in a small greased skillet over medium heat.

DIY Additions
· *Add 6 ounces of baby spinach to the skillet at the end of Step 2 and toss until completely wilted.*

· *Add leftover cooked ground or chopped protein of choice at the end of Step 2 and toss until warm. Chopped Garlic & Herb Breakfast Sausage (page 130) is an excellent option.*

· *Add 1 pound of trimmed and quartered Brussels sprouts to the skillet at the beginning of Step 2 for some extra green.*

· *Add 2 teaspoons of finely chopped fresh rosemary at the beginning of Step 2 for an extra boost of flavor.*

· *For a zesty Mediterranean take on morning hash, add ¼ cup of Orange & Olive Tapenade (page 276) and leftover shredded Classic Roast Chicken (page 224) at the end of Step 2 and omit the salt in Step 3.*

· *Drizzle the hash with Cilantro Chimichurri (page 116) or Garlic Sauce (page 106) for a big flavor boost.*

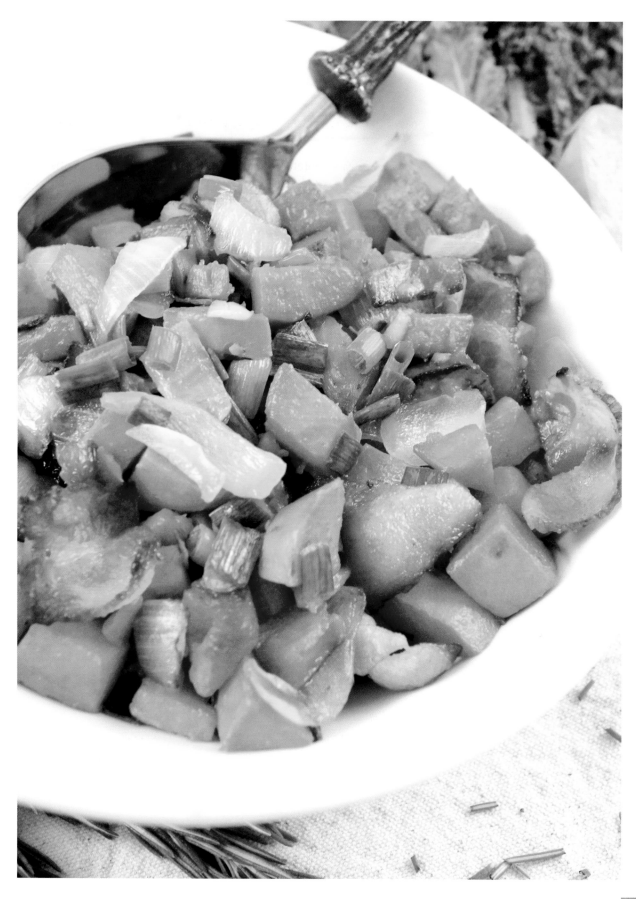

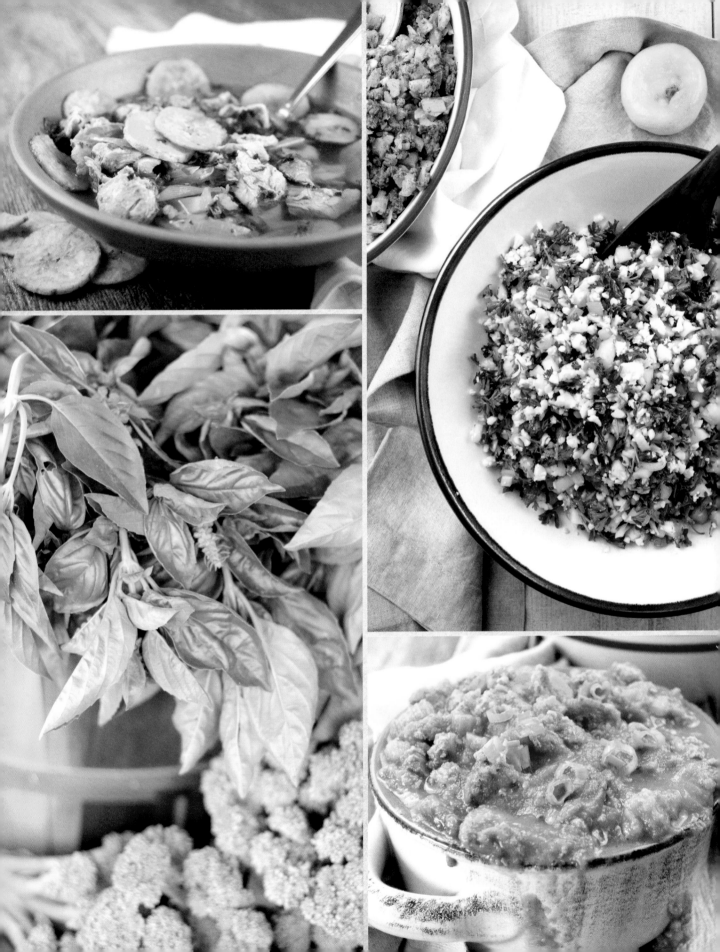

vibrant healing soup base

Makes 5 cups | Prep Time: 7 minutes | Cook Time: 28 minutes | Total Time: 35 minutes

1 tablespoon extra-virgin olive oil

2 cups chopped yellow onions

2 cloves garlic, chopped

½ teaspoon fine sea salt

4 cups Chicken Broth (page 108)

2 orange sweet potatoes (about ¾ pound), peeled and cubed

2 bay leaves

4 sprigs fresh thyme

1 tablespoon fresh lemon juice

½ cup coconut cream

Store & Reheat

Once cool, store in a sealed glass container in the refrigerator for up to 1 week or in the freezer for up to 3 months. Reheat in a saucepan over medium-low heat until warm.

Change It Up

For a coconut-free version, omit the coconut cream and increase the amount of sweet potatoes to 1 pound.

1. Heat the olive oil in a medium saucepan over medium heat. Sweat the onions, garlic, and salt in the oil for 6 to 8 minutes, until the onions have softened.

2. Add the broth, sweet potatoes, bay leaves, and thyme to the pan. Cover with a lid and bring to a boil over medium-high heat. Cook for 15 minutes or until the potatoes are very tender. Stir in the lemon juice and coconut cream.

3. Transfer the entire contents of the saucepan to a blender and blend on high speed until pureed and smooth.

Leftover Chicken & Veggie Soup. Simmer leftover Classic Roast Chicken (page 224) or Mojo Pulled Chicken (page 214) in the soup base with leftover Roasted Roots with Garlic Sauce (page 260) or the roasted vegetables of your choice.

Extra-Creamy Sweet Potato Soup. Puree leftover Silky Potato Puree (page 258) with the soup base ingredients for a thicker pureed soup as a starter or light meal.

Chicken Noodle or Chicken & Rice Soup. Simmer shredded Classic Roast Chicken (page 224) or plain cooked chicken with julienned zucchini noodles or uncooked riced cauliflower and 5 cups of spinach in the soup base until the vegetables are tender and the spinach has wilted.

Healing Morning Beverage. Warm 1 cup of soup base with a teaspoon of fresh lemon juice for a nourishing coffee replacement.

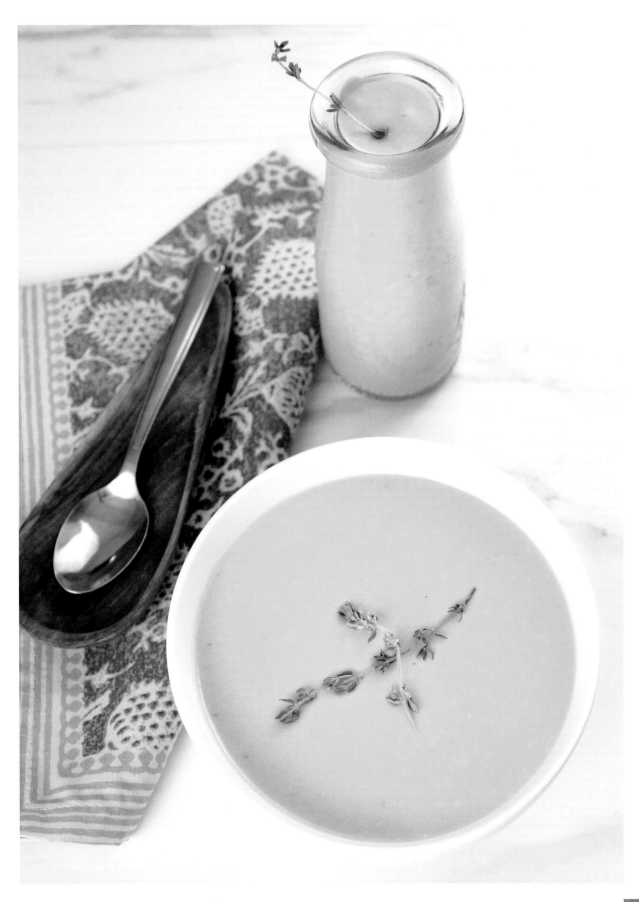

hamburger stew

Serves 5 to 6 | Prep Time: 15 minutes | Cook Time: 50 minutes | Total Time: 1 hour 5 minutes

3 tablespoons extra-virgin olive oil, divided

2 zucchini, peeled and roughly chopped

3 cups Beef Broth (page 109)

1 white onion, roughly chopped

3 carrots, peeled and sliced into ½-inch rounds

3 stalks celery, sliced into ½-inch pieces

1 bay leaf

1 sprig fresh rosemary

5 sprigs fresh thyme

2 pounds ground beef

2 teaspoons fine sea salt

8 ounces mushrooms, sliced

2 green plantains, peeled and cut into ½-inch dice

Chopped fresh parsley, for garnish (optional)

Store & Reheat

Once cool, store in a sealed glass container in the refrigerator for up to 4 days or in the freezer for up to 3 months. Reheat in a saucepan over medium heat until warm.

Change It Up

Replace the plantains with sweet potatoes, parsnips, turnips, or rutabaga. For chicken stew, use ground chicken or turkey in place of the ground beef and chicken broth in place of the beef broth.

1. Heat 2 tablespoons of the olive oil in a large stockpot or Dutch oven over medium-high heat. Add the zucchini and sauté, stirring frequently, until browned and soft, 8 to 10 minutes.

2. Remove the zucchini from the pot and place it in a blender with the broth. Blend on high speed until completely smooth, 1 to 2 minutes. Set aside.

3. Add the remaining 1 tablespoon of olive oil to the pot. Add the onion, carrots, and celery and sauté, stirring frequently, until the onion is starting to caramelize, 7 to 8 minutes. Add the bay leaf, rosemary, and thyme.

4. Add the ground beef to the pot with the vegetables, break it up into large chunks with a spoon or spatula, and season it with the salt. Cook for 8 to 10 minutes, stirring infrequently to avoid breaking the meat up into too-small pieces.

5. Add the mushrooms, plantains, and zucchini puree to the pot. Bring to a simmer, then reduce the heat to medium-low and cook uncovered for 20 minutes, stirring occasionally.

6. Remove the thyme and rosemary sprigs and bay leaf before serving. Garnish with chopped parsley, if desired.

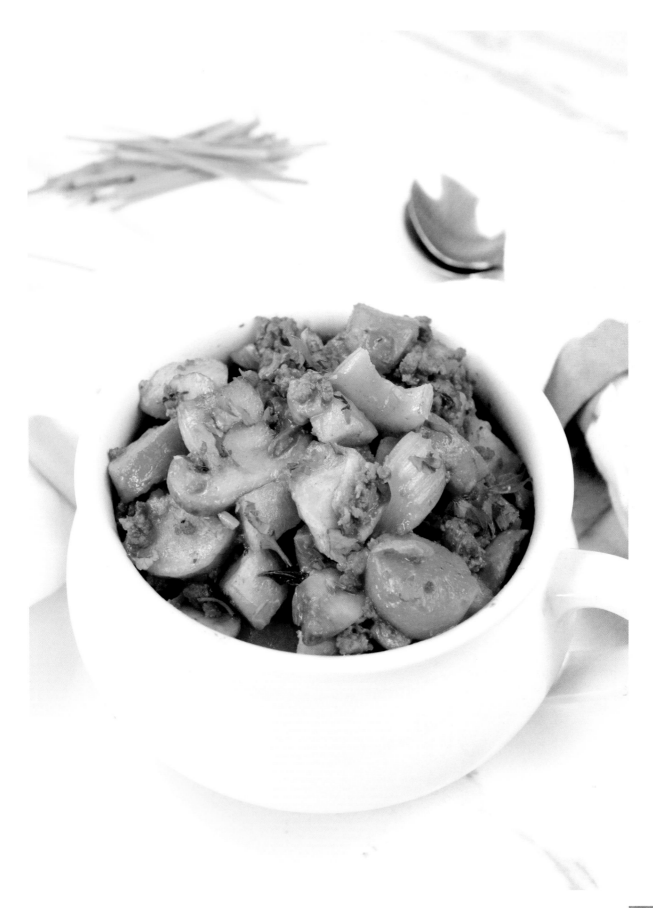

bacon & salmon chowder

Serves 3 to 4 | Prep Time: 10 minutes | Cook Time: 25 minutes | Total Time: 35 minutes

5 slices bacon

1 leek, thoroughly cleaned and thinly sliced (see Tip)

4 cups Beef Broth (page 109)

1½ pounds white sweet potatoes, peeled and diced

3 stalks celery, chopped

1 bay leaf

1 pound skinless wild-caught salmon fillets, pin bones removed (see Tip, page 230), cut into 1-inch pieces

Juice of ½ lemon

Fresh dill, for garnish (optional)

1. Cut the bacon into ½-inch pieces using kitchen shears or a sharp knife. Place the bacon and leek in a large saucepan over medium-high heat and cook until the bacon is crispy and the leek has softened, 6 to 8 minutes. Transfer to a medium bowl and set aside.

2. In the same saucepan, combine the broth, sweet potatoes, celery, and bay leaf. Bring to a boil, cover, and cook until the potatoes are fork-tender, 6 to 7 minutes. Transfer the broth, bay leaf, and half of the potatoes and celery to a blender and puree until smooth to create a creamy soup base. Transfer the remaining potatoes and celery to the bowl with the bacon and leek.

3. Add the pureed soup base and salmon to the saucepan and cook uncovered over medium heat for 3 to 5 minutes, until the salmon is opaque throughout. To avoid overcooking the salmon, do not bring the soup past a low simmer.

4. Stir in the lemon juice and the reserved sweet potatoes, celery, bacon, and leek into the soup and serve warm. Garnish with dill, if desired.

Tip
To clean the leek, slice off the root and the dark green portion, leaving only the white stalk. Slice the stalk in half lengthwise and rinse each half under warm running water until clean.

Make Ahead
Cut the bacon, leek, sweet potatoes, and celery up to 3 days in advance and store them separately in plastic bags or glass containers in the refrigerator until ready to make the soup.

Store & Reheat
Once cool, store in a sealed glass container in the refrigerator for up to 4 days or in the freezer for up to 3 months. Reheat by bringing the soup to a simmer over medium-low heat.

Change It Up
Substitute another mild white root vegetable, such as parsnip or celery root, for the white sweet potatoes.

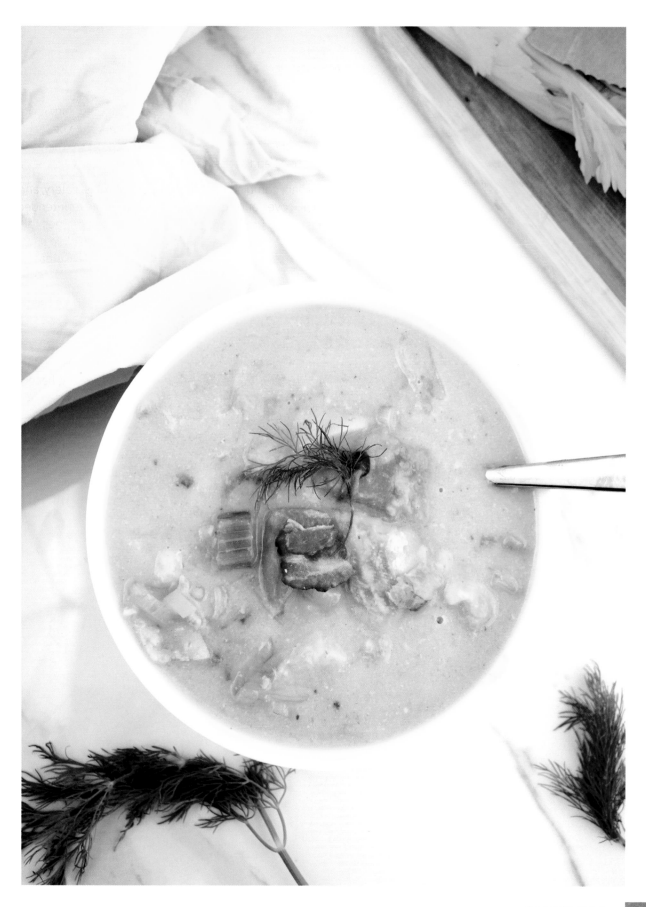

roasted fennel & parsnip soup with citrus drizzle

Serves 6 to 8 | Prep Time: 15 minutes | Cook Time: 1 hour | Total Time: 1 hour 15 minutes

2 fennel bulbs with fronds (about 1 ½ pounds), chopped into 1-inch pieces (reserve fronds for garnish)

2 tablespoons coconut oil, melted, divided

1 teaspoon fine sea salt, divided

2 pounds parsnips, peeled and chopped into ½-inch pieces

1 head garlic

7 cups Chicken or Beef Broth (pages 108–109)

1 cup water

CITRUS DRESSING

2 tablespoons extra-virgin olive oil

2 tablespoons fresh lemon juice

FOR GARNISH

1 tablespoon grated orange zest

¾ cup chopped fennel fronds (from bulbs above)

Make Ahead

Complete Steps 1 through 4 up to 2 days in advance and store the roasted vegetables in a sealed container in the refrigerator until ready to continue with Step 5.

Store & Reheat

Once cool, store in a sealed glass container in the refrigerator for up to 5 days or in the freezer for up to 6 months. Reheat in a saucepan over medium-low heat until warm.

1. Preheat the oven to 400 degrees.

2. On a rimmed baking sheet, toss together the fennel, 1 tablespoon of the melted coconut oil, and ¼ teaspoon of the salt.

3. On a second rimmed baking sheet, toss together the remaining 1 tablespoon of coconut oil, ¼ teaspoon of the salt, the parsnips, and the whole head of garlic.

4. Place the baking sheets in the oven and roast the vegetables for 35 to 40 minutes, stirring halfway through cooking, until the fennel and parsnips are golden brown. Once the garlic has cooled, squeeze the roasted cloves out of their skin.

5. In a large stockpot, bring the broth, water, roasted vegetables and garlic cloves, and remaining ½ teaspoon of salt to a boil over medium heat. Let simmer, covered with a lid, for 15 minutes.

6. Transfer the contents of the stockpot to a high-powered blender or food processor and blend on high speed until pureed and smooth.

7. Prepare the dressing by whisking together the olive oil and lemon juice in a small bowl. Ladle the soup into individual serving bowls and drizzle the citrus dressing over the soup. Top with the orange zest and chopped fennel fronds just before serving.

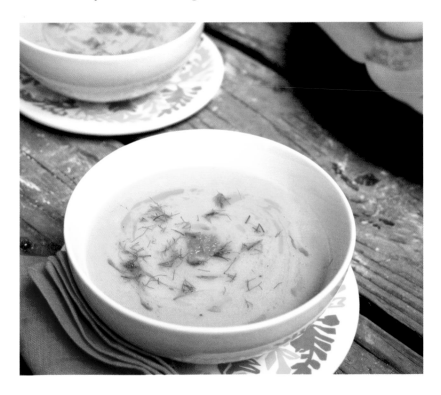

pumpkin chili

Serves 6 to 8 | Prep Time: 15 minutes | Cook Time: 1 hour 50 minutes | Total Time: 2 hours 5 minutes

2 pounds ground beef

2 teaspoons ginger powder

1 teaspoon garlic powder

1 teaspoon onion powder

1 teaspoon ground cinnamon

¼ teaspoon ground mace

2 tablespoons extra-virgin olive oil

1 large yellow onion, chopped

3 large carrots, sliced into ⅓-inch rounds

2 stalks celery, chopped

1 pound sliced mushrooms

5 cloves garlic, roughly chopped

1 teaspoon fine sea salt

2 (15-ounce) cans pumpkin puree

2 cups Beef or Chicken Broth (pages 108–109)

1 bay leaf

1 teaspoon smoked sea salt (see Tip)

2 tablespoons apple cider vinegar

Sliced green onions, for serving

1. In a large saucepan or stockpot over medium-high heat, brown the ground beef, breaking it up into small pieces with a wooden spoon, until cooked through. Stir in the ginger powder, garlic powder, onion powder, cinnamon, and mace until the meat is evenly coated in the seasonings. Transfer the mixture to a bowl and set aside.

2. Heat the olive oil in the same saucepan or stockpot over medium-high heat. Add the onion, carrots, celery, mushrooms, garlic, and salt and stir well. Cook for 10 minutes until the vegetables are softened and tender.

3. Pour in the pumpkin puree and broth and stir to incorporate into the vegetables. Add the meat back to the saucepan and bring the mixture to a boil. Add the bay leaf, reduce the heat to medium-low to maintain a simmer, and cook, covered with a lid, for 1½ hours until the vegetables are tender.

4. Stir in the smoked sea salt and vinegar and remove from the heat. The chili will be fragrant and thick like a stew.

5. Remove the bay leaf before serving. Top each bowl with a generous sprinkle of green onions.

Tip
Smoked sea salt adds a smoky finish to the soup that is reminiscent of traditional chili. If you don't have any on hand, replace the smoked sea salt with a teaspoon or two of liquid smoke (with an ingredients list of only smoke and water) or 2 to 3 tablespoons of bacon fat.

Make Ahead
Chop the onion, carrots, celery, and garlic up to 2 days in advance and store in a sealed plastic bag in the refrigerator prior to cooking the chili.

Store & Reheat
Once cool, store in a sealed glass container in the refrigerator for up to 4 days or in the freezer for up to 3 months. Reheat in a saucepan over medium heat until warm.

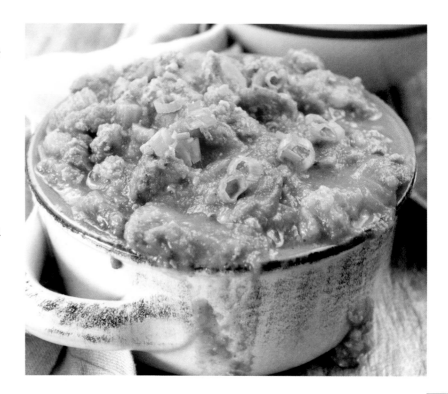

chicken "tortilla" soup

Serves 4 | Prep Time: 7 minutes | Cook Time: 15 minutes | Total Time: 22 minutes

1 tablespoon coconut oil

1 cup diced yellow onions

½ cup diced red onions

3 cloves garlic, minced

6 cups Chicken or Beef Broth (pages 108–109)

4 cups Mojo Pulled Chicken (page 214)

1 tablespoon dried oregano leaves

¾ cup chopped fresh cilantro

1 tablespoon fresh lime juice

4 ounces plantain chips (see Tip)

1. Heat the coconut oil in a large saucepan over medium heat. Add the onions and garlic and sauté until softened, 5 to 7 minutes, making sure that the garlic does not burn; reduce the heat to medium-low if needed.

2. Add the broth to the pan and bring to a boil over medium-high heat.

3. Stir in the pulled chicken and oregano. Return to a boil for 2 to 3 minutes, then remove from the heat. Stir in the cilantro and lime juice.

4. Add the plantain chips to the soup just before serving, allowing the chips to soften slightly for a few minutes.

Tip
Buy plantain chips with an ingredient list of just plantains, palm oil, and sea salt.

Store & Reheat
Once cool, store the soup without the plantain chips in a sealed glass container in the refrigerator for up to 3 days or in the freezer for up to 3 months. Reheat in a saucepan over medium heat until warm.

"cheesy" broccoli soup

Serves 4 | Prep Time: 5 minutes | Cook Time: 15 minutes | Total Time: 20 minutes

3 cups Bone Broth of choice (pages 108–109)

1 (16-ounce) bag frozen broccoli florets

1 avocado, peeled and pitted

¼ cup nutritional yeast

1½ teaspoons apple cider vinegar

½ teaspoon onion powder

½ teaspoon fine sea salt

¼ teaspoon garlic powder

1. Bring the broth and broccoli to a boil in a medium, covered saucepan over medium-high heat. Reduce the heat to medium-low and cook until the broccoli is very tender, about 10 minutes.

2. Transfer the broth and broccoli to a blender, add the remaining ingredients, and blend until smooth.

"Cheesy" Chicken & Broccoli Soup. Add 2 cups of warm chopped or shredded cooked chicken to the pureed soup.

Store & Reheat
Once cool, store in a sealed glass container in the refrigerator for up to 5 days or in the freezer for up to 6 months. Reheat in a saucepan over medium heat until warm.

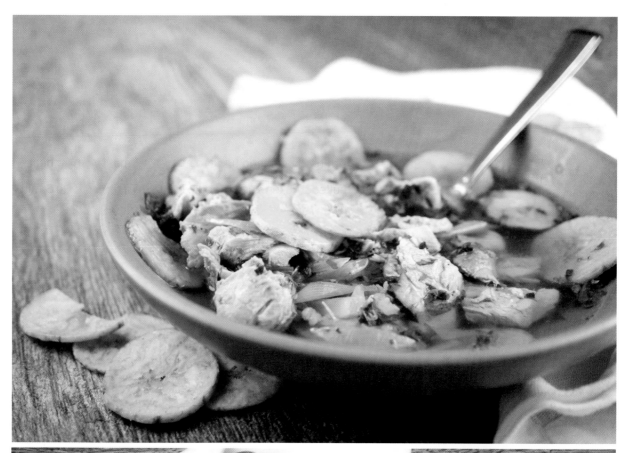

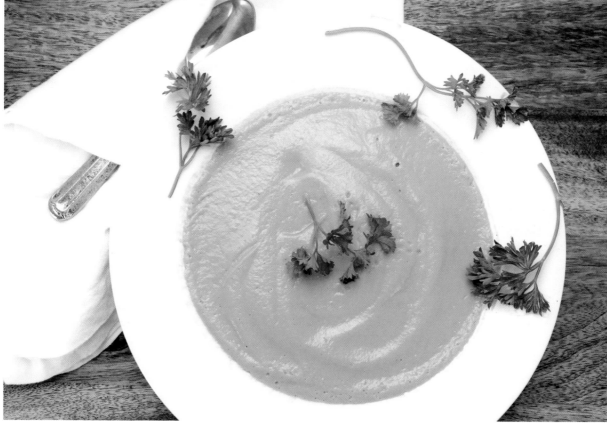

watermelon gazpacho

Serves 4 to 6 | Prep Time: 20 minutes | Total Time: 20 minutes + 2 hours to chill

5 cups cubed seedless watermelon (remove seeds if using a seeded watermelon)

2 teaspoons red or white wine vinegar

1 tablespoon extra-virgin olive oil

¼ teaspoon fine sea salt

¼ red onion, finely diced (about ½ cup)

½ cucumber, peeled and finely diced (about ¾ cup), or 1 Granny Smith apple, peeled and finely diced

½ jicama, peeled and finely diced (about 1½ cups)

2 tablespoons chopped fresh cilantro

1 tablespoon chopped fresh mint, plus additional mint leaves for garnish (optional)

Storage
Store in a sealed glass container in the refrigerator for up to 2 days.

1. Combine the watermelon, vinegar, olive oil, and salt in a blender and pulse until smooth. (It's okay if it's a little pulpy.)

2. Stir the onion, cucumber, jicama, cilantro, and mint into the watermelon mixture. Transfer to a sealed glass container.

3. Refrigerate for 2 hours (and up to overnight) before serving. Garnish with mint leaves, if desired.

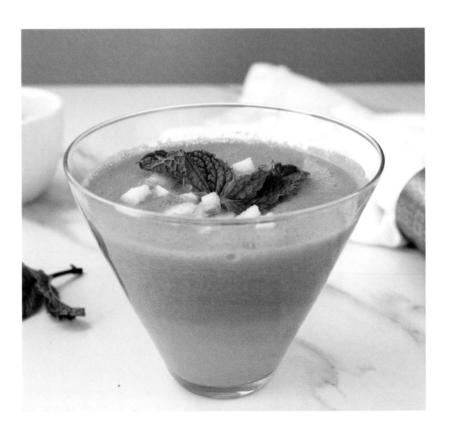

hearty healing beef stew

Serves 4 to 5 | Prep Time: 10 minutes | Cook Time: 2 hours 20 minutes | Total Time: 2 hours 30 minutes

2 tablespoons extra-virgin olive oil

2 pounds beef bottom round, cubed

1½ teaspoons fine sea salt, divided

1 large yellow onion, cut into 1-inch pieces

3 sprigs fresh thyme

1 bay leaf

1 cinnamon stick

2 (1-inch) pieces fresh orange peel

4 cups Beef Broth (page 109)

1 cup sweet potato puree (see Tip)

½ cup red wine

4 large carrots, peeled and cut into 1-inch pieces

4 stalks celery, chopped

1 bunch kale, chopped

1. Heat the olive oil in a large stockpot or Dutch oven over medium-high heat. Add the meat, sprinkle with ½ teaspoon of the salt, and brown on all sides for 8 to 10 minutes total, but avoid getting a crust on the outside.

2. Stir in the onion, thyme, bay leaf, cinnamon stick, orange peel, and remaining 1 teaspoon of salt and cook for 1 to 2 minutes, until fragrant.

3. Add the broth, sweet potato puree, and wine to the pot and bring to a boil. Reduce the heat to medium-low, cover with a lid, and cook for 1 hour.

4. Add the carrots and celery to the pot and return the stew to a boil over medium-high heat. Reduce the heat to medium-low and simmer for an additional 40 minutes. Add the chopped kale, submerging it in the liquid, and cook for 25 more minutes, until wilted and tender.

5. Remove the thyme, bay leaf, cinnamon stick, and orange peel before serving.

Tip
Buy canned sweet potato puree for quick preparation.

Serving Suggestion
Serve over a double batch of Silky Potato Puree (page 258) for a hearty and comforting meal.

Store & Reheat
Once cool, store in a sealed glass container in the refrigerator for up to 4 days or in the freezer for up to 3 months. Reheat in a saucepan or stockpot over medium heat until warm.

Change It Up
Replace the carrots with 3 cups of peeled and chopped butternut squash, the thyme with 2 sprigs of fresh rosemary, and the orange peel with an equal amount of lemon peel.

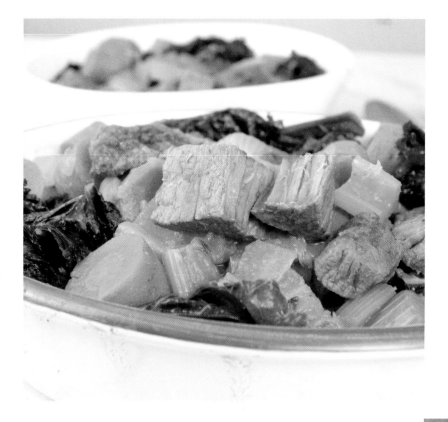

new england clam chowder

Serves 6 | Prep Time: 20 minutes | Cook Time: 35 minutes | Total Time: 55 minutes

4 thick-cut slices bacon, chopped

1 yellow onion, diced

2 to 3 stalks celery, thinly sliced

1 large carrot, peeled and diced

1 large turnip, cut into ¾-inch cubes

3 cups Chicken or Pork Broth (pages 108–109)

3 (5- to 6-ounce) cans clams, drained

1 green plantain, peeled and grated

2 bay leaves

4 to 5 sprigs fresh thyme, leaves only

2 cups coconut cream

3 tablespoons chopped fresh parsley

Fine sea salt or truffle salt (see Tip, page 122), to taste

1. Place the chopped bacon in a medium stockpot, then turn on the heat to medium-high. Cook, stirring occasionally, until the bacon is crisp.

2. Add the onion, celery, carrot, and turnip to the pot. Cook until fragrant, about 5 minutes, stirring occasionally.

3. Add the broth, clams, grated plantain, bay leaves, and thyme to the pot. Bring to a boil, then reduce the heat to maintain a simmer for 20 minutes, stirring occasionally.

4. Add the coconut cream and parsley to the soup. Taste and season with sea salt or truffle salt, if desired. Cook for 1 to 2 minutes and serve.

Store & Reheat

Once cool, store in a sealed glass container in the refrigerator for up to 4 days or in the freezer for up to 3 months. Reheat in a saucepan over medium heat until warm.

Change It Up

Add 1 to 2 tablespoons of peeled and grated fresh horseradish for some bite. Try adding copious amounts of smoked salmon or chunks of any fish you like. Add 1 to 2 sliced green onions and chopped fresh dill or tarragon with or instead of the parsley. Use smoked clams for an extra dimension of flavor.

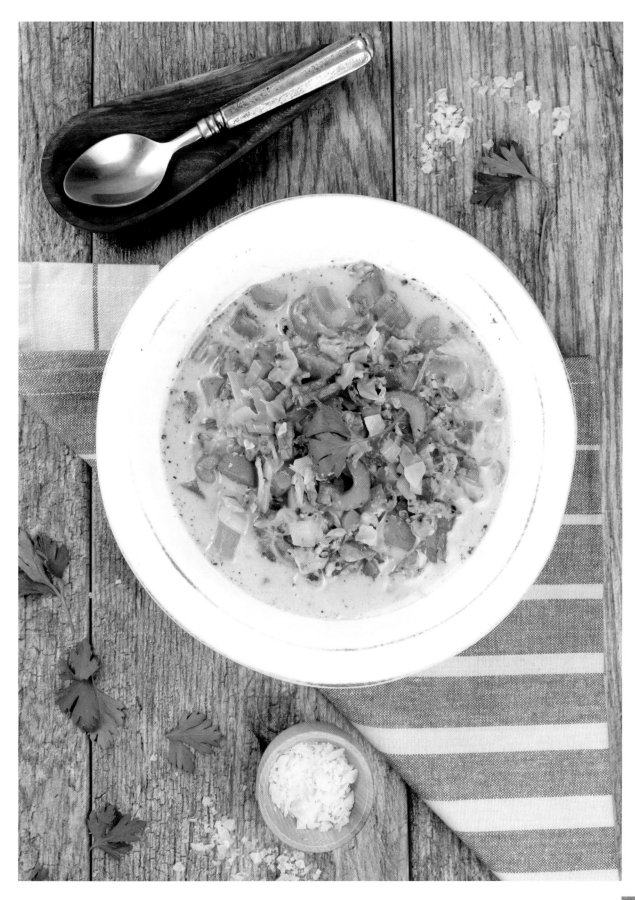

lettuce soup 🍲

Serves 2 to 4 | Prep Time: 10 minutes | Cook Time: 30 minutes | Total Time: 40 minutes

3 tablespoons extra-virgin olive oil or coconut oil

1 cup chopped shallots (about 3 large)

1 clove garlic, chopped

¾ teaspoon fine sea salt

1 pound lettuce (about 2 large heads), such as Boston or Bibb (see Tip), roughly chopped

4 cups Chicken Broth (page 108)

1 green plantain, peeled and cut into 1-inch chunks

Coconut cream, room temperature, for garnish (optional)

Tip
Boston and Bibb lettuce are the classic varieties for lettuce soup, but any sweet variety will work well.

Store & Reheat
Once cool, store in a sealed glass container in the refrigerator for up to 4 days or in the freezer for up to 6 months. Reheat in a saucepan over medium-low heat until warm.

1. Heat the olive oil in a large stockpot over medium-high heat. Add the shallots and cook, stirring frequently, until beginning to soften, about 5 minutes.

2. Add the garlic and salt. Cook, stirring frequently, for another minute, until fragrant.

3. Add the lettuce. Stir constantly for 2 to 3 minutes to wilt the lettuce.

4. Add the broth and plantain. Bring to a boil, then reduce the heat to maintain a simmer, uncovered, for 20 minutes.

5. Transfer the entire contents of the pot to a blender and blend on high speed for 1 minute (do this in batches if you have a smaller blender). You can also use an immersion blender, but it will be more difficult to get the perfect creamy consistency. Whisk the coconut cream to remove any lumps, then drizzle some on each serving of soup, if desired.

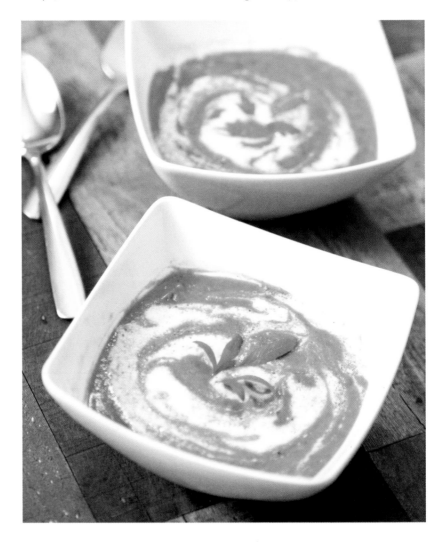

caesar salad

Serves 4 | Prep Time: 5 minutes | Total Time: 5 minutes

2 hearts romaine lettuce, roughly chopped

⅓ cup halved and thinly sliced red onion

½ cup Caesar Dressing (page 110), or more as desired

Tip

Missing croutons? Make the Everything Sweet Potatoes on page 273, let cool completely in the refrigerator, and then chop them up into crouton-size pieces and toss them in the salad.

Make Ahead

Make the salad up to 1 day in advance and store covered in the refrigerator, undressed, until ready to serve.

Toss together the romaine, onion, and dressing in a large salad bowl. Add more dressing, if desired, and serve immediately.

Chicken Caesar Salad. Add 3 cups of chopped cooked chicken and 6 slices of chopped cooked bacon to the salad. Use an additional 2 to 3 tablespoons of dressing.

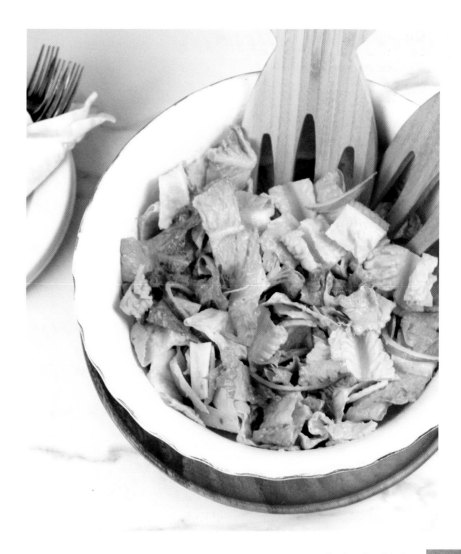

antipasto salad

Serves 4 | Prep Time: 15 minutes | Cook Time: 5 minutes | Total Time: 20 minutes

8 slices prosciutto (see Tips)

1 cup diced uncured ham (see Tips)

4 cups chopped romaine lettuce

¾ cup black olives, pitted

⅔ cup chopped hearts of palm

¼ cup fresh basil leaves, slivered

¼ cup Greek Dressing (page 110)

1. Preheat the broiler to high. Chop the prosciutto into bite-size pieces and place on a rimmed baking sheet with the diced ham. Broil for 3 to 5 minutes, until the prosciutto is crispy.

2. In a large serving bowl, toss the meat with the rest of the ingredients. Serve at room temperature or cold.

Tips
Buy prosciutto with an ingredient list of just pork and salt.

Can't find uncured ham? Use plain cooked smoked turkey or smoked chicken breast chopped into ½-inch cubes instead, or have your butcher slice deli ham (check the ingredients) into ¾-inch-thick slices for you to dice at home.

Make Ahead
Make the salad up to 2 days in advance and store covered in the refrigerator, undressed, until ready to serve.

sweet & smoky spa salad

Serves 2 | Prep Time: 7 minutes | Total Time: 7 minutes

6 cups mixed spring salad greens

6 ounces smoked salmon, chopped

1 Kirby cucumber, thinly sliced

½ cup Roasted Strawberries (page 321), cooled

1 tablespoon sliced green onion

2 to 3 tablespoons Honey Balsamic Dressing (page 110), as desired

Divide the salad greens, salmon, cucumber, strawberries, and green onion equally between two serving plates. Drizzle with the desired amount of dressing and serve cold.

Make Ahead
Make the salad up to 6 hours in advance and store covered in the refrigerator, undressed, until ready to serve.

Serving Suggestion
Serve with Smoked Salmon Potato Salad (page 175) for a light spring or summer meal.

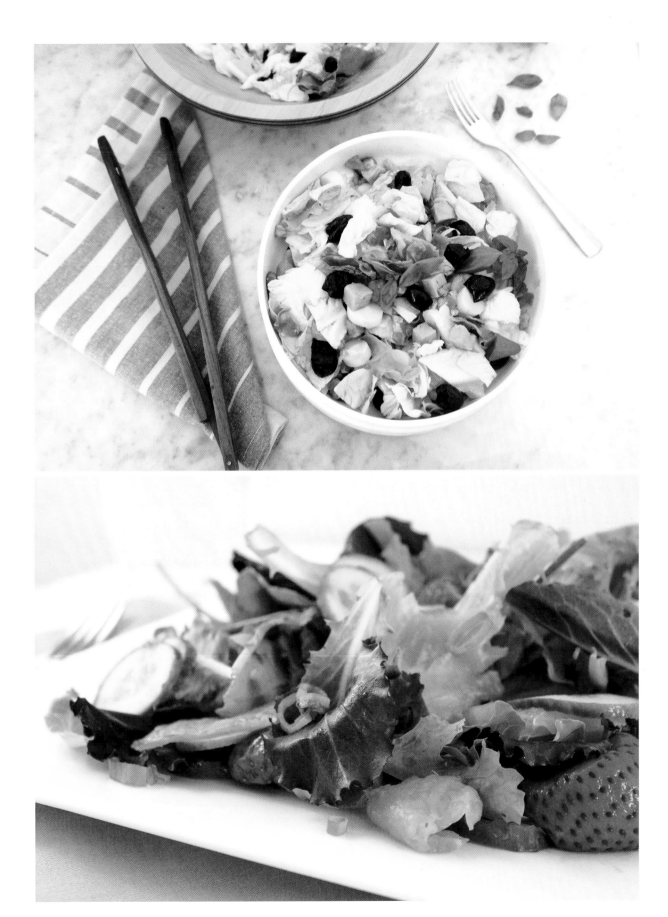

grilled chicken souvlaki salad

Serves 4 | Prep Time: 10 minutes | Cook Time: 18 minutes | Total Time: 28 minutes + 30 minutes to marinate

GRILLED CHICKEN SOUVLAKI

2 pounds boneless, skinless chicken breast

⅔ cup Greek Dressing (page 110)

½ teaspoon fine sea salt

1 large head iceberg lettuce, thinly sliced

½ cup thinly sliced red onion

1 recipe Tzatziki Sauce (page 115)

Handful of olives, pitted (optional)

Lemon wedges, for serving

1. Preheat the grill to medium-high heat.

2. Coat the chicken in the dressing and place it in a large plastic bag or sealed shallow container. While the grill preheats, let the chicken marinate on the countertop for 30 minutes.

3. Grill the chicken for 8 to 9 minutes per side, until the center is no longer pink and the outside is golden brown. Sprinkle with the salt and let rest for 5 to 10 minutes, then slice thickly.

4. Meanwhile, divide the lettuce, red onion, Tzatziki Sauce, and olives (if using) evenly among 4 bowls. Top with grilled chicken slices and serve with lemon wedges.

Serving Suggestion
Serve with Garlic-Dill Parsnip Fries (page 252), which can be baked while the chicken is on the grill.

Storage
Store undressed salad covered in the refrigerator for up to 2 days.

Greek Gyro Wraps. Layer several tablespoons of Tzatziki Sauce, sliced Grilled Chicken Souvlaki, and shredded lettuce in warmed Plantain Wraps (page 121).

roasted root, arugula & balsamic salad

Serves 4 | Prep Time: 5 minutes | Total Time: 5 minutes

6 cups arugula

⅓ cup Honey Balsamic Dressing (page 110)

4 cups Roasted Roots with Garlic Sauce (page 260)

Serving Suggestion
Serve with Classic Roast Chicken (page 224).

For warm salad: Toss the arugula with the dressing and just-roasted vegetables until the arugula begins to wilt. Serve immediately. (This version is best eaten within 1 hour of preparing to prevent the arugula from wilting too much.)

For cold salad: Chill the roasted vegetables in the refrigerator for at least 2 hours. Toss with the arugula and dressing when ready to serve.

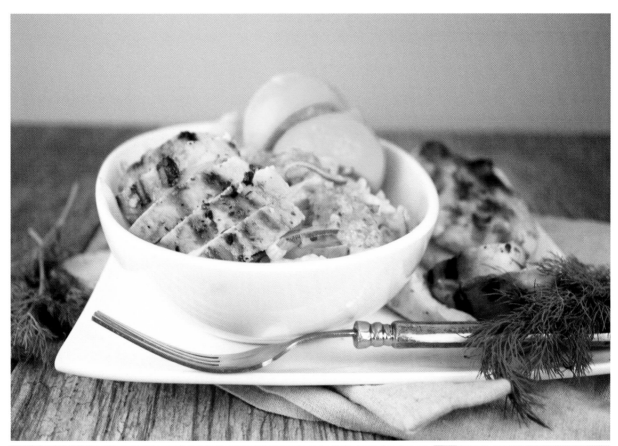

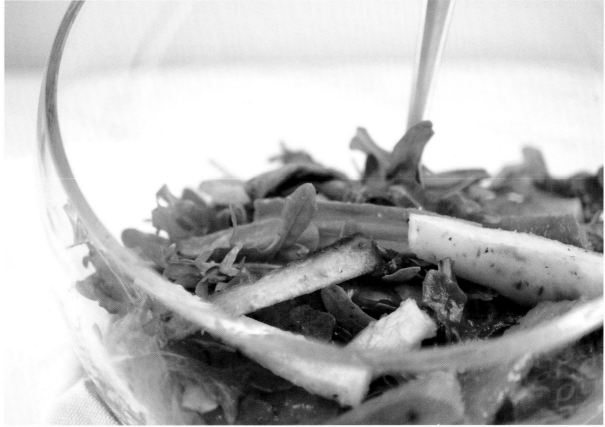

fennel mandarin slaw

Serves 6 | Prep Time: 15 minutes | Total Time: 15 minutes

2 cups thinly sliced fennel bulb

3 cups thinly sliced green cabbage

4 Mandarin oranges, peeled and segmented

¼ cup chopped fresh dill

3 tablespoons extra-virgin olive oil

2 tablespoons apple cider vinegar

¼ teaspoon fine sea salt

Make Ahead

Slice the fennel and cabbage up to 2 days in advance and store in a sealed plastic bag or container in the refrigerator until ready to use.

Serving Suggestions

Serve with Wild Salmon with Roasted Raspberries (page 234) or Honey-Garlic Drumsticks (page 218).

Storage

Store covered in the refrigerator for up to 2 days if dressed or up to 5 days if undressed.

1. Combine the fennel, cabbage, orange segments, and dill in a large serving bowl.

2. In a small bowl, whisk together the olive oil, vinegar, and salt. Pour over the slaw and toss well to combine.

3. Serve immediately or let marinate in the fridge for 1 to 2 hours to allow the flavors to marry before serving.

Shredded Chicken & Fennel Mandarin Slaw. Toss 3 cups of shredded cooked chicken and ¼ cup of sliced green onions with the slaw. You may increase the amount of dressing, if desired.

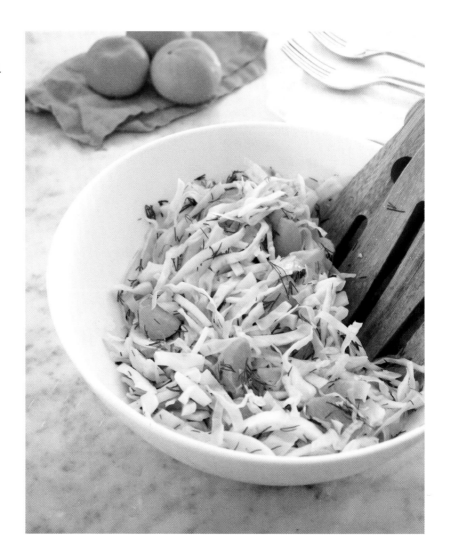

honey-lime chicken & strawberry salad

Serves 4 to 6 | Prep Time: 15 minutes | Cook Time: 10 minutes | Total Time: 25 minutes

1 tablespoon coconut oil

1 teaspoon fine sea salt, divided

2 pounds boneless, skinless chicken breast, cut into ½-inch pieces

2 tablespoons fresh lime juice

2 tablespoons honey, liquid

2 romaine hearts, chopped

1 cup strawberries, sliced

½ English cucumber, peeled and chopped

2 avocados, peeled, pitted, and diced

2 tablespoons sliced fresh mint

¾ cup Strawberry Lime Dressing (page 110), for serving

Make Ahead

Prepare the chicken through Step 3. Store in a sealed glass container in the refrigerator for up to 2 days. When ready to serve the salad, rewarm the chicken and proceed with Step 4.

Storage

Store undressed salad covered in the refrigerator for up to 2 days.

1. Heat the coconut oil in a large skillet over medium-high heat until hot.

2. Sprinkle ½ teaspoon of the salt on the chicken and add the chicken to the skillet. Do not overcrowd the pan, or the chicken will not brown. Cook, undisturbed, for at least 3 minutes, until golden brown. Flip the chicken and continue cooking for about 2 minutes, until cooked through but still moist.

3. In a small bowl, whisk together the lime juice, honey, and remaining ½ teaspoon of salt. Pour over the chicken and cover with a lid slightly ajar to let steam escape. Cook on medium-low heat until a thickened glaze has formed. Remove from the heat.

4. Toss together the romaine, strawberries, cucumber, avocados, and mint in a large serving bowl. Top with the warm chicken and serve with Strawberry Lime Dressing.

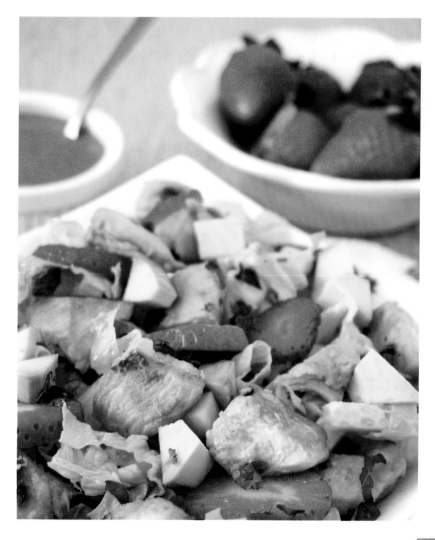

chunky tuna salad

Serves 2 to 3 | Prep Time: 12 minutes | Total Time: 12 minutes

1 (10-ounce) can albacore tuna, no salt added

⅔ cup quartered red grapes

⅔ cup diced celery

½ cup diced dried apricots

¼ cup chopped green onions

3 tablespoons diced shallots

½ teaspoon fine sea salt

½ cup Avocado Mayo (page 113) or Garlic-Dill Ranch Dressing (page 112)

Mixed spring salad greens or baby spinach, for serving

In a bowl, mix together the tuna, grapes, celery, dried apricots, green onions, shallots, and salt until well combined. Toss with the dressing. Serve cold over spring mix or baby spinach.

Storage

Store the tuna salad separate from the greens in a sealed glass container in the refrigerator for up to 3 days.

toasted coconut, fig & kale salad 🍲

Serves 4 | Prep Time: 10 minutes | Cook Time: 15 minutes | Total Time: 25 minutes

⅓ cup unsweetened shredded coconut

2 large bunches curly kale, ribs removed, leaves torn into 2-inch pieces

¼ cup water

3 tablespoons extra-virgin olive oil

2 teaspoons apple cider vinegar

1½ teaspoons grated fresh ginger

¼ teaspoon fine sea salt

1 Granny Smith apple, cored and thinly sliced

4 dried Turkish figs, diced

1. Preheat the oven to 325 degrees. Spread the coconut on a rimmed baking sheet and bake for 4 to 5 minutes, until golden brown, stirring halfway through cooking. Set aside.

2. Meanwhile, bring the kale and water to a boil in a large pot over medium-high heat. Reduce the heat to medium-low, cover with a lid, and steam the kale until the leaves are tender with a slight crunch, 8 to 10 minutes. Drain the kale.

3. While the kale steams, whisk together the olive oil, vinegar, ginger, and salt in a small bowl to make a dressing.

4. Toss the warm kale, apple slices, and figs in a large salad bowl with the dressing to coat evenly. Stir in the toasted coconut. Serve warm.

Serving Suggestions

Serve with Bacon-Date Crusted Salmon (page 230) or Honey-Garlic Drumsticks (page 218).

Store & Reheat

Store in a sealed glass container in the refrigerator for up to 1 week. Reheat by warming gently in a pot with 1 tablespoon of coconut oil.

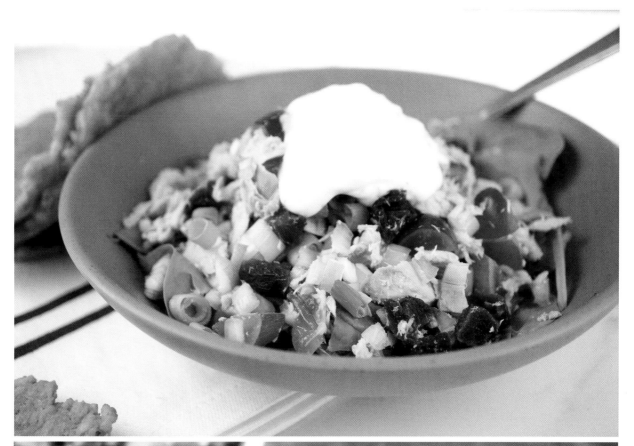

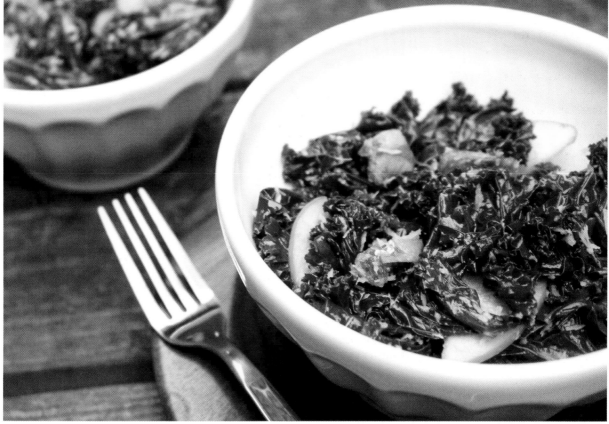

peach & kale summer salad

Serves 4 | Prep Time: 10 minutes | Total Time: 10 minutes

1 large bunch curly kale, ribs removed, leaves chopped into 1-inch pieces

2 tablespoons extra-virgin olive oil

2 peaches, sliced

2 tablespoons minced shallot

2 tablespoons Honey Balsamic Dressing (page 110)

Storage
Store in a sealed glass container in the refrigerator for up to 2 days.

1. Measure 7 to 8 cups of the chopped kale and place in a large serving bowl. Pour the olive oil over the kale and massage the leaves with your hands for 5 minutes to break down the tough fibers, until the kale is softened and wilted.

2. Toss the peaches and shallot with the massaged kale and serve at room temperature or cold, drizzled with the dressing.

Chicken, Peach, & Kale Summer Salad. Toss 2 cups of cooled and shredded Classic Roast Chicken (page 224) into the salad for two entrée-size salads.

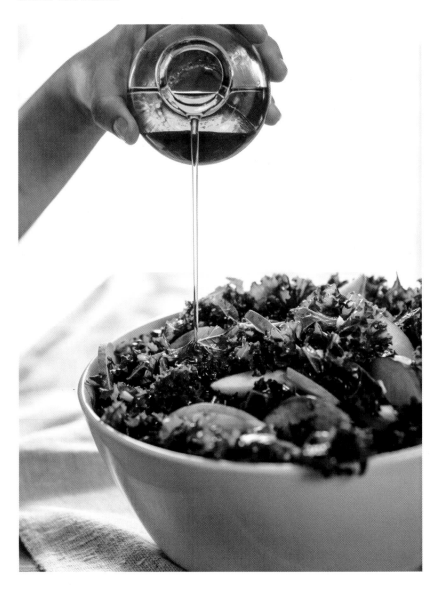

smoked salmon potato salad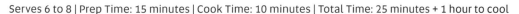

Serves 6 to 8 | Prep Time: 15 minutes | Cook Time: 10 minutes | Total Time: 25 minutes + 1 hour to cool

2 pounds white sweet potatoes

1½ teaspoons fine sea salt, divided

¼ cup extra-virgin olive oil

3 tablespoons apple cider vinegar

2 cups chopped cucumber

1 cup chopped celery

⅓ cup sliced green onions

4 ounces smoked salmon, chopped

¼ cup chopped fresh dill

Make Ahead
Peel and chop the sweet potatoes up to 3 days in advance and store wrapped in paper towels in a plastic bag in the refrigerator until ready to use.

Serving Suggestion
Serve with BBQ Pulled Pork (page 206).

Storage
Store in a sealed glass container in the refrigerator for up to 3 days. Do not freeze.

1. Peel the sweet potatoes and chop them into ¾-inch chunks.

2. Place the sweet potatoes in a large pot and add water to cover. Sprinkle 1 teaspoon of the salt into the pot. Bring to a boil and cook, covered with a lid, for 3 to 5 minutes, until the potatoes are fork-tender but still firm. Drain the water and place the potatoes in a large serving bowl. Let cool in the refrigerator for about 1 hour.

3. In a small bowl, whisk together the olive oil, vinegar, and remaining ½ teaspoon of salt to make a dressing. Add the dressing and the remaining ingredients to the bowl with the sweet potatoes and toss to coat evenly. Serve at room temperature or cold.

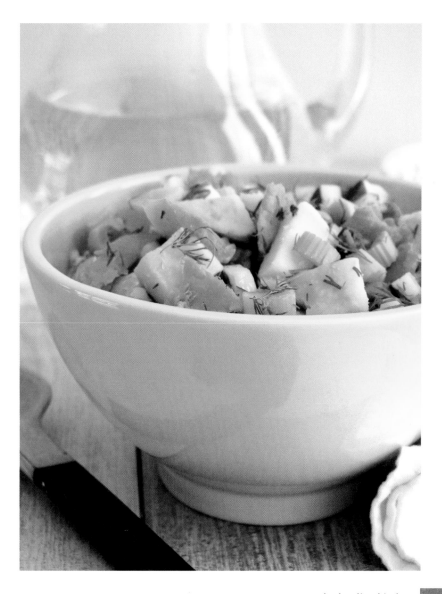

grain-free tabbouleh

Serves 4 | Prep Time: 15 minutes | Total Time: 15 minutes

1 head cauliflower (about 1½ pounds), cored and cut into florets, or 2 (12-ounce) bags cauliflower florets

3 cups finely chopped curly parsley (see Tip)

2 cups peeled and diced English cucumber

¾ cup sliced green onions, white and light green parts only

¼ cup chopped fresh mint leaves

3 tablespoons extra-virgin olive oil

2 tablespoons fresh lemon juice

½ teaspoon fine sea salt

1. Place the cauliflower florets in a food processor or high-powered blender and pulse until finely chopped to the size of rice grains (work in two batches if using a blender).

2. Toss together the riced cauliflower, parsley, cucumber, green onions, and mint in a large serving bowl.

3. In a small bowl, whisk together the olive oil, lemon juice, and salt to make a dressing. Toss the salad with the dressing until evenly incorporated.

Tip
Curly parsley is traditionally used in tabbouleh. Avoid using flat-leaf Italian parsley as a replacement.

Make Ahead
Chop the cauliflower up to 2 days in advance, wrap in paper towels, and store in a plastic bag in the refrigerator until ready to use.

Serving Suggestion
Serve with Classic Roast Chicken (page 224), Lebanese Beef & Rice Stuffing (page 246), and Smoky Artichoke Baba Ghanoush (page 275) for a traditional Middle Eastern meal.

Storage
Store in a sealed glass container in the refrigerator for up to 3 days.

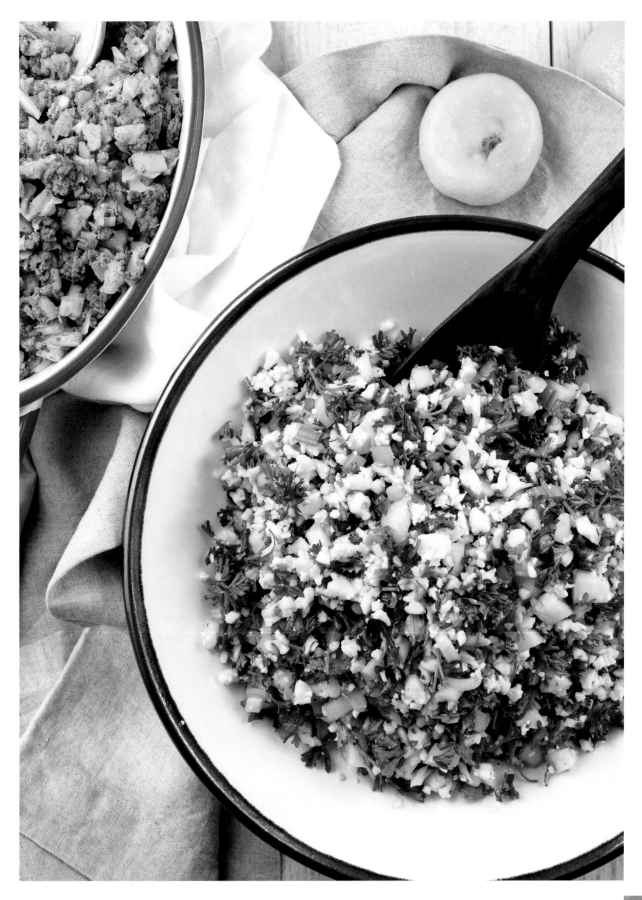

thai green mango salad

Serves 2 to 3 | Prep Time: 12 minutes | Total Time: 12 minutes

1 green mango, peeled and chopped into ½-inch pieces (see Tip)

2 avocados, peeled and diced

⅓ cup finely diced red onion

⅓ cup finely chopped fresh cilantro

1 tablespoon fresh lime juice

1 teaspoon honey

¾ teaspoon fish sauce

½ teaspoon ginger powder

¼ teaspoon fine sea salt

Tip

A green mango is an unripe mango that is medium green in color and firm to the touch. It is much tangier and less sweet than a ripe mango, which has a mostly orange and red skin and is soft to the touch. You may use ripe mango in this recipe, but it will result in a sweeter flavor that transforms this salad into a perfect accompaniment for grilled or baked fish or pork, such as the variation for baked salmon at right.

Make Ahead

Make the recipe as directed, but do not add the diced avocados until ready to serve. It will keep for up to 8 hours in the refrigerator without the avocados.

Storage

Store in a sealed glass container in the refrigerator for up to 1 day.

1. In a large bowl, toss together the mango, avocados, red onion, and cilantro.

2. In a small bowl, whisk together the remaining ingredients to make a dressing. Toss the salad with the dressing until evenly coated. Serve immediately.

Baked Salmon with Mango Salsa. Remove the pin bones from a 1-pound wild-caught salmon fillet (see Tip, page 230, or ask your fishmonger to remove them for you). Marinate the fillet in 1 tablespoon of olive oil, 1 tablespoon of balsamic vinegar, and ¼ teaspoon of fine sea salt or truffle salt for 4 to 6 hours. Bake in a 400-degree oven for 8 to 12 minutes, depending on the thickness of the salmon, until the center is a light translucent pink and the rest of the salmon is cooked through. Meanwhile, prepare the recipe as directed above, but use a ripe mango instead of a green one and cut it into ¼-inch dice to make a salsa. Serve the salmon topped with the mango salsa, with a side of Toasted Lime Cilantro Cauli-Rice (page 188), for a tropical-inspired meal.

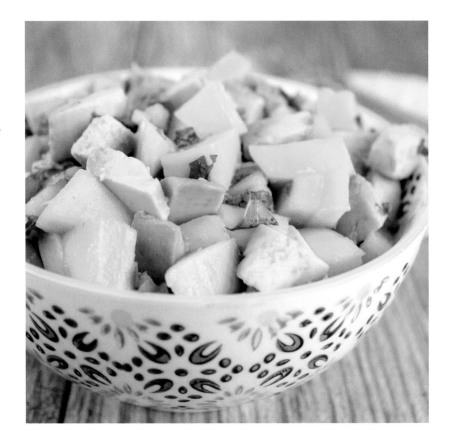

tropical broccoli salad

Serves 4 | Prep Time: 12 minutes | Total Time: 12 minutes + 1 hour to chill

1 medium head broccoli (about 1½ pounds), chopped into florets, or 1 (12-ounce) bag broccoli florets

1 cup diced pineapple

½ cup raisins

½ cup Avocado Mayo (page 113)

1½ teaspoons apple cider vinegar

½ teaspoon onion powder

¼ teaspoon garlic powder

¼ teaspoon fine sea salt

1. Working in two batches, pulse the broccoli florets in a food processor or in a blender using a tamper until very finely chopped.

2. Combine the chopped broccoli, pineapple, and raisins in a large serving bowl.

3. To make the dressing, stir together the mayo, vinegar, onion powder, garlic powder, and salt in a small bowl. Toss with the broccoli mixture until well combined.

4. Refrigerate for at least 1 hour before serving.

Make Ahead

Chop the broccoli up to 2 days in advance and store in a plastic bag in the refrigerator until ready to use.

Storage

Store in a sealed glass container in the refrigerator for up to 2 days.

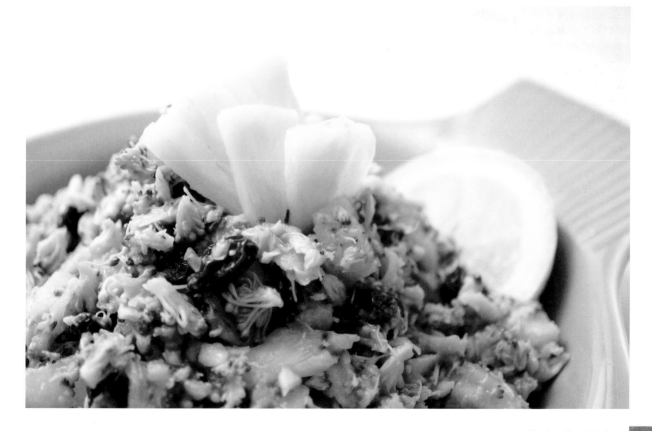

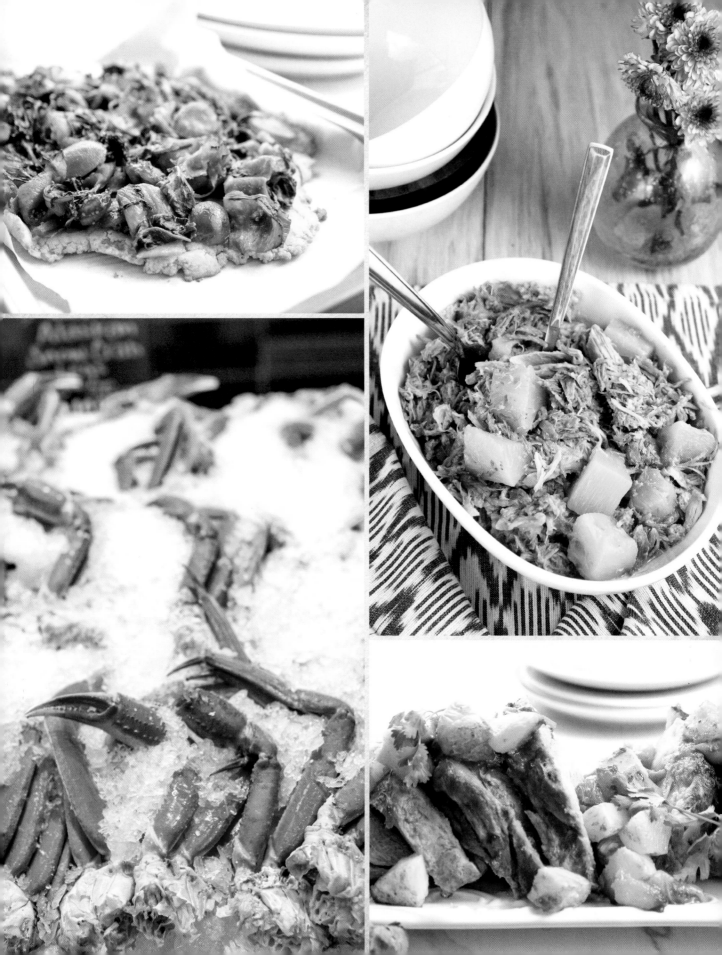

CHAPTER 8

easy-peasy mains

beef pot pie

Serves 4 to 5 | Prep Time: 15 minutes | Cook Time: 50 minutes | Total Time: 1 hour 5 minutes

4 carrots, peeled and chopped into ½-inch pieces

1 green plantain, peeled and chopped into ½-inch pieces

1 cup Beef or Chicken Broth (pages 108–109)

1½ cups Country Herb Gravy (page 134)

1 pound ground beef

½ teaspoon garlic powder

¼ teaspoon sea salt

CRUST

2 green plantains, peeled and chopped

3 tablespoons olive oil

2 tablespoons warm water

1 tablespoon coconut flour

1 tablespoon arrowroot starch

1 teaspoon apple cider vinegar

½ teaspoon baking soda

¼ teaspoon fine sea salt

Store & Reheat

Once cool, cover the pie dish and store in the refrigerator for up to 3 days or in the freezer for up to 3 months. Reheat covered with foil in a 300-degree oven or in the microwave in 30-second increments until warm.

Change It Up

Omit the crust and bake covered with a lid for 15 to 20 minutes, then uncover and broil for a few minutes until the top is browned.

1. Preheat the oven to 375 degrees.

2. To make the filling: Combine the carrots, plantain, and broth in a large saucepan and bring to a boil over medium heat. Cover with a lid and cook until the vegetables are tender and easily pierced with a fork, about 8 minutes. Drain the liquid from the pan and stir in the gravy until well combined. Set aside.

3. Cook the ground beef in a skillet over medium heat until cooked through, stirring to break it up into crumbles as it cooks. Season with the garlic powder and salt, then stir into the vegetable-gravy mixture in the saucepan. Pour the filling into a 9-inch glass pie dish in an even layer.

4. To make the crust: Puree all the ingredients together in a blender on high speed until very smooth. You may add an additional tablespoon of water to keep the mixture going, if needed. Using a spatula, spread the dough evenly on top of the filling.

5. Bake for 30 to 35 minutes, until the crust is firm to the touch and cooked through. Let cool for several minutes before serving.

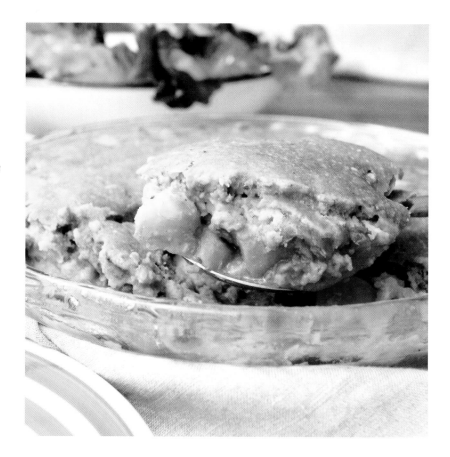

west coast burritos
with cucumber pico de gallo

Serves 4 | Prep Time: 15 minutes | Total Time: 15 minutes

2 cups Beef or Pork Carnitas (page 186)

4 large leaves iceberg lettuce

1 avocado, sliced

CUCUMBER PICO DE GALLO

¾ cup peeled, diced, and seeded cucumber

⅔ cup diced radish

¼ cup chopped fresh cilantro leaves

2 cloves garlic, pressed

2 teaspoons fresh lime juice

1 teaspoon grated lime zest

¼ teaspoon ginger powder

¼ teaspoon fine sea salt

1. Drain the carnitas in a colander set over the sink and discard any liquid. Spoon ½ cup of the meat onto the center of each lettuce leaf. Top with the sliced avocado.

2. Prepare the pico de gallo by combining the remaining ingredients in a bowl. Let marinate on the counter for 10 minutes, then drain the liquid into the sink. Spoon ¼ cup of the pico de gallo onto each burrito.

3. Fold the short sides of each lettuce leaf into the center of the burrito, then roll tightly so that the seam side faces down. If desired, slice the burritos in half with a sharp serrated knife. Alternatively, you can serve the burritos open-faced, as shown in the photo.

Tip

The carnitas can be warmed or remain cold for this recipe. Excess moisture will be less of an issue if the meat remains cold.

Make Ahead

The pico de gallo can be made up to 1 day in advance. Be sure to drain the liquid prior to serving. Do not assemble the burritos until ready to serve or they will become soggy.

Change It Up

Rather than making burritos, thinly slice 6 cups of iceberg lettuce and divide among 4 bowls. Top each bowl with the beef, avocado, and pico de gallo for a Mexican-inspired salad. Serve with sliced limes for dressing.

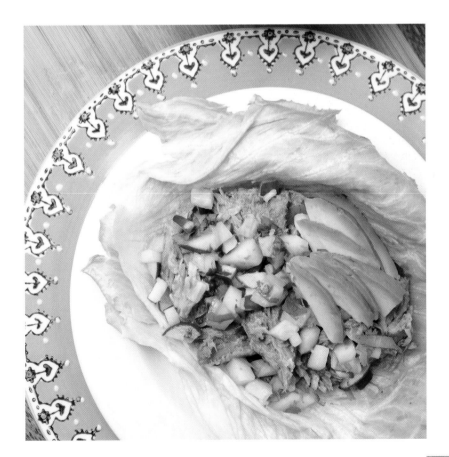

brisket & gravy

Serves 4 to 5 | Prep Time: 8 minutes | Cook Time: 3 hours 10 minutes | Total Time: 3 hours 18 minutes

2 pounds beef brisket (thin fat cap on)

2 tablespoons coconut sugar

1 tablespoon garlic powder

1 teaspoon onion powder

1 teaspoon smoked sea salt, coarsely ground

½ teaspoon dried rubbed sage

¼ teaspoon ground cinnamon

Fine sea salt

1 tablespoon cold water

1 teaspoon arrowroot starch

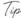

Tip

Feeding a larger crowd? Increase the dry rub proportionally and increase the initial baking time by 1 hour for every additional pound of meat. For example, for a 4-pound brisket, double the dry rub ingredients and bake covered for 4 hours instead of 2 hours. Then bake uncovered for 1 hour, as called for in Step 6.

Make Ahead

Season the brisket with the dry rub up to 24 hours in advance and store wrapped tightly in foil in the refrigerator.

Serving Suggestions

Serve with Silky Potato Puree (page 258), Toasted Coconut, Fig & Kale Salad (page 172), or Smoked Salmon Potato Salad (page 175).

Store & Reheat

Once cool, store the gravy in a sealed glass container in the refrigerator for up to 4 days. Store the cooled brisket tightly wrapped in foil in the refrigerator for up to 4 days to make for easy reheating. To reheat, pour several tablespoons of beef broth or gravy over the brisket and rewrap tightly. Reheat in a 250-degree oven for 20 to 30 minutes, until warm in the center.

1. Preheat the oven to 250 degrees.

2. Place the brisket in a large glass baking dish.

3. Make a dry rub by whisking together the coconut sugar, garlic and onion powders, smoked sea salt, sage, and cinnamon in a small bowl. Take a couple minutes to rub the blend into all sides of the brisket to ensure that it adheres to the meat well.

4. Cover the dish tightly with foil or with a lid if your baking dish has one.

5. Bake for 2 hours, until tender enough to easily slice. The brisket should be sitting in a pool of brown liquid, which you want for the gravy.

6. Remove the foil or lid and continue baking for an additional hour to brown the top.

7. Remove the brisket to a large cutting board and tent with foil for at least 10 minutes to allow the juices to be reabsorbed. Slice the meat against the grain into ½-inch-thick slices to serve. Season with salt to taste.

8. Make the gravy by transferring all the liquid from the baking dish to a small saucepan. You should have at least 1 cup of flavorful liquid. Bring the liquid to a low boil over medium heat. Simmer for 10 minutes until the liquid is reduced by half.

9. Meanwhile, whisk together the water and arrowroot starch to make a paste. Remove the saucepan from the heat and quickly whisk in the arrowroot paste to thicken the gravy.

10. Pour the gravy over the sliced brisket or serve on the side to make it easier to store separately.

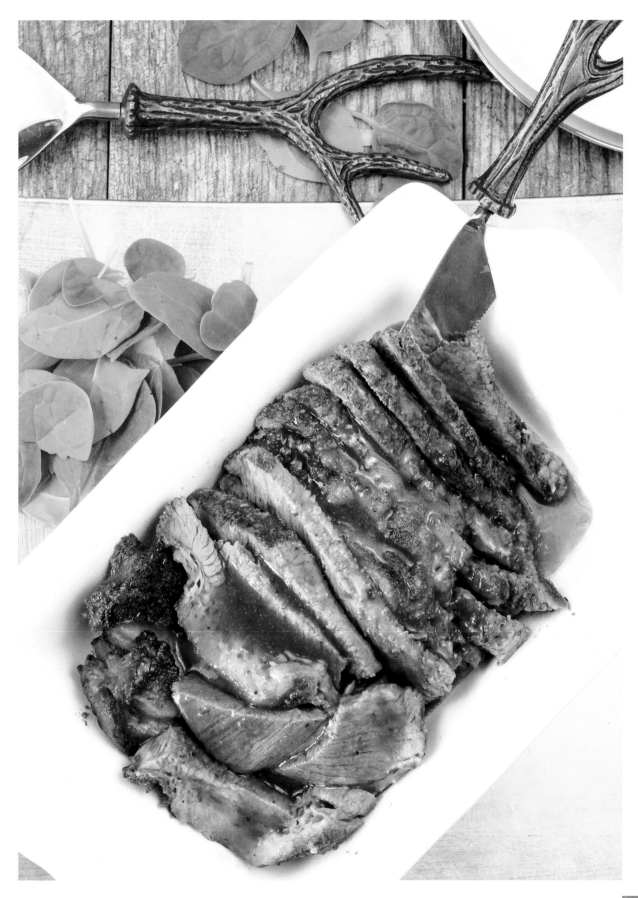

beef or pork carnitas 🍲

Serves 6 to 8 | Prep Time: 5 minutes | Cook Time: 1 hour 40 minutes to 9 hours, depending on cooking method | Total Time: 1 hour 45 minutes to 9 hours 5 minutes, depending on cooking method

½ cup Beef or Pork Broth (pages 108–109)

2 bay leaves

3 pounds boneless beef chuck roast or boneless pork shoulder such as Boston butt or picnic roast, trimmed of excess fat

¼ cup fresh lime juice

1 tablespoon dried thyme leaves

2 teaspoons fine sea salt

1 teaspoon onion powder

6 cloves garlic, minced

1 teaspoon House Rub (page 122)

Serving Suggestion
Serve in a bowl with sliced jicama, carrot ribbons, chopped cabbage, sliced green onions, and lime wedges.

Store & Reheat
Once cool, store in a sealed glass container or lidded cooker insert in the refrigerator for up to 4 days or in the freezer for up to 3 months. Reheat in a saucepan over medium heat until warm.

Slow cooker instructions

1. Put the broth and bay leaves in the slow cooker insert and lay the meat on top.

2. Pour the lime juice over the meat and rub the meat with the thyme, salt, onion powder, and garlic on all sides.

3. Cook on high for 1 hour, then on low for 7 to 8 hours, until the meat is tender enough to be shredded easily. Shred the meat well with two forks by pulling the forks in opposite directions to pull the meat apart.

4. Sprinkle the shredded meat with the House Rub and keep it in the cooking juices to maintain the moisture.

Pressure cooker instructions (see Tip, page 108)

1. Put the broth and bay leaves in the pressure cooker insert and lay the meat on top.

2. Pour the lime juice over the meat and rub the meat with the thyme, salt, onion powder, and garlic on all sides.

3. Seal the lid and set the pressure cooker's manual timer to 100 minutes.

4. When the timer goes off, release the pressure and remove the meat to a large serving dish. If the meat does not shred easily with two forks, use a knife to cut the roast into large chunks and return them to the pressure cooker for an additional 15 minutes of cooking. Shred the meat well with two forks by pulling the forks in opposite directions to pull the meat apart.

5. Sprinkle the shredded meat with the House Rub and keep it in the cooking juices to maintain the moisture.

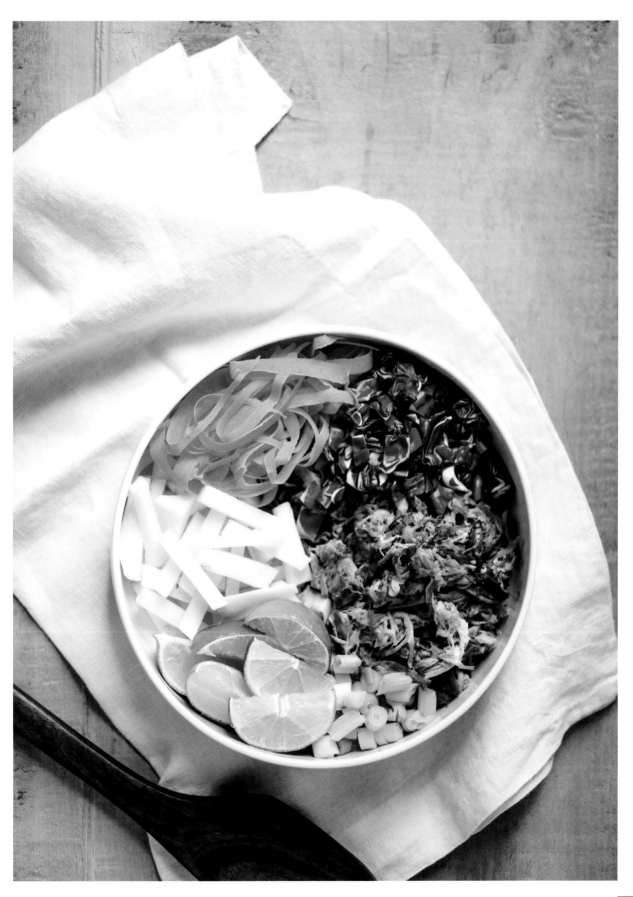

taco night

Serves 3 to 4 | Prep Time: 20 minutes | Cook Time: 20 minutes | Total Time: 40 minutes

TOASTED LIME CILANTRO CAULI-RICE

1 head cauliflower (about 1½ pounds), cored and cut into florets, or 2 (12-ounce) bags cauliflower florets

2 teaspoons fat of choice

⅔ cup Chicken Broth (page 108) or water, divided

1 tablespoon plus 1 teaspoon fresh lime juice

1 teaspoon grated lime zest

¼ teaspoon fine sea salt

2 tablespoons finely chopped fresh cilantro

TACO BEEF

1 pound ground beef

½ cup Chicken or Beef Broth (pages 108–109)

1 teaspoon dried oregano leaves

½ teaspoon garlic powder

½ teaspoon onion power

½ teaspoon dried thyme leaves

½ teaspoon ginger powder

½ teaspoon fish sauce

¼ teaspoon turmeric powder

⅛ teaspoon ground cinnamon

½ teaspoon fine sea salt

EASY GUACAMOLE

1 large ripe avocado

2 teaspoons fresh lime or lemon juice

¼ teaspoon garlic powder

¼ teaspoon fine sea salt

8 to 10 large lettuce leaves, such romaine, Bibb, or iceberg, for serving

1. To make the cauli-rice: Place the cauliflower florets in a food processor or high-powered blender and pulse until finely chopped to the size of rice grains (work in two batches if using a blender). Heat the fat in a large skillet over medium-high heat. Add the cauliflower, flatten down firmly with a spatula, and allow it to toast in the pan for 3 minutes. Stir in ⅓ cup of the broth, lime juice, zest, and salt and cook for 4 to 5 minutes, until the liquid has been absorbed. Add the remaining ⅓ cup of broth and the cilantro and continue cooking for 2 to 3 more minutes, until absorbed again. Transfer to a serving dish and keep warm.

2. To make the seasoned taco beef: Brown the ground beef in the same skillet over medium-high heat, breaking it up into very small pieces with a wooden spoon as it cooks. Pour in the broth and bring to a boil. Stir in the remaining taco beef ingredients and cook, stirring continuously, until the majority of the liquid has evaporated. Remove from the heat and keep warm.

3. To make the guacamole: Using a potato masher or fork, mash all the guacamole ingredients together in a bowl to the desired smoothness or chunkiness.

4. To serve: Divide the cauli-rice, taco beef, and guacamole among large lettuce leaves, or make taco salads over shredded lettuce.

Store & Reheat

Once cool, store the components separately in sealed glass containers in the refrigerator for up to 3 days. Reheat the taco beef and cauli-rice in a skillet over medium-low heat, or serve cold.

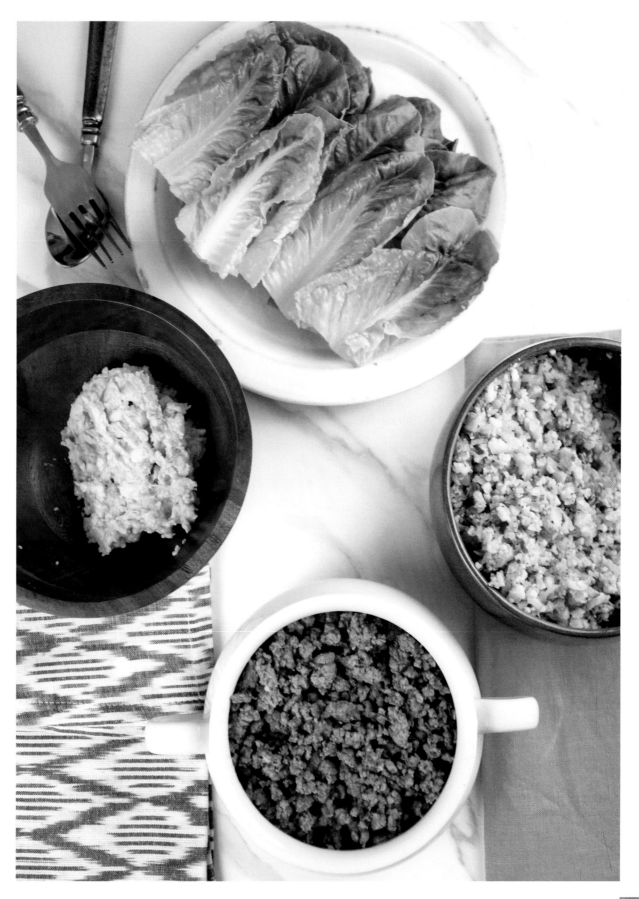

grilled steak cucumber noodle bowl

Serves 4 | Prep Time: 10 minutes | Cook Time: 8 minutes | Total Time: 18 minutes

1½ pounds skirt steak

2 large English cucumbers

1 teaspoon fine sea salt, divided

2 tablespoons extra-virgin olive oil

2 teaspoons grated fresh ginger

1 tablespoon coconut aminos

1 tablespoon fresh lime juice

½ cup sliced fresh mint

Make Ahead

Make the steak up to 2 days in advance and serve it warm or cold over the cucumber noodles. Do not prepare the cucumber noodles until you are ready to serve the meal.

1. Remove the steak from the refrigerator 30 minutes prior to cooking. Preheat the grill to medium-high heat or place an oven rack in the top position and turn your oven's broiler setting to high.

2. Spiral-slice or julienne the cucumbers into long, thin noodles. Toss with ½ teaspoon of the salt and let sweat in a colander set over the sink for 10 minutes as the steak cooks and rests. Squeeze the noodles gently with a paper towel or tea towel to absorb any excess moisture.

3. Rub the steak with the olive oil and the remaining ½ teaspoon of salt. Grill for 3 to 4 minutes per side or broil for 2 to 3 minutes per side. Let rest for 5 minutes before slicing thinly against the grain.

4. In a bowl, toss the cucumber noodles with the ginger, coconut aminos, lime juice, and mint. Top with the steak and serve immediately.

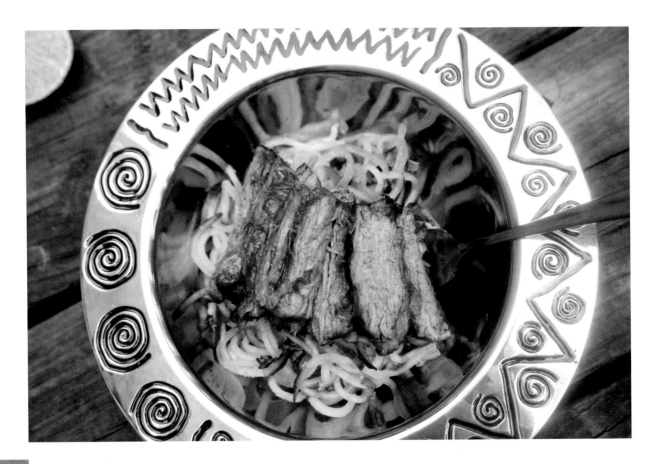

caramelized onion & herb meatloaf

Serves 6 | Prep Time: 5 minutes | Cook Time: 50 minutes | Total Time: 55 minutes

1 pound ground beef

1 pound ground pork

1 tablespoon dried thyme leaves

1½ teaspoons dried rubbed sage

1¼ teaspoons fine sea salt, divided

1 recipe Caramelized Onions (page 107), divided

2 tablespoons water

Store & Reheat

Once cool, store in a sealed glass container in the refrigerator for up to 3 days. To freeze, slice and place between layers of parchment paper in a freezer-safe bag or container for up to 3 months. Reheat wrapped tightly in foil in a 300-degree oven until warm in the center.

1. Preheat the oven to 375 degrees. Grease a 9 by 5-inch loaf pan with your choice of fat.

2. In a large mixing bowl, use your hands to combine the beef, pork, thyme, sage, and 1 teaspoon of the salt.

3. Finely chop ¾ cup of the caramelized onions and mix into the meatloaf mixture. Transfer the mixture to the prepared loaf pan. Bake for 40 to 45 minutes, until the meatloaf has pulled away from the sides of the pan and the internal temperature has reached 150 degrees. Be sure not to overcook, or the meatloaf will dry out.

4. Meanwhile, place the remaining caramelized onions, remaining ¼ teaspoon of salt, and water in a blender and pulse until a chunky puree forms. Top the cooked meatloaf with the onion puree and broil on high for 5 minutes until the onions are a deep golden brown. Let rest for 10 minutes to let the juices reabsorb before slicing.

Serving Suggestions

Serve with Silky Potato Puree (page 258) or Carrot Pilaf with Lemon & Parsley (page 242).

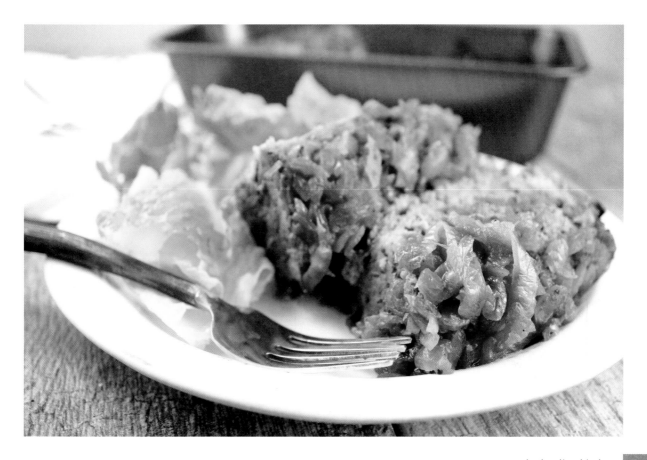

sweet & savory shepherd's pie

Serves 4 to 5 | Prep Time: 12 minutes | Cook Time: 48 minutes | Total Time: 1 hour

MASHED SWEET POTATO TOPPING

1½ pounds orange sweet potatoes, peeled and chopped

2 tablespoons coconut oil

½ teaspoon dried rubbed sage

½ teaspoon fine sea salt

¼ teaspoon ground cinnamon

FILLING

5 slices bacon, chopped

1 large yellow onion, halved and thinly sliced

1 tablespoon minced fresh sage or 1 teaspoon dried rubbed sage

2 pounds ground beef or lamb

½ teaspoon garlic powder

½ teaspoon ground cinnamon

1 tablespoon Worcestershire Sauce (page 106) or 1½ teaspoons blackstrap molasses

1. Place an oven rack in the center of the oven and preheat the broiler to high.

2. To make the topping: Place the sweet potatoes in a medium saucepan and add enough water to cover. Cover with the lid, bring to a boil, and cook for 10 minutes, until the potatoes are fork-tender. Drain well and return the potatoes to the pan. Add the coconut oil and mash well with a potato masher until smooth. Stir in the dried sage, salt, and cinnamon.

3. Meanwhile, make the filling: Cook the bacon in a large skillet over medium heat until the fat has rendered and the bacon is crispy. Stir in the sliced onion and fresh sage and cook for 10 to 12 minutes, until the onion has softened and caramelized. Drain any liquid from the pan and transfer the bacon-onion mixture to a deep 8-inch glass casserole dish.

4. In the same skillet, cook the ground beef with the garlic powder and cinnamon until the meat is light pink in the center, breaking it up into small pieces as it cooks. Transfer to the casserole dish and add the Worcestershire Sauce. Mix the filling ingredients together until well combined.

5. Spoon the mashed sweet potatoes on top and smooth with your hands or the back of a spoon to completely cover the top.

6. Broil for 10 to 15 minutes, until the top begins to brown and the meat mixture is bubbling. Let cool for 5 minutes before serving.

Make Ahead
Prepare the mashed sweet potatoes up to 3 days in advance. You may also assemble the pie as directed, cover with a lid, and place in the refrigerator for up to 2 days prior to broiling. Bring to room temperature before placing in the oven.

Serving Suggestion
Serve with a simple spinach side salad dressed with Honey Balsamic Dressing (page 110).

Store & Reheat
Once cool, cover the casserole dish and store in the refrigerator for up to 3 days or in the freezer for up to 3 months. Reheat covered with foil in a 300-degree oven or in the microwave in 30-second increments until warm.

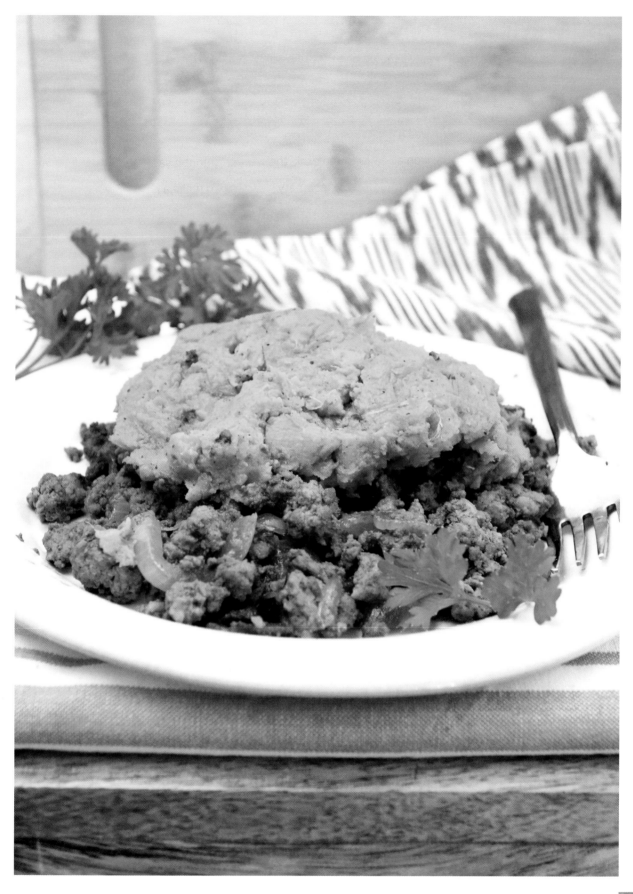

anti-inflammatory meatballs

Makes 12 meatballs, serves 2 to 3 | Prep Time: 10 minutes | Cook Time: 18 minutes | Total Time: 28 minutes

1 pound lean ground beef

¼ cup chopped fresh cilantro leaves

3 cloves garlic, minced

1 teaspoon grated lime zest

1 teaspoon grated fresh ginger or ½ teaspoon ginger powder

½ teaspoon fine sea salt, plus more for serving

¼ teaspoon turmeric powder

Tip

You can batch cook these meatballs by doubling the ingredients, baking the meatballs on two sheets, and freezing one sheet's worth for a future meal.

1. Preheat the oven to 350 degrees. Line a rimmed baking sheet with parchment paper.

2. Mix all the ingredients together in a medium bowl. Form into 12 meatballs, about 1⅓ ounces (1½ tablespoons) each, and place on the prepared baking sheet, leaving space between the meatballs. Bake for 16 to 18 minutes, until light pink in the center. Sprinkle with more salt before serving, if desired.

Serving Suggestion
Serve on top of Spaghetti Squash Noodles (page 238) with Pronto Pesto (page 116) for a full meal.

Store & Reheat
Once cool, store in a sealed glass container in the refrigerator for up to 3 days. To freeze, place the baking sheet in the freezer until the meatballs are frozen, then transfer the meatballs to a freezer-safe container and freeze for up to 3 months. Reheat in a saucepan over medium heat until warm.

mediterranean lamb meatballs

Makes 20 meatballs, serves 6 | Prep Time: 7 minutes | Cook Time: 18 minutes | Total Time: 25 minutes

2 pounds ground lamb

½ cup Smoky Artichoke Baba Ghanoush (page 275)

½ cup chopped black olives, drained if canned

2 tablespoons dried oregano leaves

2 teaspoons grated lemon zest

Make Ahead

Make the meat mixture up to 1 day in advance and store it in the refrigerator until ready to cook.

1. Preheat the oven to 375 degrees. Line two rimmed baking sheets with parchment paper.

2. Mix all the ingredients together in a large bowl. Form into 20 meatballs, about 1½ ounces (2 tablespoons) each, and place on the prepared baking sheets, leaving space between the meatballs. Bake for 18 minutes or until light pink in the center, rotating the pans halfway through cooking.

Serving Suggestions
Serve with Garlic-Dill Parsnip Fries (page 252) or as "sliders" drizzled with Tzatziki Sauce (page 115) or additional Smoky Artichoke Baba Ghanoush on top of peeled and thickly sliced cucumber.

Store & Reheat
Once cool, store in a sealed glass container in the refrigerator for up to 3 days. To freeze, place the baking sheet in the freezer until the meatballs are frozen, then transfer the meatballs to a freezer-safe container and freeze for up to 3 months. Reheat in a saucepan over medium heat until warm.

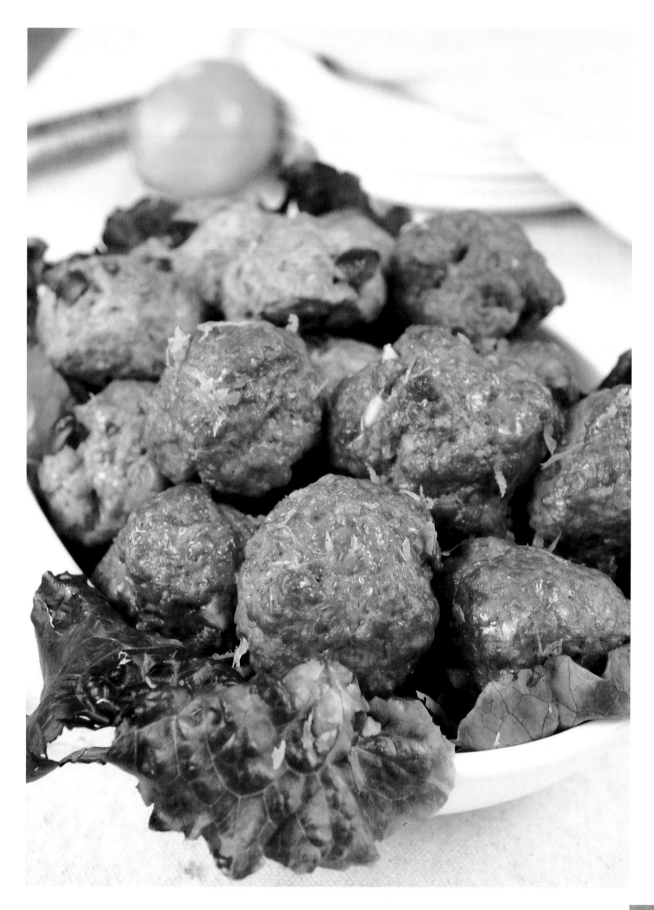

meat sauce & spaghetti 🍲

Serves 6 | Prep Time: 17 minutes | Cook Time: 43 minutes | Total Time: 1 hour

2 tablespoons extra-virgin olive oil

1½ cups chopped yellow onions

1½ cups chopped celery

8 cloves garlic, sliced

4 cups Beef Broth (page 109)

1⅓ cups butternut squash puree (see Tip)

2 pounds ground beef

2 teaspoons dried oregano leaves

2 teaspoons dried thyme leaves

1½ teaspoons sea salt

1 teaspoon dried marjoram leaves

½ teaspoon dried rubbed sage

⅔ cup sliced fresh basil

3 zucchini, par-boiled and julienned or spiral-sliced, or 1 recipe Spaghetti Squash Noodles (page 238), for serving

1. Heat the olive oil in a large pot or saucepan over medium heat. Add the onions, celery, and garlic and sauté for a few minutes until softened and fragrant.

2. Add the broth and bring to a boil. Simmer uncovered for 8 to 10 minutes, until the vegetables are very tender.

3. Transfer the entire contents of the pot to a blender with the butternut squash and puree until smooth. Set aside.

4. Cook the ground beef in the same pot over medium heat until browned and cooked through. Stir in the dried herbs and seasonings, then add the vegetable puree back to the pot. Simmer for 15 to 20 minutes, until the sauce has reduced to the desired consistency. Remove from the heat and stir in the basil until wilted.

5. Serve with the zucchini noodles.

Tip
Buy canned butternut squash puree for quick preparation. You can also buy it frozen; look for winter squash puree in the frozen foods aisle.

Make Ahead
Chop the onions, celery, and garlic up to 5 days in advance and store in a sealed plastic bag in the refrigerator until ready to use.

Store & Reheat
Once cool, store in a sealed glass container in the refrigerator for up to 4 days or in the freezer for up to 3 months. Reheat in a saucepan over medium-low heat until warm.

Change It Up
Use canned or homemade sweet potato puree in place of the butternut squash. Replace the dried herbs with 2 tablespoons of Herbes de Provence, but ensure that the store-bought blend does not contain any seeds.

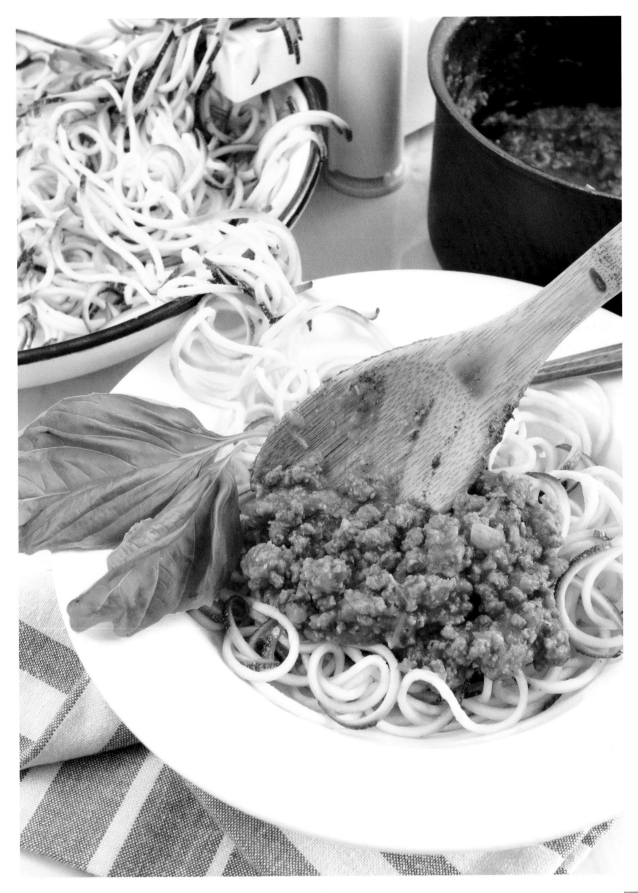

beef & mushroom risotto

Serves 3 | Prep Time: 20 minutes | Cook Time: 20 minutes | Total Time: 40 minutes

1 pound London broil, about 2 inches thick

1 tablespoon plus 2 teaspoons balsamic vinegar, divided

½ teaspoon garlic powder

1¼ teaspoons fine sea salt, divided

2 pounds sliced mushrooms

1 pound green plantains (about 2 medium), peeled and chopped

1½ cups Beef or Chicken Broth (pages 108–109)

3 cloves garlic

1 teaspoon dried oregano leaves

2 tablespoons extra-virgin olive oil

1 teaspoon nutritional yeast

1 teaspoon fish sauce

Make Ahead

The risotto can be made up to 2 days in advance and rewarmed in a saucepan over medium heat, thinned with additional broth, if needed, while you broil the beef.

Store & Reheat

Once cool, store the meat and risotto in separate sealed glass containers in the refrigerator for up to 3 days. Reheat the meat under a low broil for a few minutes just until warm while you heat the risotto as described under "Make Ahead" above.

1. Remove the London broil from refrigerator 20 minutes prior to cooking. Place an oven rack in the second-highest position and preheat the broiler to high.

2. Place the meat in a glass baking dish and rub the meat on all sides with 1 tablespoon of the vinegar, the garlic powder, and ½ teaspoon of the salt.

3. Broil for 6 minutes per side. Let rest for 5 minutes, then thinly slice against the grain. The meat should be tender, juicy, and medium-done. Sprinkle with ¼ teaspoon of the salt and allow the salt to melt into the meat.

4. Meanwhile, pulse the sliced mushrooms in a blender or food processor in two batches until very finely chopped to the size of rice grains. Set aside in a bowl.

5. Place the plantains, broth, garlic, oregano, and remaining ½ teaspoon of salt in the blender or food processor and puree until smooth.

6. Heat the olive oil in a large saucepan over medium-high heat. Add the mushrooms and stir to coat in the oil. Stir in ½ cup of the plantain puree and simmer for 1 minute until the mushrooms absorb the liquid. Repeat 2 or 3 more times until the risotto is the texture of stovetop oatmeal, stirring often to prevent sticking. You may have leftover puree, which you can use to thin the risotto, if desired.

7. Cover the saucepan with a lid and reduce the heat to medium. Cook for 5 more minutes until the risotto has the soft texture of traditional risotto.

8. Remove from the heat and stir in the remaining 2 teaspoons of vinegar, nutritional yeast, and fish sauce. Serve ladled into bowls with thinly sliced London broil on top.

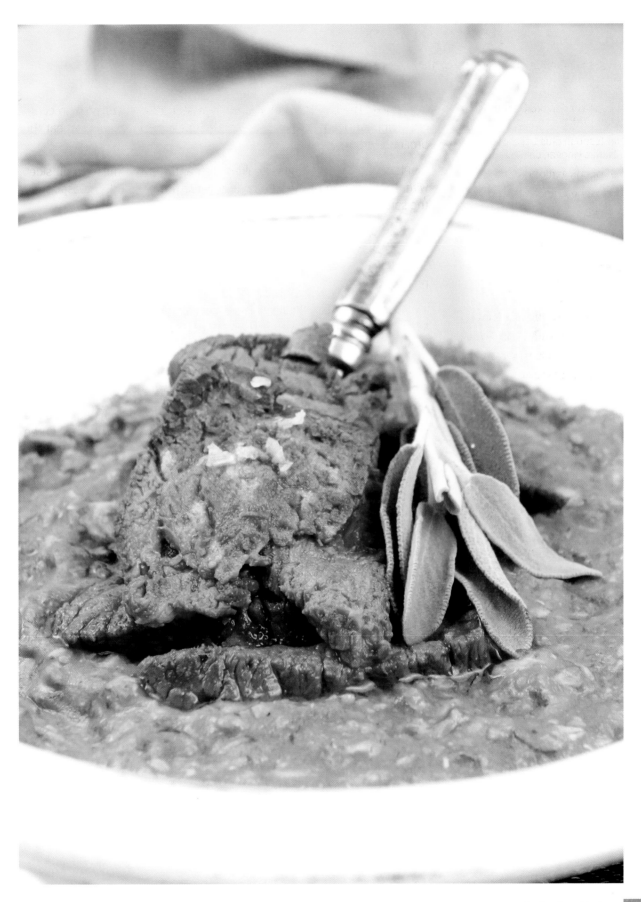

classic american hamburgers

Serves 4 to 6 | Prep Time: 5 minutes | Cook Time: 10 minutes | Total Time: 15 minutes

2 pounds ground beef

2 tablespoons fresh thyme leaves, chopped

1 tablespoon Worcestershire Sauce (page 106)

1 teaspoon fine sea salt

SUGGESTED TOPPINGS

Caramelized Onions (page 107)

Lettuce

Sliced red onion

Sliced avocado

1. Preheat the grill to medium-high and brush the grates with olive oil.

2. Mix all the ingredients together in a bowl. Form the mixture into 6 to 8 equal-size patties and, using your finger, make a small indentation on top of each patty to allow the meat to rise as it cooks.

3. Grill for 4 to 5 minutes per side, until the internal temperature reaches 160 degrees for medium-done meat with a light pink center. Let rest for 5 minutes before serving on top of salad or wrapped in lettuce leaves, with the toppings of your choice.

greek lamb burgers

Serves 4 to 6 | Prep Time: 5 minutes | Cook Time: 10 minutes | Total Time: 15 minutes

2 pounds ground lamb

2 tablespoons finely chopped Kalamata olives

2 teaspoons dried dill weed

1 teaspoon fine sea salt

½ teaspoon garlic powder

½ teaspoon onion powder

SUGGESTED TOPPINGS

Tzatziki Sauce (page 115)

Orange & Olive Tapenade (page 276)

Smoky Artichoke Baba Ghanoush (page 275)

Lettuce

Sliced red onion

1. Preheat the grill to medium-high and brush the grates with olive oil.

2. Mix all the ingredients together in a bowl. Form the mixture into 6 to 8 equal-size patties.

3. Grill for 4 to 5 minutes per side, until the internal temperature reaches 160 degrees for medium-done meat with a light pink center. Let rest for a few minutes before serving on top of salad or wrapped in lettuce leaves, with the toppings of your choice.

bbq chicken burgers

Serves 4 to 6 | Prep Time: 5 minutes | Cook Time: 14 minutes | Total Time: 19 minutes

2 pounds ground chicken, preferably thighs

⅓ cup Tangy Carolina BBQ Sauce (page 118)

SUGGESTED TOPPINGS

Tangy Carolina BBQ Sauce (page 118)

Iceberg lettuce

Sliced red onion

Green onion

Crispy bacon

1. Preheat the grill to medium-high and brush the grates well with olive oil.

2. Mix all the ingredients together in a bowl. Form the mixture into 6 to 8 equal-size patties. They will be more moist than traditional burgers.

3. Grill for 6 to 7 minutes per side, until the internal temperature reaches 165 degrees and the juices run clear. Let rest for a few minutes before serving on top of salad or wrapped in lettuce leaves, with the toppings of your choice.

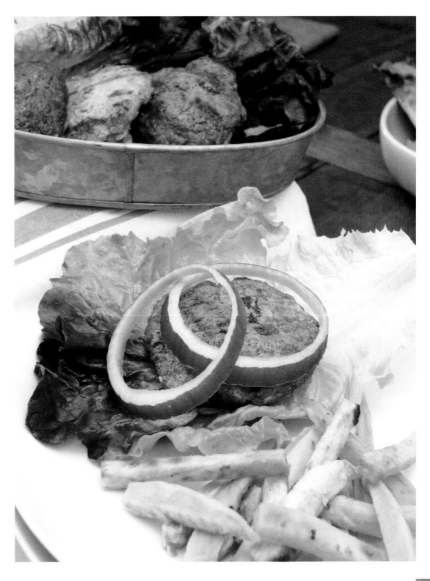

island roasted pork

Serves 8 | Prep Time: 10 minutes | Cook Time: 1 hour 12 minutes | Total Time: 1 hour 22 minutes + 10 minutes to rest

2 tablespoons extra-virgin olive oil, divided

1 teaspoon fine sea salt

4 pounds boneless pork shoulder such as Boston butt or picnic roast

¼ cup pineapple juice

2 tablespoons fresh lime juice

2 tablespoons grated fresh ginger, or 2 teaspoons ginger powder

1 teaspoon ground cinnamon

1 teaspoon garlic powder

3 cups pineapple chunks (about 1 inch), fresh or canned

1 large peach, chopped into ¾-inch pieces

1 large pear, chopped into ¾-inch pieces

¼ cup fresh cilantro leaves, chopped

1. Preheat the oven to 375 degrees.

2. In a large, deep, oven-safe skillet or cast-iron pan, heat 1 tablespoon of the olive oil over medium-high heat. Salt all sides of the pork roast. Sear the pork for 2 to 3 minutes per side, until browned.

3. While the pork is searing, whisk together the pineapple and lime juices, ginger, cinnamon, and garlic powder in a small bowl.

4. Position the chopped fruit around and on top of the roast in the skillet. Pour the juice mixture over the pork and fruit. Roast in the oven until the internal temperature reaches 155 degrees, about 1 hour.

5. Let rest for at least 10 minutes before slicing thickly and serving sprinkled with chopped cilantro.

Make Ahead
Up to 1 day in advance, chop the fruit, toss with 1 teaspoon of fresh lemon juice, and store in a sealed container in the refrigerator. Whisk together the juices, ginger, cinnamon, and garlic powder and store in a sealed container in the refrigerator.

Serving Suggestions
Serve with Toasted Lime Cilantro Cauli-Rice (page 188), Caribbean Plantain Rice (page 239), Garlic-Rubbed Tostones (page 248), or Garlic Roasted Broccoli (page 264).

Store & Reheat
Once cool, store in a sealed glass container in the refrigerator for up to 4 days or in the freezer for up to 3 months. If planning to freeze, do not add the cilantro until the pork is reheated and ready to serve. Reheat in a covered glass or ceramic dish in a 300-degree oven or in a large skillet over medium heat until warm in the center.

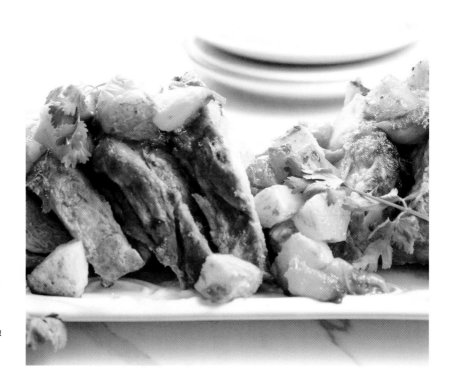

rosemary & prosciutto stromboli

Serves 2 | Prep Time: 10 minutes | Cook Time: 35 minutes | Total Time: 45 minutes

1 cup cooked and mashed white sweet potato (about 1 medium; see Tip)

½ cup tapioca starch

¼ teaspoon fine sea salt

1 teaspoon finely chopped fresh rosemary

4 slices prosciutto

1 tablespoon bacon fat or duck fat, divided

Sweet Marinara Sauce (page 114), for serving (optional)

Tip
Bake or steam a large white sweet potato until the potato can be easily pierced with a fork. It must be fully cooked to mash smoothly.

Serving Suggestions
Serve with Antipasto Salad (page 166), Caesar Salad (page 165), or Spinach with Alliums & Lemon (page 242).

Store & Reheat
Once cool, store in a sealed glass container in the refrigerator for up to 3 days. To reheat, place under a low broil until crispy on both sides.

1. Place an oven rack in the center of the oven and preheat the oven to 375 degrees. Line a rimmed baking sheet with parchment paper.

2. In a medium bowl, combine the mashed sweet potato with ¼ cup of the tapioca starch at a time to create a thick ball of dough. Season the dough with the salt.

3. Place the dough on the prepared baking sheet and use your hands to spread it into a rectangle about ¼ inch thick.

4. Sprinkle the rosemary evenly over the dough and lay the prosciutto slices in a single layer over the rosemary.

5. Starting at one of the short ends, roll the dough into a log shape with the seam side down.

6. Brush with 1½ teaspoons of the bacon fat and bake for 30 minutes. Remove the stromboli from the oven and brush with the remaining 1½ teaspoons of fat. Broil on high for 2 to 3 minutes and carefully flip over to broil the underside for an additional 1 to 2 minutes, until the outside is crispy.

7. Let cool for several minutes, then slice in half. Serve with marinara sauce on the side for dipping, if desired.

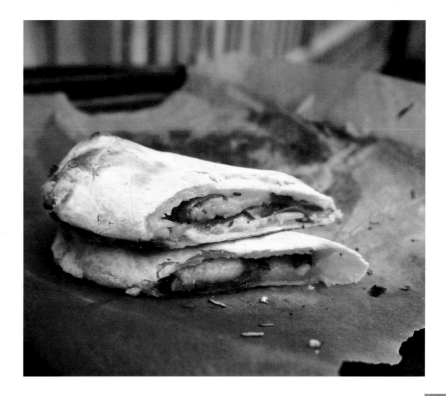

hawaiian pulled pork

Serves 6 to 8 | Prep Time: 10 minutes | Cook Time: 1½ to 9 hours, depending on cooking method | Total Time: 1 hour 40 minutes to 9 hours 10 minutes, depending on cooking method

3 pounds boneless pork shoulder such as Boston butt or picnic roast

1 (14-ounce) can pineapple chunks in juices

3 tablespoons apple cider vinegar

1 teaspoon fine sea salt

3 slices bacon

Serving Suggestions

Serve with Toasted Lime Cilantro Cauli-Rice (page 188) or make an island-inspired bowl by layering shredded romaine lettuce, Toasted Lime Cilantro Cauli-Rice (page 188), Hawaiian Pulled Pork, and Easy Guacamole (page 188) in a bowl.

Store & Reheat

Once cool, store in a sealed glass container in the refrigerator for up to 4 days or in the freezer for up to 3 months. Reheat in a saucepan or skillet over medium heat until warm.

Slow cooker instructions

1. Place the pork in the slow cooker insert and pour the pineapple and vinegar over the pork. Sprinkle the salt on the meat and top with the bacon slices.

2. Cook on high for 1 hour, then on low for 6 to 8 hours, until the pork is tender and can be easily shredded with two forks.

3. Shred the pork and bacon by pulling two forks in opposite directions to pull the meat apart. Shred the pineapple if desired, or leave it whole, as pictured.

4. Transfer the pulled pork to a serving dish and stir in at least ¾ cup of the cooking liquid.

Pressure cooker instructions (see Tip, page 108)

1. Place the pork in the pressure cooker insert and pour the pineapple and vinegar over the pork. Sprinkle the salt on the meat and top with the bacon slices.

2. Seal the lid and set the pressure cooker's manual timer for 90 minutes. When the timer goes off, release the pressure. If the meat does not shred easily with two forks, use a knife to cut the roast into large chunks and return them to the pressure cooker for an additional 15 minutes of cooking.

3. Shred the pork and bacon by pulling two forks in opposite directions to pull meat apart. Shred the pineapple, if desired, or leave it whole, as pictured.

4. Transfer the pulled pork to a serving dish and stir in at least ¾ cup of the cooking liquid.

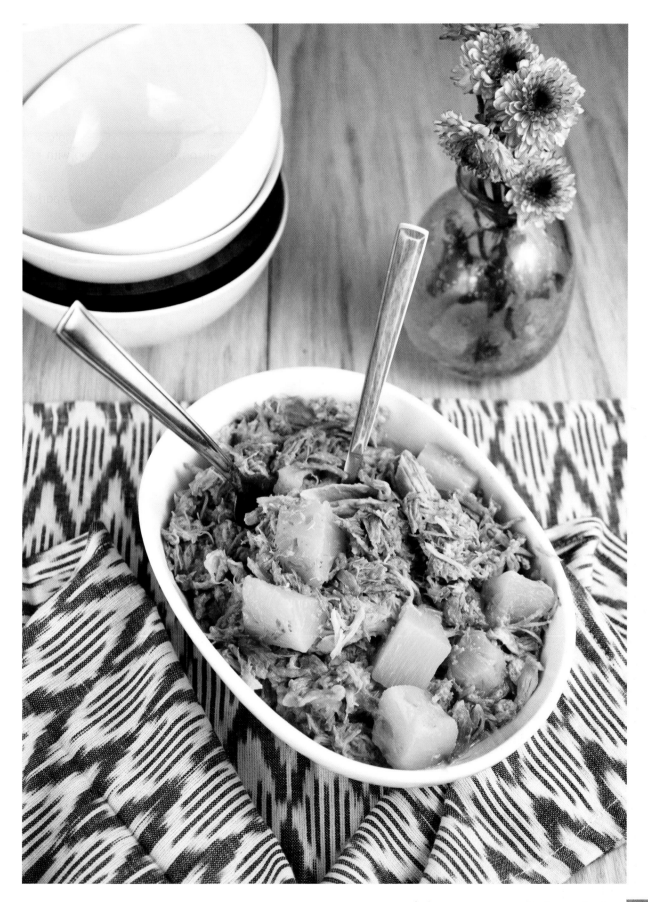

bbq pulled pork

Serves 8 to 10 | Prep Time: 10 minutes | Cook Time: 1 hour 40 minutes to 8 hours, depending on cooking method | Total Time: 1 hour 50 minutes to 8 hours 10 minutes, depending on cooking method

3 pounds boneless pork shoulder, such as Boston butt

4 cloves garlic, peeled

1 tablespoon coconut sugar or maple sugar

1 teaspoon ginger powder

1 teaspoon smoked fine sea salt or fine sea salt

½ teaspoon ground cinnamon

1 cup Bone Broth of choice (pages 108–109)

1 cup thinly sliced yellow onions

3 slices bacon

¾ cup Tangy Carolina BBQ Sauce (page 118)

Serving Suggestion
Use in Pulled Pork Sliders (page 271).

Store & Reheat
Once cool, cover the cooker insert with the lid and store in the refrigerator for up to 4 days or transfer to a freezer-safe glass container and freeze for up to 3 months. Reheat in a saucepan or skillet over medium heat until warm.

Slow cooker instructions

1. Slice 4 slits in the top of the meat and stuff a garlic clove in each slit. Rub the entire surface of the meat with the sugar, ginger, salt, and cinnamon. Put the broth and onions in the slow cooker insert, then lay the meat on top of the onions. Lay the bacon slices on top of the meat.

2. Cook on high for 1 hour, then on low for 6 to 7 hours, until the pork can be easily shredded with two forks.

3. Transfer the meat to a cutting board. Drain the liquid from the cooking pot, but reserve the onions. Shred the pork and bacon by pulling two forks in opposite directions to pull the meat apart. Transfer the meat back to the pot with the onions and stir in the BBQ sauce, tasting and adding more sauce or salt as desired.

Pressure cooker instructions (see Tip, page 108)

1. Slice 4 slits in the top of the meat and stuff a garlic clove in each slit. Rub the entire surface of the meat with the sugar, ginger, salt, and cinnamon. Put the broth and onions in the pressure cooker insert, then lay the meat on top of the onions. Lay the bacon slices on top of the meat.

2. Seal the lid and set the pressure cooker's manual timer for 90 minutes. When the timer goes off, release the pressure. If the meat does not shred easily with two forks, use a knife to cut the roast into large chunks and return them to the pressure cooker for an additional 15 minutes of cooking.

3. Transfer the meat to a cutting board. Drain the liquid from the cooking pot, but reserve the onions. Shred the pork and bacon by pulling two forks in opposite directions to pull the meat apart. Transfer the meat back to the pot with the onions and stir in the BBQ sauce, tasting and adding more sauce or salt as desired.

BBQ Pulled Pork Stromboli. Replace the filling in the Rosemary & Prosciutto Stromboli (page 203) with 1 cup of BBQ Pulled Pork and increase the broil time to 5 minutes per side until crispy.

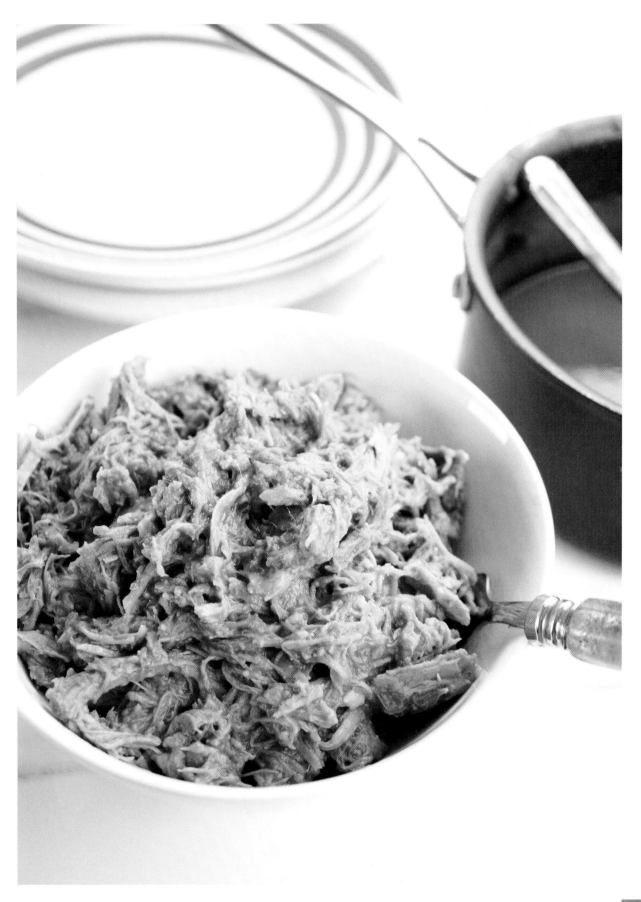

garlic & rosemary crusted pork loin

Serves 6 | Prep Time: 7 minutes | Cook Time: 58 minutes | Total Time: 1 hour 5 minutes + 15 minutes to rest

2½ pounds boneless pork loin roast, fat cap on

1 tablespoon extra-virgin olive oil

1½ teaspoons fine sea salt

1 tablespoon finely chopped fresh rosemary

1 tablespoon pressed garlic

Make Ahead

Prepare the pork through Step 3. Cover and place in the refrigerator overnight. Let sit at room temperature for 30 minutes before roasting.

Serving Suggestions

Serve with Spinach with Alliums & Lemon (page 242), Silky Potato Puree (page 258), or Carrot Pilaf with Lemon & Parsley (page 242), or serve leftover cold chopped pork loin in a large dinner salad with romaine lettuce, diced avocado, thinly sliced red onion, and Greek Dressing (page 110).

Store & Reheat

Slice the pork and let cool completely before transferring to a sealed glass container. Store in the refrigerator for up to 4 days or in the freezer for up to 3 months. Reheat covered in a glass dish or wrapped in foil in a 300-degree oven for 20 to 30 minutes, until warm in the center.

1. Remove the pork from the refrigerator 30 minutes prior to roasting. Preheat the oven to 450 degrees. Line a rimmed baking sheet with parchment paper and place a roasting rack on top.

2. Rub the olive oil on all sides of the pork, then repeat with the salt.

3. In a small bowl, mix together the rosemary and garlic to make a paste. Position the pork roast so that the fat cap is facing up. Rub the rosemary paste on just the top side of the roast. If you wish to cover all sides of the pork, triple the amount of rosemary and garlic, which will make for an extra-flavorful dish. Carefully place the roast on the roasting rack.

4. Roast for 15 to 18 minutes, until the top is lightly browned. Reduce the oven temperature to 325 degrees and continue roasting for about 40 minutes, until the internal temperature reaches 155 degrees.

5. Remove from the oven and let rest for 15 minutes prior to slicing crosswise into 1-inch-thick slices. To make homemade deli meat, use an electric knife to thinly slice the roast.

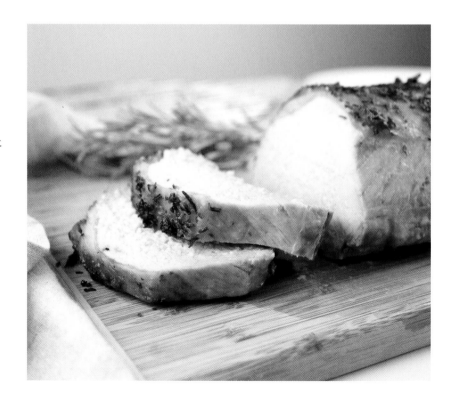

speedy shanghai stir-fry

Serves 3 to 4 | Prep Time: 8 minutes | Cook Time: 12 minutes | Total Time: 20 minutes

1 pound ground pork

¼ teaspoon fine sea salt

6 cups shredded green cabbage (about 1 pound)

1 tablespoon coconut oil

STIR-FRY SAUCE

¼ cup coconut aminos

1 tablespoon fresh lime juice

1 teaspoon ginger powder

1 teaspoon honey

½ teaspoon garlic powder

½ teaspoon arrowroot starch

¼ cup sliced green onions, for garnish

Make Ahead

Slice the cabbage up to 2 days in advance and store in a sealed container or bag in the refrigerator. Make a double batch of the sauce and store in a glass jar in the refrigerator for up to 2 weeks.

Store & Reheat

Once cool, store in a sealed glass container in the refrigerator for up to 3 days or in the freezer for up to 3 months. Reheat in a skillet over medium heat until warm.

1. In a large, deep skillet or wok, cook the ground pork over medium heat until no longer pink. Season with the salt and transfer to a fine-mesh strainer set over the sink to drain. Wipe the skillet clean.

2. In the same skillet, sauté the cabbage in the coconut oil over medium-high heat until wilted but still crunchy, 6 to 7 minutes.

3. In a small bowl, whisk together the ingredients for the sauce.

4. Return the pork to the pan and combine well with the cabbage. Add the sauce and continuously toss the pork with the cabbage until the sauce has thickened slightly and the cabbage is translucent, 1 to 2 minutes. Serve immediately, topped with the green onions.

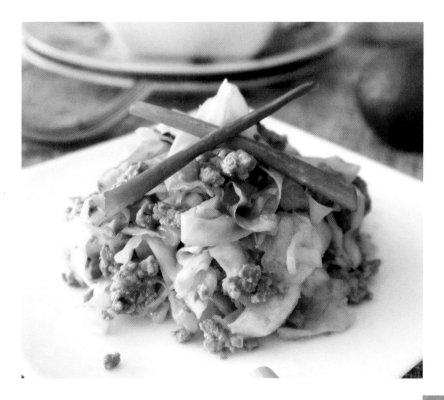

cinnamon pork & applesauce

Serves 4 to 6 | Prep Time: 5 minutes | Cook Time: 6 minutes | Total Time: 11 minutes

2 pounds boneless pork loin cutlets (about ½ inch thick)

1 teaspoon fine sea salt

½ teaspoon ground cinnamon

2 tablespoons bacon fat or coconut oil

Homemade Applesauce (recipe below), warmed

2 teaspoons minced fresh sage, for garnish

1. Season the pork on both sides with the salt and cinnamon.

2. Heat the bacon fat in a large skillet over medium-high heat. Cook the pork for 2 to 3 minutes per side, until the internal temperature reaches 150 degrees, making sure not to overcook it, as pork loin dries out quickly. You may need to cook the pork in two batches, depending on the size of your skillet.

3. Spoon a few tablespoons of applesauce over the pork and sprinkle the sage on top. Serve immediately.

Serving Suggestions
Serve with Cinnamon Mashed Carrots (page 254) or Silky Potato Puree (page 258).

Store & Reheat
Once cool, store the pork in a sealed glass container separate from the applesauce. To reheat, wrap the pork in foil and warm in a 300-degree oven or quickly sear in a greased skillet over medium heat until warm. Serve with the reheated applesauce.

homemade applesauce

Makes 2 cups | Prep Time: 8 minutes | Cook Time: 20 minutes | Total Time: 28 minutes

2 Gala apples, peeled, cored, and chopped

2 Golden Delicious apples, peeled, cored, and chopped

¾ cup water

2 cinnamon sticks

¼ teaspoon fine sea salt

1. Place all the ingredients in a medium saucepan, making sure to submerge the cinnamon sticks under the apples. Cook over medium heat for 20 minutes, being careful not to scorch the applesauce, until the apples are tender and cooked through. Remove from the heat.

2. Mash with a potato masher to the desired chunkiness and stir well to incorporate any liquid. Alternatively, you can place in a blender and puree for a thinner sauce.

Serving Suggestions
Use in Cinnamon Pork & Applesauce (above) or, for an easy weeknight treat, bake in small ramekins with the crumble topping from the Apple Crumble (page 316) in a 350-degree oven for 8 to 10 minutes, until the tops are browned.

Storage
Once cool, store in a sealed glass container in the refrigerator for up to 6 weeks or in the freezer for up to 1 year.

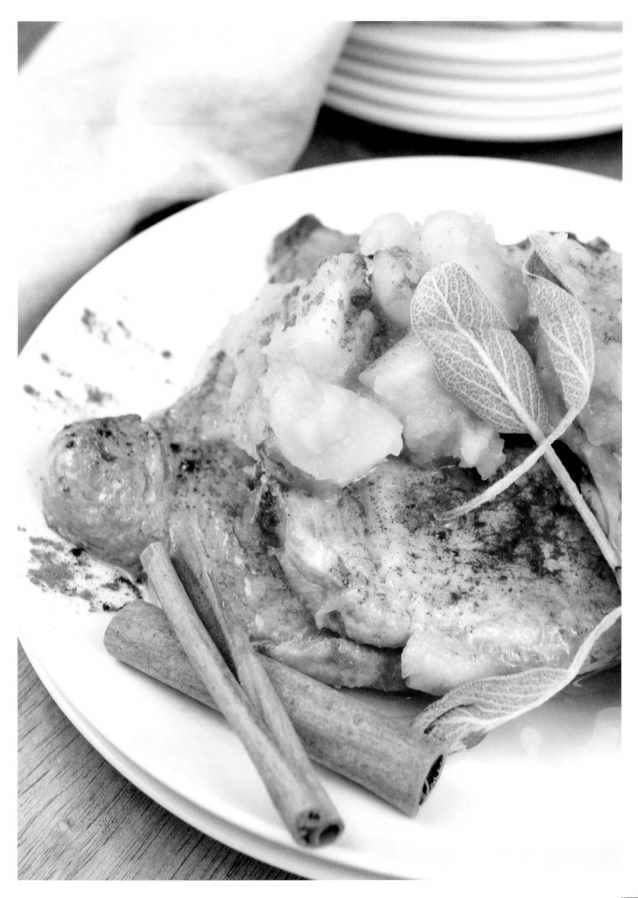

ham & pineapple pizza ⏲

Makes one 10-inch pizza, serves 2 to 3 | Prep Time: 8 minutes | Cook Time: 10 minutes | Total Time: 18 minutes

1 recipe Thin Pizza Crust (page 120), prebaked

1 tablespoon extra-virgin olive oil

⅔ cup thinly sliced yellow onions

3 cloves garlic, minced

1 cup diced pineapple (canned or fresh)

1 cup shredded spinach (optional)

6 ounces uncured ham or Canadian bacon, diced

1½ teaspoons fresh thyme leaves

1. Place an oven rack in the center of the oven and preheat the broiler to high. Place the prebaked pizza crust on a cookie sheet.

2. Heat the olive oil in a medium skillet over medium heat. Add the onions and garlic and sauté for a few minutes until softened and fragrant. Add the remaining ingredients to the skillet and cook for 2 to 3 more minutes, until the pineapple begins to release some of its juice.

3. Spoon the topping onto the pizza crust using a slotted spoon, leaving as much juice in the pan as possible. Press the toppings down into the crust lightly with the back of the spoon.

4. Broil for 3 to 4 minutes, until the ham begins to turn golden brown with crisp edges. Let rest for a few minutes, then slice with a rocker knife or sharp pizza cutter. Serve immediately.

Store & Reheat
Store cooled and sliced pizza in a sealed glass container in the refrigerator for up to 3 days or in the freezer for up to 3 months. To keep the crust from getting soggy when reheating, place the pizza directly on an oven rack and warm under a low broil.

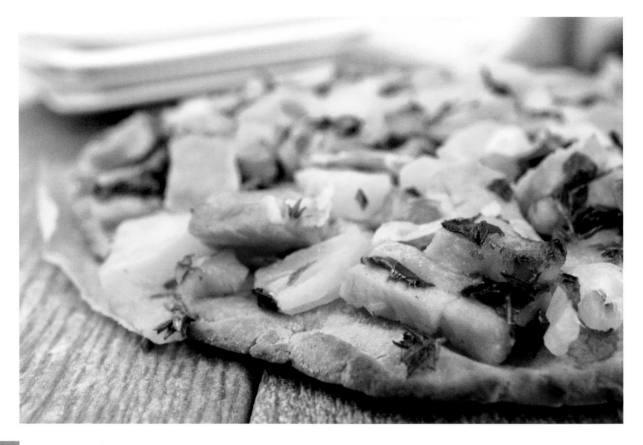

prosciutto & fig bistro pizza

Makes one 10-inch pizza, serves 2 to 3 | Prep Time: 5 minutes | Cook Time: 12 minutes | Total Time: 17 minutes

1 recipe Thin Pizza Crust (page 120), prebaked

1 tablespoon extra-virgin olive oil

6 slices prosciutto, chopped

½ cup chopped dried Turkish figs

½ cup halved red grapes

5 ounces arugula

½ teaspoon garlic powder

1. Preheat the oven to 350 degrees. Place the prebaked pizza crust on a cookie sheet.

2. Heat the olive oil in a large skillet over medium-high heat. Add the chopped prosciutto, figs, and grapes to the pan and cook for 2 to 3 minutes, until the prosciutto is crispy.

3. Add the arugula and stir continuously until completely wilted, about 2 minutes.

4. Top the pizza crust with the prosciutto and arugula mixture. Bake for 5 to 7 minutes, until the top layer is golden brown and crispy.

Serving Suggestion
Serve with Antipasto Salad (page 166).

Store & Reheat
Store cooled and sliced pizza in a sealed glass container in the refrigerator for up to 3 days or in the freezer for up to 3 months. To keep the crust from getting soggy when reheating, place the pizza directly on an oven rack and warm under a low broil.

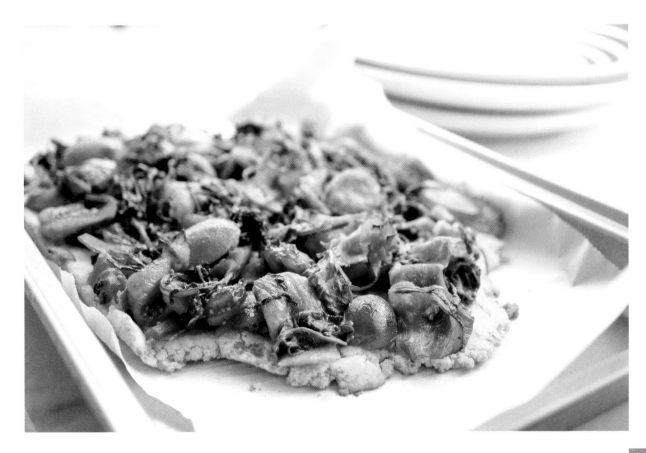

mojo pulled chicken 🍲

Serves 10 | Prep Time: 10 minutes | Cook Time: 30 minutes to 5 hours, depending on cooking method |
Total Time: 40 minutes to 5 hours 10 minutes, depending on cooking method

3 pounds boneless, skinless chicken thighs

2 pounds boneless, skinless chicken breast

1 cup fresh orange juice

¼ cup fresh lime juice

10 cloves garlic, pressed

1 tablespoon dried oregano leaves

1½ teaspoons dried thyme leaves

2½ teaspoons fine sea salt

1 teaspoon ginger powder

½ teaspoon ground cinnamon

1 cup finely chopped fresh cilantro (see Store & Reheat)

Make Ahead

Combine all the ingredients except the cilantro in the cooking vessel and let marinate overnight in the refrigerator.

Store & Reheat

Once cool, store in a sealed glass container in the refrigerator for up to 4 days or in the freezer for up to 3 months. If planning to freeze, do not add the cilantro until the chicken is reheated and ready to serve. Reheat in a saucepan on the stovetop over medium heat until warm.

Slow cooker instructions

1. Spread the chicken evenly in the slow cooker insert.

2. In a bowl, whisk together the remaining ingredients except the cilantro. Pour over the chicken and toss to coat the chicken evenly.

3. Cook on low for 4 to 5 hours, until the chicken can be easily shredded with two forks.

4. Transfer the chicken to a large serving bowl. Shred the chicken by pulling two forks in opposite directions to pull the meat apart. Stir in the cilantro.

5. Pour the desired amount of cooking liquid from the pot over the shredded chicken and combine to flavor and moisten the meat.

Pressure cooker instructions (see Tip, page 108)

1. Spread the chicken evenly in the pressure cooker insert.

2. In a bowl, whisk together the remaining ingredients except the cilantro. Pour over the chicken and toss to coat the chicken evenly.

3. Seal the lid and set the pressure cooker's manual timer for 30 minutes. When the timer goes off, release the pressure.

4. Transfer the chicken to a large serving bowl. Shred the chicken by pulling two forks in opposite directions to pull the meat apart. Stir in the cilantro.

5. Pour the desired amount of cooking liquid from the pot over the shredded chicken and combine to flavor and moisten the meat.

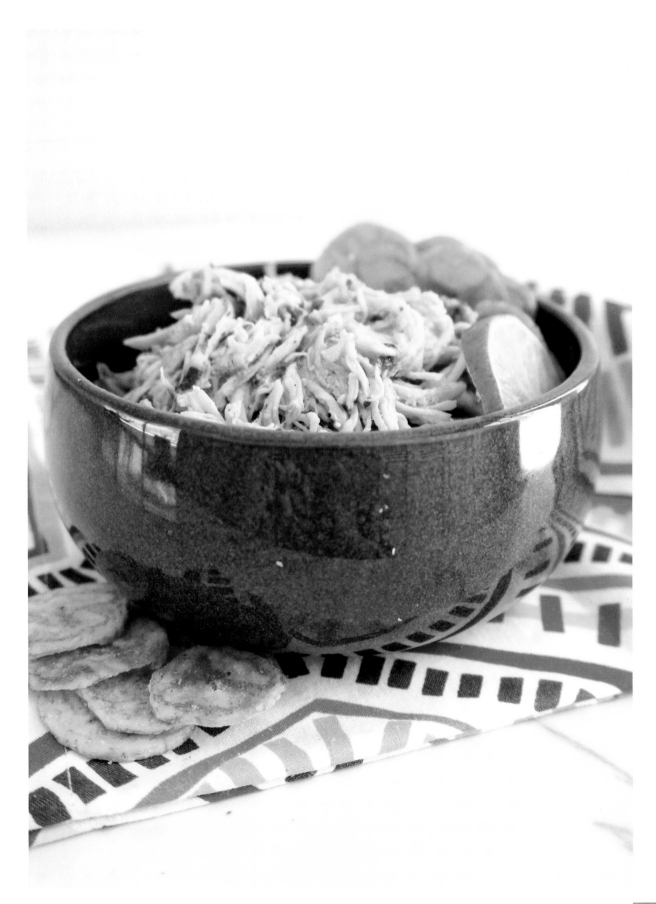

oven-fried chicken

Serves 4 to 6 | Prep Time: 15 minutes | Cook Time: 25 minutes | Total Time: 40 minutes

4 cups salted plantain chips (see Tip)

1 teaspoon garlic powder

1 teaspoon onion powder

1 teaspoon fine sea salt

2 pounds boneless, skinless chicken thighs

¼ cup full-fat coconut milk

Tip
Purchase plantain chips with an ingredient list of just plantains, palm oil, and sea salt.

Make Ahead
Up to 1 day ahead, prepare the plantain breading mixture and store in a plastic bag on the countertop until ready to use.

Serving Suggestions
Serve with Silky Potato Puree (page 258), Creamy Herb Mushrooms (page 248), or Smoked Salmon Potato Salad (page 175), or top with Country Herb Gravy (page 134).

Store & Reheat
Once cool, store in a sealed glass container in the refrigerator for up to 3 days, or wrap the chicken thighs individually in parchment paper, place in a freezer bag, and freeze for up to 2 months. Reheat under a low broil, 6 inches from the broiler, for 5 to 7 minutes, until warm.

1. Preheat the oven to 425 degrees. Line a rimmed baking sheet with aluminum foil and place a baking rack on top. (This allows the underside of the chicken to crisp up.)

2. In a food processor, process the plantain chips, garlic powder, onion powder, and salt for 60 to 90 seconds, until the chips are ground into small pieces, but not so long that they turn into flour. You want the texture to be similar to a coarse meal; if the chips are too coarsely ground, they will not easily adhere to the chicken. Transfer the plantain breading to a large, shallow bowl or plate.

3. Place the chicken thighs and coconut milk in a resealable plastic bag, seal it closed, and toss until the chicken is evenly coated.

4. Coat each piece of chicken thoroughly in the plantain breading mixture. Transfer the coated thighs to the baking rack, laying them flat and leaving plenty of space between them.

5. Bake for 20 to 23 minutes, until the juices run clear when pierced with a fork. Then broil on high for 2 to 3 minutes, until crisp and golden brown.

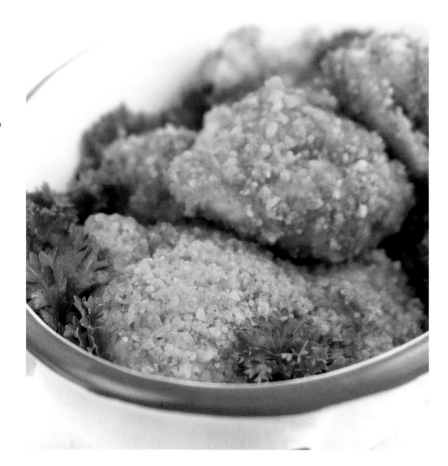

pesto chicken pasta

Serves 3 to 4 | Prep Time: 10 minutes | Total Time: 10 minutes

1 recipe Spaghetti Squash Noodles (page 238), precooked and cooled

3 cups coarsely shredded cooked chicken breast (see Tip)

1 recipe Pronto Pesto (page 116)

⅓ cup sliced black olives

¼ teaspoon fine sea salt

Mix together all the ingredients in a serving bowl and serve cold or at room temperature.

Tip

Use precooked rotisserie chicken, chicken breast, or Classic Roast Chicken (page 224).

Make Ahead

Shred a whole rotisserie chicken up to 3 days in advance, reserving 3 cups of chicken breast for this recipe. The pesto can be made up to 2 days in advance.

Storage

Store in a sealed glass container in the refrigerator for up to 2 days.

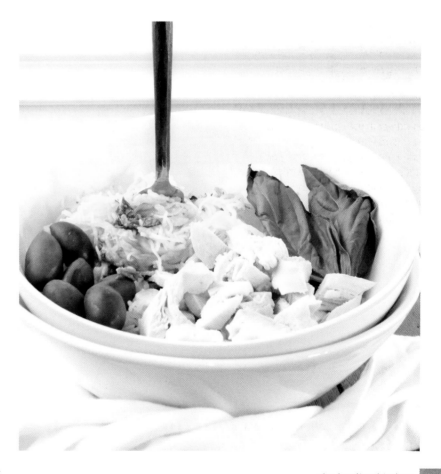

honey-garlic drumsticks

Serves 4 to 6 | Prep Time: 5 minutes | Cook Time: 48 minutes | Total Time: 53 minutes + 3 hours to marinate

12 skin-on chicken drumsticks

½ cup Garlic Sauce (page 106)

¼ cup honey

½ teaspoon fine sea salt

Make Ahead
The chicken can be marinated up to 24 hours in advance.

Serving Suggestions
Serve with Caribbean Plantain Rice (page 239), Sweet Potato & Kale "Rice" Salad (page 244), or Cinnamon Mashed Carrots (page 254).

Store & Reheat
Once cool, cover the baking dish and store in the refrigerator for up to 3 days or in the freezer for up to 3 months. Reheat uncovered in a 350-degree oven until warm.

1. Place the drumsticks in a large glass baking dish in a single layer. In a bowl, whisk together the Garlic Sauce and honey until combined. Pour over the chicken and let marinate in the fridge for 2 to 3 hours.

2. Place an oven rack in the middle of the oven and preheat the oven to 400 degrees.

3. Bake the chicken uncovered for 20 minutes. Flip and bake for an additional 25 minutes until golden brown and cooked through. Then broil for 2 to 3 minutes, until the skin has caramelized into a deeper golden brown.

4. Sprinkle with the salt and let rest for 5 to 10 minutes to allow the juices to be reabsorbed before serving.

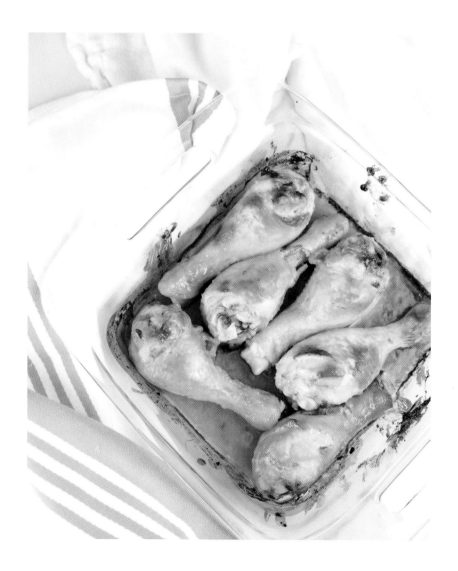

mojo-mango stuffed sweet potatoes

Serves 4 | Prep Time: 5 minutes | Cook Time: 10 minutes | Total Time: 15 minutes

4 baked orange sweet potatoes, each 6 inches long

2 cups Mojo Pulled Chicken (page 214)

⅔ cup Mango Guacamole (page 116)

Serving Suggestions
Serve with Fennel Mandarin Slaw (page 170) or Spicy Carrots (page 244).

Store & Reheat
Once cool, store the stuffed sweet potatoes (without the guacamole) in a sealed glass container or wrapped in foil in the refrigerator for up to 3 days. Reheat according to the directions in Step 2, then top with the guacamole.

1. Slice each sweet potato in half lengthwise. Divide the pulled chicken evenly among the potato halves.

2. Either warm the stuffed potatoes in the microwave for 1 minute or place them in a glass baking dish and warm in a 350-degree oven for 5 to 10 minutes. Top with the guacamole and serve immediately.

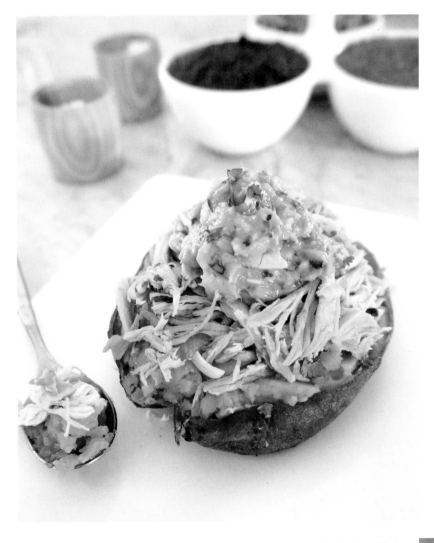

teriyaki chicken & fried rice

Serves 3 to 4 | Prep Time: 15 minutes | Cook Time: 20 minutes | Total Time: 35 minutes

1 tablespoon coconut oil

1 pound boneless, skinless chicken breast, cut into 1-inch pieces

TERIYAKI SAUCE

3 tablespoons coconut aminos

1 tablespoon blackstrap molasses

1 teaspoon fish sauce

½ teaspoon ginger powder

½ teaspoon arrowroot starch

¼ teaspoon garlic powder

¼ teaspoon onion powder

FRIED RICE

1 head cauliflower (about 1½ pounds), cored and cut into florets, or 2 (12-ounce) bags cauliflower florets

4 slices bacon, diced

2 carrots, peeled and finely diced

1 cup finely diced yellow onions

2 tablespoons extra-virgin olive oil

4 tablespoons coconut aminos, divided

1 tablespoon fresh lime juice

1 teaspoon fish sauce

½ teaspoon fine sea salt

⅓ cup sliced green onions

1. To make the teriyaki chicken: Heat the coconut oil in a medium skillet over medium-high heat. Add the chicken and sauté until golden brown and cooked through, 5 to 7 minutes.

2. Meanwhile, whisk together the ingredients for the sauce in a small bowl. Once the chicken is cooked, pour the sauce into the skillet. Immediately remove from the heat and continue stirring the chicken and sauce until thickened. Set aside at the back of the stove with the lid ajar to keep warm while you prepare the rice.

3. To make the fried rice: Place the cauliflower florets in a food processor or high-powered blender and pulse until finely chopped to the size of rice grains (work in two batches if using a blender). Cook the diced bacon in a large, deep pan or wok until crispy. Add the carrots and onions to the pan and cook in the rendered bacon fat until softened, about 5 minutes. Stir in the cauliflower rice and olive oil. Cook for 3 to 4 minutes, until the cauliflower is softened but not mushy.

4. Meanwhile, whisk together 3 tablespoons of the coconut aminos, the lime juice, fish sauce, and salt and stir into the fried rice. Turn the heat up to medium-high and cook for 1 minute more to allow some of the liquid to evaporate. Remove from the heat and stir in the green onions and remaining tablespoon of coconut aminos.

5. Divide the rice among 3 or 4 plates and top with the chicken and pan sauce.

Store & Reheat
Once cool, store in a sealed glass container in the refrigerator for up to 3 days or in the freezer for up to 3 months. Reheat in a greased skillet over medium heat until just warm.

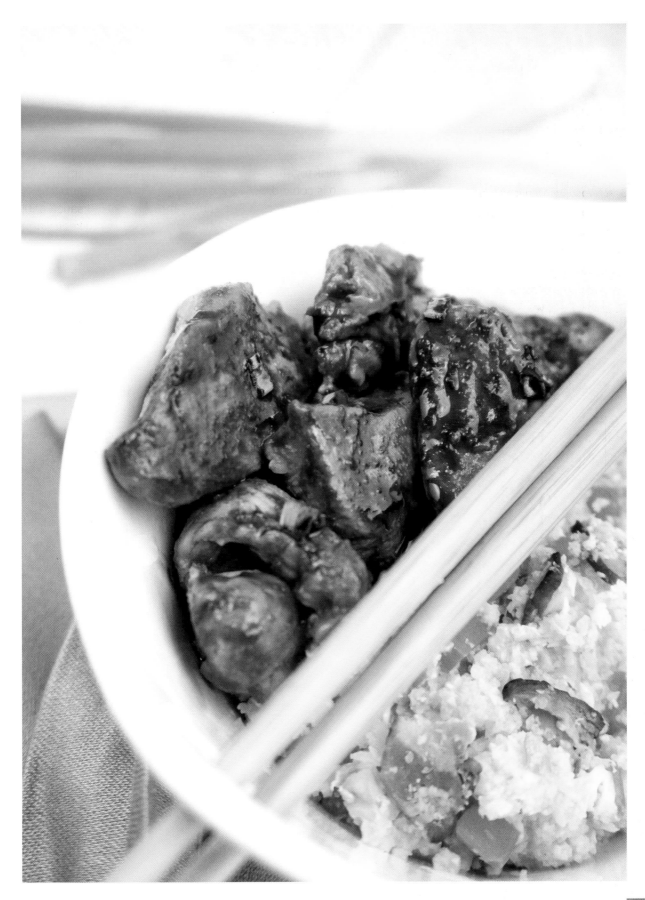

coconut-crusted chicken tenders with pineapple dipping sauce

Serves 2 to 3 | Prep Time: 10 minutes | Cook Time: 6 minutes | Total Time: 16 minutes + 1½ hours to marinate

1 (14-ounce) can pineapple chunks

1 tablespoon blackstrap molasses

1 tablespoon honey

1 teaspoon fish sauce

1 tablespoon fresh lime juice

½ teaspoon fine sea salt

1 pound chicken tenders

1 cup unsweetened shredded coconut

¼ cup coconut oil

Make Ahead

Make the dipping sauce up to 4 days in advance and store in the refrigerator until ready to use.

Store & Reheat

Once cool, store in a sealed glass container in the refrigerator for up to 3 days. To reheat, place the chicken tenders on a broiler rack and broil for 2 to 3 minutes, until warm and crispy.

1. Prepare the dipping sauce: Drain the pineapple and reserve the juice. Transfer the pineapple chunks to a blender with the molasses, honey, fish sauce, and 2 tablespoons of the reserved juice, setting the rest of the juice aside for use in Step 2. Blend on high speed until a smooth, thin sauce forms. Set this dipping sauce aside in a small serving bowl.

2. Whisk together ⅓ cup of the remaining pineapple juice, lime juice, and salt. Marinate the chicken in the liquid in a large plastic bag in the refrigerator for 1 to 1½ hours.

3. Remove the chicken from the marinade and place on a work surface. Spread the shredded coconut on a shallow plate. Roll each chicken tender in the coconut until coated on all sides.

4. Heat the coconut oil in a very large skillet over medium-high heat. Ideally, you want to cook all the chicken in one batch to prevent the coconut oil from burning, but avoid crowding the pan. Fry the chicken tenders for 2 to 3 minutes per side, until cooked through. If cooking in two batches, wipe out the skillet between batches and then add additional coconut oil to the skillet.

5. Serve the chicken tenders immediately with the pineapple dipping sauce.

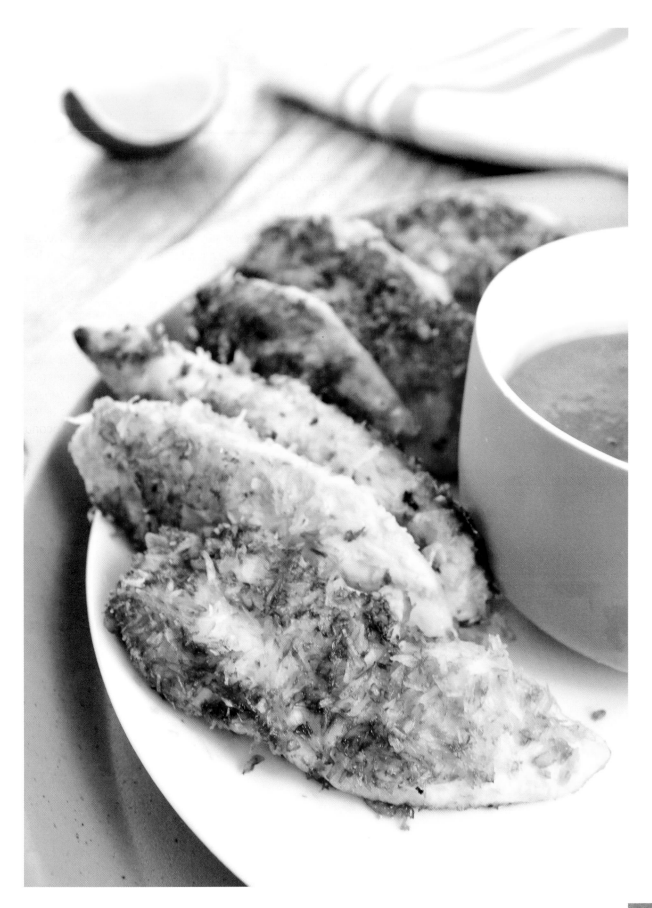

classic roast chicken

Serves 6 | Prep Time: 8 minutes | Cook Time: 1 hour | Total Time: 1 hour 8 minutes + 20 minutes to rest

1 (4-pound) whole chicken, giblets removed

5 large carrots, peeled and ends removed

2 teaspoons extra-virgin olive oil

1¼ teaspoons fine sea salt, divided

1 lemon, halved

5 sprigs fresh thyme

2 sprigs fresh rosemary

1. Remove the chicken from the refrigerator 30 minutes prior to roasting. Preheat the oven to 400 degrees. Line a large rimmed baking sheet with parchment paper.

2. Toss the carrots with the olive oil and ¼ teaspoon of the salt on the baking sheet. Place one half of the lemon on the sheet as well.

3. Set a small roasting rack on top of the carrots, which will allow the underside of the chicken to crisp.

4. Rinse the chicken and pat it dry with paper towels both on the outside and inside the cavity until the skin is dry to the touch. Drying it thoroughly ensures the crispiest skin.

5. Place the chicken breast side up on the roasting rack. Rub the remaining teaspoon of salt on the skin. Stuff the remaining half of the lemon and all of the fresh herbs in the cavity and tie the legs together with kitchen string or twine.

6. Roast for 1 hour or until the internal temperature in the breast reads 170 degrees. Turn the oven off and let the chicken rest in the oven with the door closed for 10 minutes. Remove the chicken from the oven and let it rest on the countertop, tented with foil, for 10 more minutes before slicing. After slicing, squeeze the roasted lemon over the chicken and serve warm.

Tip
This recipe can easily be doubled. If both chickens do not fit on the same oven rack, rotate the pans halfway through cooking.

Serving Suggestions
Serve with Lebanese Beef & Rice Stuffing (page 246), Carrot Pilaf with Lemon & Parsley (page 242), or Creamy Bacon Scalloped Sweet Potatoes (page 250). Use leftover chicken to top salads or soups or in wraps made from large lettuce leaves or Plantain Wraps (page 121).

Store & Reheat
Once cool, store in a sealed glass container in the refrigerator for up to 3 days or in the freezer for up to 3 months. Reheat in a 350-degree oven until warm. To crisp the skin, broil on high for a few minutes. If the meat has been removed from the bones, reheat in a skillet over medium heat until warm.

Change It Up
Add 3- to 4-inch chunks of chopped root vegetables tossed in olive oil and salt to the pan around the chicken and roast for the entire hour.

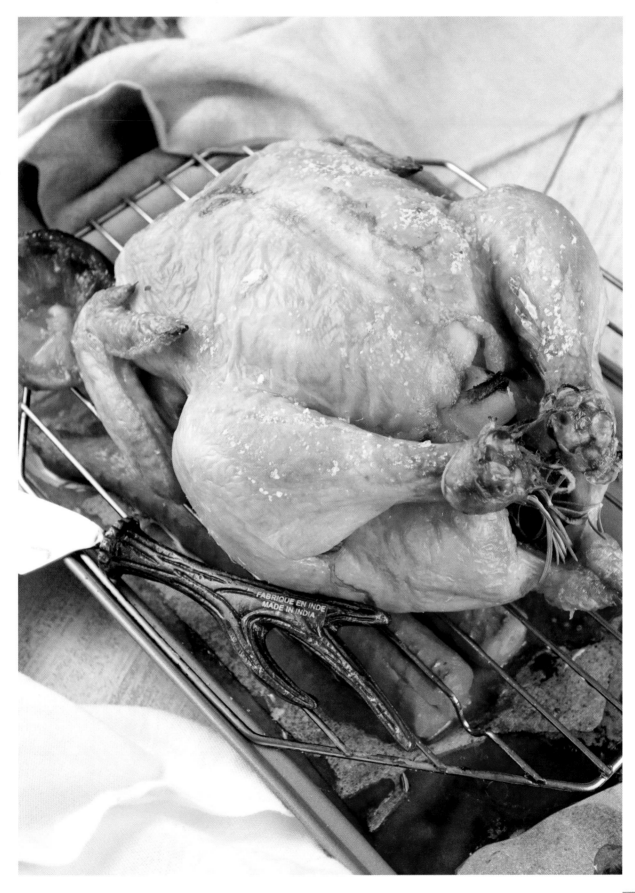

raisin & spice meatballs

Serves 5 | Prep Time: 8 minutes | Cook Time: 20 minutes | Total Time: 28 minutes

2 pounds ground chicken, preferably thighs

½ cup raisins

2 tablespoons coconut flour

1 teaspoon ground cinnamon

1 teaspoon ginger powder

1 teaspoon fine sea salt

½ teaspoon ground mace

½ teaspoon garlic powder

Make Ahead

Complete the recipe through Step 2. Cover the baking sheet with plastic wrap and refrigerate for up to 24 hours before baking.

Serving Suggestions

Serve with Sweet Potato & Kale "Rice" Salad (page 244) or Cinnamon Mashed Carrots (page 254).

Store & Reheat

Once cool, store in a sealed glass container in the refrigerator for up to 3 days. To freeze, place the baking sheet in the freezer until the meatballs are frozen, then transfer the meatballs to a freezer-safe container and freeze for up to 3 months. Reheat in a skillet over medium heat until warm.

1. Preheat the oven to 400 degrees. Line a rimmed baking sheet with parchment paper.

2. Mix together all the ingredients in a medium bowl until well combined. Scoop up 2 tablespoons of the mixture, roll into a ball, and place on the prepared baking sheet. Repeat this step until all the meat is used up. You should end up with about 20 meatballs.

3. Bake for 18 to 20 minutes, until the chicken is cooked through. Serve warm.

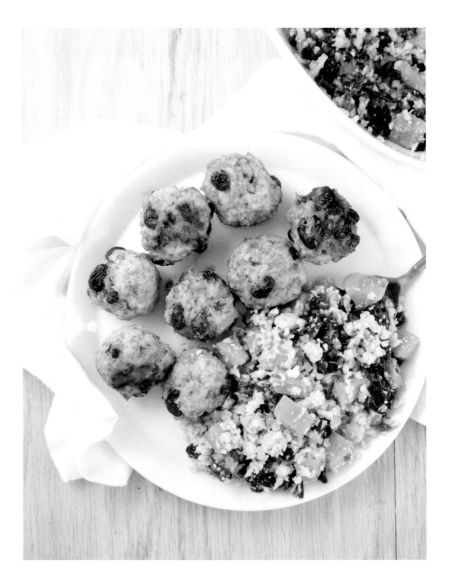

pesto chicken pizza

Makes one 10-inch pizza, serves 2 to 3 | Prep Time: 10 minutes | Cook Time: 10 minutes | Total Time: 20 minutes

1 recipe Thin Pizza Crust (page 120), prebaked

1 recipe Pronto Pesto (page 116)

1¼ cups shredded cooked chicken (see Tip)

¼ cup sliced black olives

¼ cup sliced canned artichoke hearts

¼ teaspoon truffle salt (see Tip, page 122) or fine sea salt

Tip
To save time, use shredded meat from a store-bought plain rotisserie chicken.

Serving Suggestions
Serve with Peach & Kale Summer Salad (page 174) or Antipasto Salad (page 166).

Store & Reheat
Store cooled and sliced pizza in a sealed glass container in the refrigerator for up to 3 days or in the freezer for up to 3 months. To keep the crust from getting soggy when reheating, place the pizza directly on an oven rack and warm under a low broil.

1. Preheat the oven to 425 degrees.

2. Place the prebaked pizza crust on a cookie sheet or pizza pan. Spread the pesto evenly on the crust, reserving a few tablespoons for garnish, if desired. Top with the chicken, olives, artichoke hearts, and salt.

3. Bake for 8 to 10 minutes, until the crust is crispy and the edges of the toppings are lightly browned. Let rest for a few minutes, then slice the pizza using a rocker knife or sharp pizza cutter. Garnish with a drizzle of the reserved pesto, if desired.

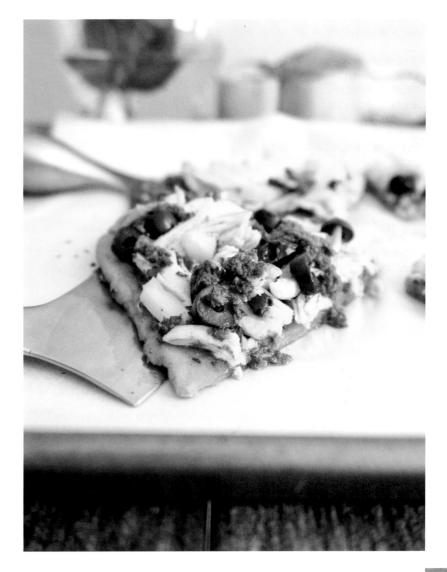

spinach & garlic lover's pizza 🕐

Makes one 10-inch pizza, serves 2 to 3 | Prep Time: 5 minutes | Cook Time: 10 minutes | Total Time: 15 minutes

1 recipe Thin Pizza Crust (page 120), prebaked

1 tablespoon extra-virgin olive oil

8 ounces spinach

1¼ cups cooked and coarsely chopped chicken breast

¼ cup plus 2 tablespoons Garlic Sauce (page 106), divided

¼ teaspoon fine sea salt

¾ teaspoon nutritional yeast, for cheeselike flavor (optional)

Serving Suggestion
Serve with Caesar Salad (page 165).

Store & Reheat
Store cooled and sliced pizza in a sealed glass container in the refrigerator for up to 3 days or in the freezer for up to 3 months. To reheat, place the pizza directly on an oven rack and warm under a low broil.

1. Place an oven rack in the top third of the oven and preheat the broiler to high.

2. Place the prebaked pizza crust on a cookie sheet or pizza pan.

3. Heat the olive oil in a large, deep skillet over medium-high heat. Add half of the spinach and stir continuously to cook and wilt the spinach. Once wilted, add the rest of the spinach, the chicken, and ¼ cup of the Garlic Sauce and cook until all of the spinach has wilted.

4. Transfer the mixture to a fine-mesh strainer placed in the sink and use a potato masher to press the excess liquid out of the spinach. This will prevent the crust from getting soggy.

5. Spoon the mixture on top of the pizza crust, drizzle on the remaining 2 tablespoons of Garlic Sauce, and sprinkle with the salt and nutritional yeast, if using.

6. Broil for 2 to 3 minutes, until the chicken begins to lightly brown.

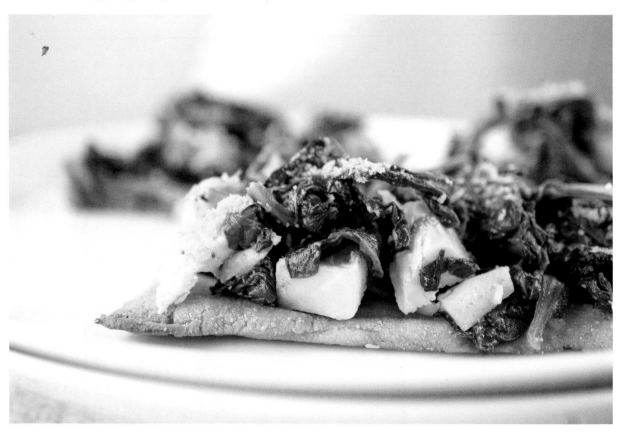

lamb with olive-butternut rice

Serves 3 | Prep Time: 10 minutes | Cook Time: 10 minutes | Total Time: 20 minutes

1½ pounds butternut squash, peeled, seeded, and chopped (see Tip)

¾ cup pitted Kalamata olives

¼ cup chopped fresh oregano leaves, divided

1 pound ground lamb, crumbled

½ cup raisins

½ teaspoon ground cinnamon

½ teaspoon fine sea salt

Tip
It will be easier to peel and chop the squash if it is microwaved first for 3 minutes to soften. To save time, buy 1 pound prechopped fresh (not frozen) butternut squash.

Make Ahead
Chop the squash up to 1 week in advance and store in a plastic bag or sealed container in the refrigerator until ready to use.

Store & Reheat
Once cool, store in a sealed glass container in the refrigerator for up to 3 days or in the freezer for up to 3 months. Reheat in a saucepan or skillet over medium heat until warm.

1. Rice the butternut squash by running it through the shredder attachment of your food processor. Alternatively, you may pulse the chopped squash in batches in a blender until very finely chopped to the size of rice grains. Set the squash aside.

2. Pulse the olives and 2 tablespoons of the oregano leaves in the food processor or blender until finely chopped.

3. Heat a large skillet over medium-high heat. Add the lamb and cook, breaking up the meat with a wooden spoon, until browned and no longer pink.

4. Add the butternut squash rice, olive-oregano mixture, raisins, and cinnamon to the skillet, tossing continuously for 5 to 6 minutes, until the squash is tender but still has a firm bite. Remove from the heat and stir in the remaining 2 tablespoons of oregano leaves and salt. Serve warm.

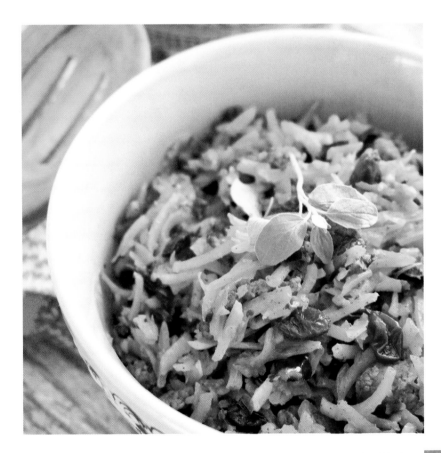

bacon-date crusted salmon

Serves 4 | Prep Time: 5 minutes | Cook Time: 20 minutes | Total Time: 25 minutes

6 slices bacon

8 Medjool dates, pitted

2 tablespoons minced garlic

1 tablespoon plus 1 teaspoon minced fresh rosemary

4 (6-ounce) wild-caught salmon fillets, pin bones removed (see Tip)

2 tablespoons fresh lemon juice

1. Preheat the oven to 400 degrees. Lightly grease a large glass baking dish with olive oil.

2. Cook the bacon in a skillet over medium heat until crispy. Reserve the bacon fat and finely mince the cooked bacon using a chef's knife or rocker knife. Set both the bacon fat and the bacon aside.

3. Place the dates in a small glass bowl, cover with water, and microwave for 1 minute until soft. Alternatively, the dates can be softened in just-boiled water for 10 to 15 minutes. Drain the liquid and mash the dates into a smooth paste using a fork. Stir in the cooked bacon, reserved bacon fat, garlic, and rosemary.

4. Pat the salmon dry and lay it skin side down in the prepared baking dish. Sprinkle the lemon juice over the salmon. Spread the bacon-date mixture on the salmon fillets to cover the top surface entirely.

5. For medium-done salmon, bake for 10 to 12 minutes, until the salmon flakes easily with a fork yet is still a dark pink in the center. For well-done salmon, which will be opaque in the center, bake for up to 15 minutes.

Tip

If you're buying fresh salmon, ask your fishmonger to remove the pin bones for you. To remove them yourself, starting at the thick end of the fillet and going about halfway down, feel along the center of the fillet to locate the pin bones and gently pull them out, in the direction of where the fish's head would be, with a pair of needle-nose pliers or tweezers. This portion of the fillet corresponds to the top front half of the fish, where the pin bones are located. Pin bones are generally already removed from frozen salmon.

Make Ahead

Prepare the bacon-date mixture up to 3 days in advance and store in the refrigerator until ready to use.

Serving Suggestions

Serve with Silky Potato Puree (page 258), Carrot Pilaf with Lemon & Parsley (page 242), or Toasted Coconut, Fig & Kale Salad (page 172).

Store & Reheat

Once cool, store in a sealed glass container in the refrigerator for up to 3 days. Do not freeze. Reheat in a 300-degree oven until warm throughout.

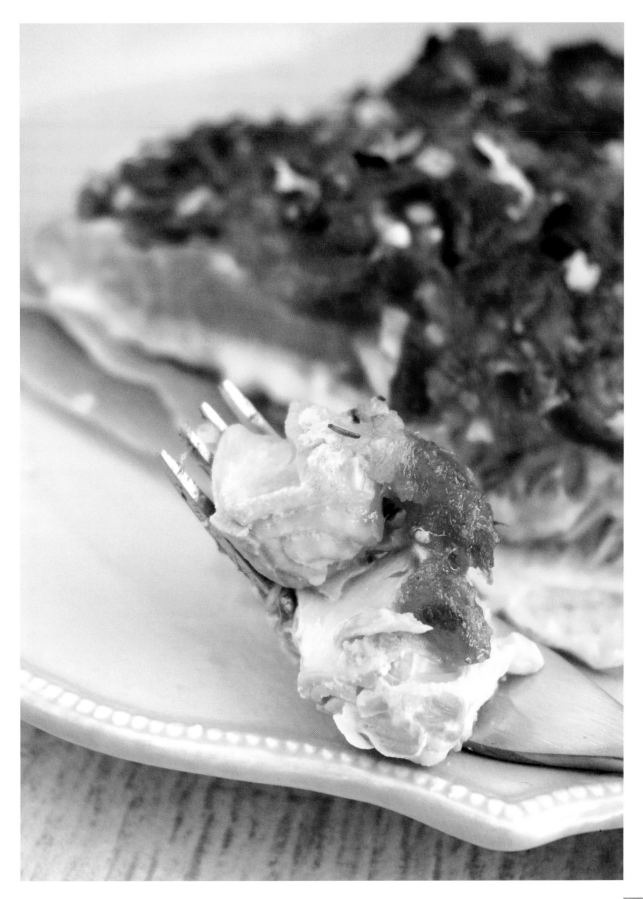

shrimp n' cauli-grits 🍲

Serves 3 | Prep Time: 10 minutes | Cook Time: 20 minutes | Total Time: 30 minutes

1 large head cauliflower (about 2 pounds), cored and cut into florets

5 slices bacon, chopped

1 cup diced yellow onions

1 pound medium shrimp, peeled and deveined

1 teaspoon dried oregano leaves

1 teaspoon dried parsley

½ teaspoon garlic powder

¼ teaspoon ginger powder

1 cup Bone Broth of choice (pages 108–109)

2 tablespoons solid fat like duck fat, lard, or tallow

1 tablespoon fresh lemon juice

¼ cup chopped fresh basil

½ teaspoon fine sea salt

Sliced green onion, for garnish

Make Ahead

Complete Step 1 up to 3 days in advance. Store the cauliflower rice wrapped in paper towels in a sealed plastic bag in the refrigerator until ready to use.

Store & Reheat

Once cool, store in a sealed glass container in the refrigerator for up to 4 days or in the freezer for up to 3 months. Reheat in a skillet over medium heat until warm.

1. Place the cauliflower florets in a food processor or high-powered blender and pulse until finely chopped to the size of rice grains (work in two batches if using a blender). Set aside.

2. Sauté the bacon and onions in a large, deep skillet between medium and medium-high heat until the onions are softened and the bacon has rendered its fat and is slightly crispy, 8 to 10 minutes.

3. Increase the heat to medium-high and add the shrimp, oregano, parsley, garlic powder, and ginger. Continue cooking until the shrimp is opaque throughout, 3 to 4 minutes. Set aside in a serving dish.

4. Add the cauliflower rice and broth to the pan. Bring to a boil and cook, stirring continuously, until the cauliflower has absorbed all the liquid and has softened, about 5 minutes. Remove from the heat.

5. Using a potato masher, lightly mash the cauliflower rice to break up the pieces slightly with the solid fat and lemon juice. Stir in the basil and salt.

6. Serve the cauliflower "grits" with the shrimp and bacon mixture while still warm, topped with green onions.

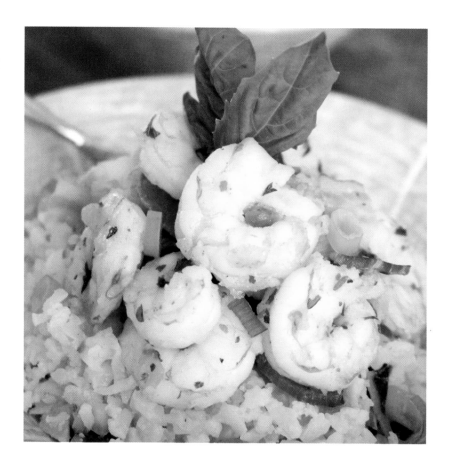

seared shrimp pasta with white sauce

Serves 4 | Prep Time: 5 minutes | Cook Time: 5 minutes | Total Time: 10 minutes

1 tablespoon extra-virgin olive oil

½ cup minced shallots

1½ pounds medium shrimp, peeled, deveined, and cooked (see Tip)

¾ teaspoon fine sea salt

1 recipe Spaghetti Squash Noodles (page 238), precooked

1 recipe Cauli'fredo Sauce (page 119)

½ cup loosely packed fresh basil leaves, sliced

1. Heat the olive oil in a large sauté pan over medium-high heat. Add the shallots and sauté for 1 minute until fragrant, then add the precooked shrimp and salt to the pan. Heat the shrimp with the shallots for about 2 minutes.

2. Reduce the heat to medium-low. Using tongs, quickly stir in the spaghetti squash, sauce, and basil until heated through. Serve immediately or serve cold.

Tip
To save time, buy fresh precooked peeled and deveined shrimp.

Store & Reheat
Once cool, store in a sealed glass container in the refrigerator for up to 3 days. Reheat in a pan over medium heat until warm.

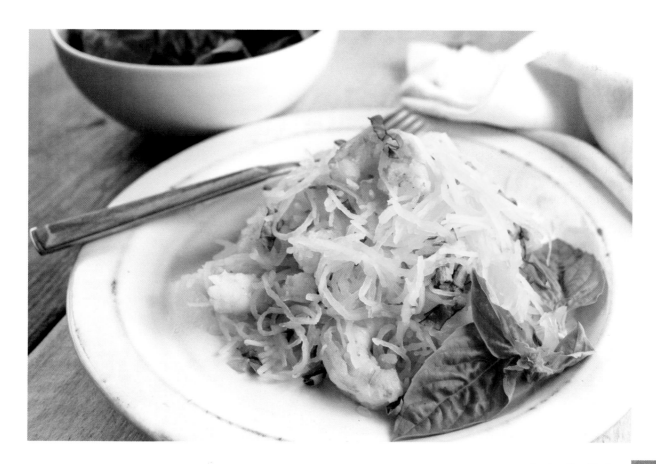

wild salmon with roasted raspberries

Serves 3 | Prep Time: 5 minutes | Cook Time: 13 minutes | Total Time: 18 minutes

3 (6-ounce) wild-caught salmon fillets, pin bones removed (see Tip, page 230)

2 cloves garlic, pressed

½ teaspoon fine sea salt

1 tablespoon minced fresh ginger

1 pint raspberries

1 teaspoon balsamic vinegar

1. Preheat the oven to 400 degrees. Line a rimmed baking sheet with parchment paper.

2. Rub the tops of the salmon fillets with the garlic and salt. Sprinkle with the minced ginger and place on the prepared baking sheet.

3. Toss the raspberries with the balsamic vinegar and place around the salmon on the baking sheet.

4. Bake for 12 to 13 minutes, until the salmon flakes easily with a fork and is a medium pink in the center. Gently spoon the roasted raspberries on top and serve immediately.

Serving Suggestions
Serve with Peach & Kale Summer Salad (page 174) or Caribbean Plantain Rice (page 239).

Store & Reheat
Once cool, store in a sealed glass container in the refrigerator for up to 3 days. You may store the roasted raspberries separately or on top of the salmon. Reheat in a 300-degree oven until just warm.

Change It Up
Raspberries have seeds and will be a bit crunchy. If you prefer a seedless berry topping, top the salmon with the same amount of Roasted Strawberries (page 321) or replace the raspberries in this recipe with blueberries.

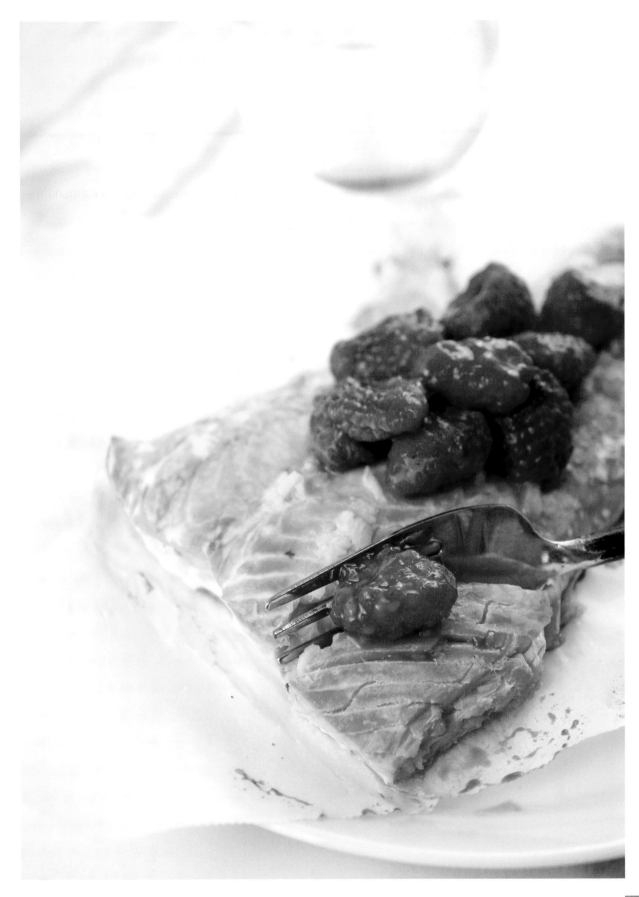

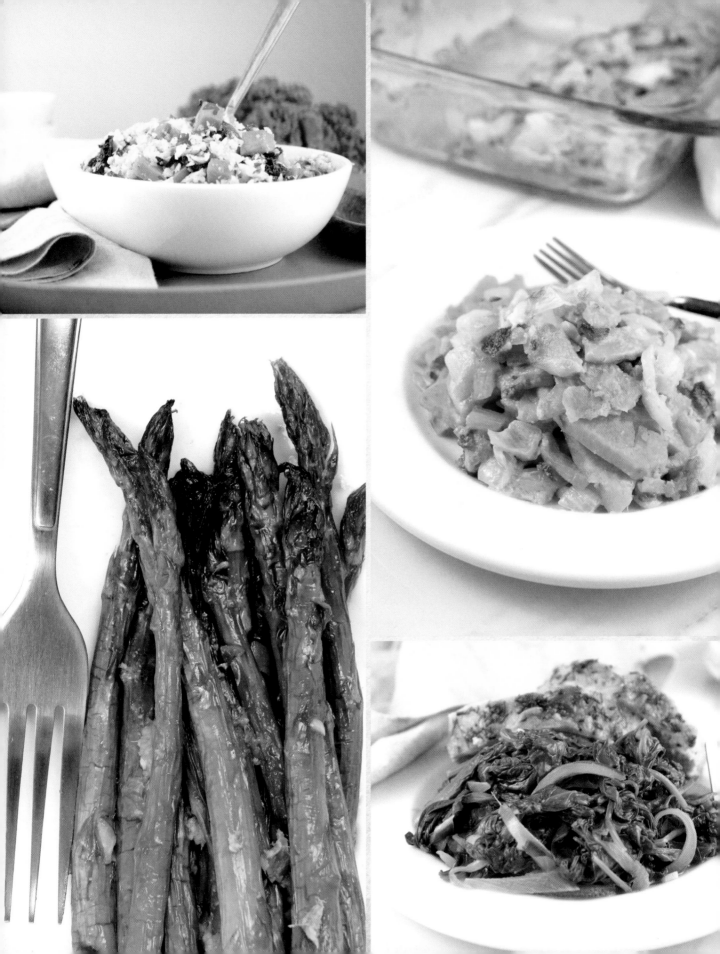

CHAPTER 9

simple sides

spaghetti squash noodles

Makes 6 cups, serves 6 | Prep Time: 5 minutes | Cook Time: 10 to 40 minutes, depending on cooking method | Total Time: 15 to 45 minutes, depending on cooking method

1 (4-pound) spaghetti squash

Store & Reheat
Once cool, store in a sealed glass container in the refrigerator for up to 1 week or in the freezer for up to 6 months. Reheat in the microwave or in a saucepan on the stovetop until warm.

Microwave instructions: Place the squash on a microwave-safe plate and cook for 10 to 12 minutes until easily pierced with a fork. Let cool for 5 minutes before slicing lengthwise.

Oven instructions: Preheat the oven to 400 degrees. Using a sharp knife, slice the squash in half lengthwise and place facedown on a lightly greased rimmed baking sheet. Roast for 40 to 45 minutes, until the squash can be easily pierced with a fork and the "noodles" separate easily from the skin.

Pressure cooker instructions (see Tip, page 108): Place the squash in the pressure cooker insert with ½ cup water. Seal the lid and set the pressure cooker's manual timer for 12 minutes. When the timer goes off, release the pressure.

For all methods: Dispose of the seeds. Scoop the "noodles" into a serving dish by scraping the flesh from all angles with a fork.

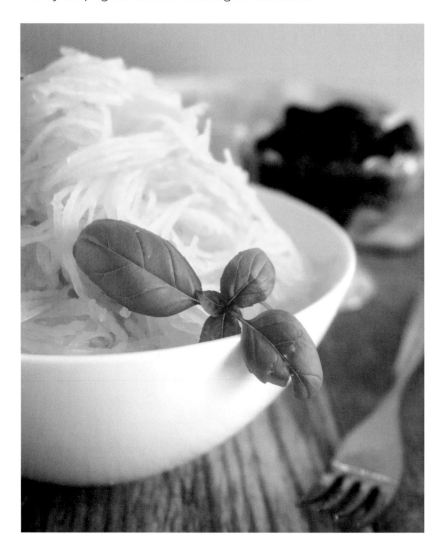

caribbean plantain rice

Serves 4 | Prep Time: 10 minutes | Cook Time: 10 minutes | Total Time: 20 minutes

3 green plantains, peeled and chopped

1 tablespoon extra-virgin olive oil

⅓ cup finely diced red onions

3 cloves garlic, pressed

Grated zest of 1 lime

2 teaspoons dried oregano leaves

1 cup Bone Broth of choice (pages 108–109), divided

⅓ cup fresh cilantro leaves

1 tablespoon fresh lime juice

¼ teaspoon fine sea salt

Store & Reheat
Once cool, store in a sealed glass container in the refrigerator for up to 1 week or in the freezer for up to 3 months. Reheat in a skillet over medium heat until warm.

1. Run the plantains through the shredder attachment of your food processor. Alternatively, pulse the plantains in a blender until finely chopped. Do not overpulse, or the starch will begin to break down and the plantains will become mushy.

2. Heat the olive oil in a large, deep skillet over medium heat. Add the onions and garlic and sauté for 3 to 4 minutes, until fragrant.

3. Stir in the shredded plantains, lime zest, oregano, and ½ cup of the broth. Increase the heat to medium-high and continuously stir the mixture until the broth evaporates and the plantains begin to soften, 3 to 4 minutes. Add the remaining ½ cup broth and cook until all the liquid has been absorbed and the color has deepened to a golden yellow. Remove from the heat.

4. Stir in the cilantro, lime juice, and salt. Serve warm.

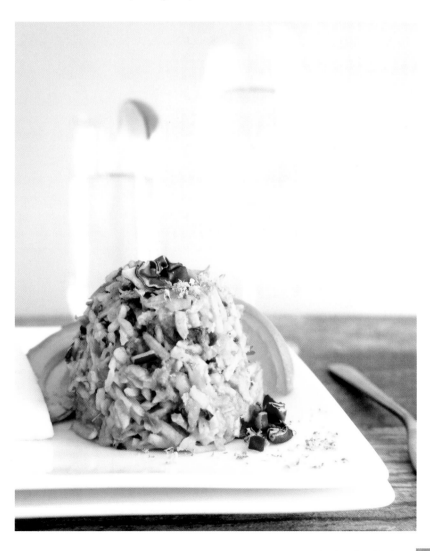

mac n' cheese

Serves 3 to 4 | Prep Time: 7 minutes | Cook Time: 6 minutes | Total Time: 13 minutes

2 pounds green plantains (about 4 medium)

1 cup plus 2 tablespoons coconut cream, divided

1 cup Chicken Broth (page 108; see Tip)

½ teaspoon garlic powder

½ teaspoon onion powder

1 teaspoon fine sea salt, divided

¼ teaspoon turmeric powder (for color)

2 teaspoons arrowroot starch

2 tablespoons minced fresh chives, for garnish

Tip

You must use homemade broth to get the "cheese" flavor here. Store-bought broth is not going to cut it.

Store & Reheat

Once cool, store in a sealed glass container in the refrigerator for up to 2 days. Reheat in a small saucepan over medium heat just until warm, or microwave on high for 30 seconds.

1. Peel and slice the plantains into ¼-inch-thick coins. Slice each coin lengthwise 4 times to make short rectangle-shaped "noodles." Place in a small saucepan with 1 cup of the coconut cream, broth, garlic powder, onion powder, ½ teaspoon of the salt, and turmeric. Bring to a boil uncovered over medium-high heat. Reduce the heat to medium and maintain a low boil for a few minutes to cook the plantains until tender.

2. Remove from the heat. Quickly whisk together the remaining 2 tablespoons of coconut cream and arrowroot starch until smooth. Stir into the saucepan with the remaining ½ teaspoon of salt until the sauce begins to thicken. Serve immediately with a sprinkle of chives, or make one of the variations below.

Bacon & Green Onion Mac n' Cheese (pictured). Prepare the recipe as directed, but cook 4 slices of finely chopped bacon in the saucepan first. Set the bacon aside and drain out all but 2 teaspoons of the bacon fat, then proceed with Step 1. Stir in the cooked bacon and ¼ cup of sliced green onions at the end of Step 2.

Smoky Truffle Mac n' Cheese. Prepare the recipe as directed, but replace the unflavored sea salt with ½ teaspoon of smoked sea salt and ½ teaspoon of truffle salt. Stir in the smoked salt during Step 1 and the truffle salt during Step 2.

Italian Mac n' Cheese. Prepare the recipe as directed, but stir in ½ cup of finely sliced fresh basil leaves and ½ teaspoon of dried oregano leaves at the end of Step 2.

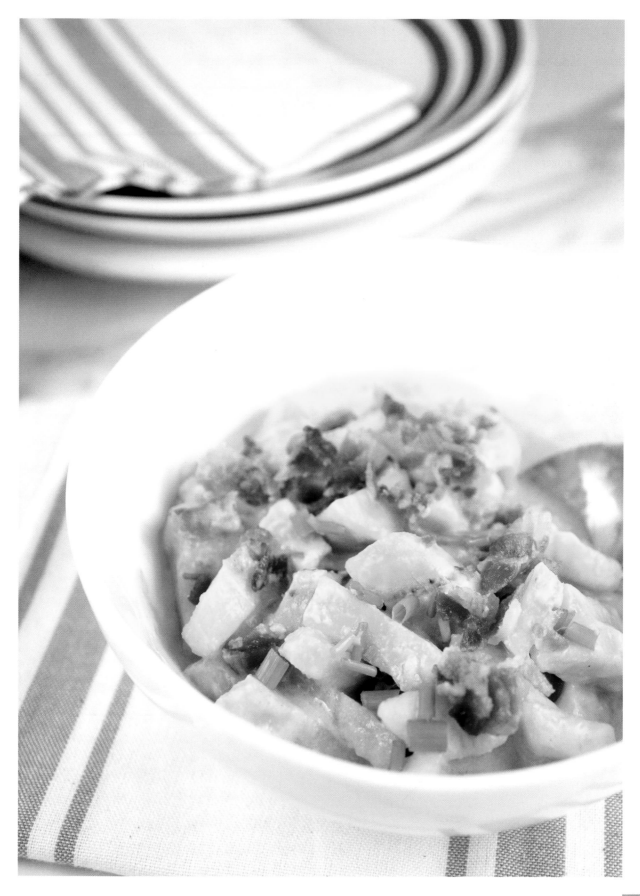

carrot pilaf with lemon & parsley

Serves 2 to 3 | Prep Time: 5 minutes | Cook Time: 23 minutes | Total Time: 28 minutes

1 tablespoon extra-virgin olive oil

⅓ cup diced yellow onions

2 tablespoons diced shallots

1 (10-ounce) bag shredded carrots or ⅔ pound carrots, peeled and shredded

¾ cup Chicken Broth (page 108)

¼ cup finely chopped fresh parsley

1 teaspoon grated lemon zest

1 teaspoon fresh lemon juice

¼ teaspoon fine sea salt

1. Heat the olive oil in a medium saucepan over medium heat. Add the onions and shallots and sauté for a few minutes until fragrant and slightly softened.

2. Add the carrots and broth to the pan and bring to a boil. Cover with a lid slightly ajar to allow steam to escape and cook for 15 to 20 minutes, until the carrots are very tender.

3. Remove from the heat and stir in the parsley, lemon zest and juice, and salt. Serve warm.

Serving Suggestions
Serve with Classic Roast Chicken (page 224) or Spicy African Kale (page 256) for a light meal.

Store & Reheat
Once cool, store in a sealed glass container in the refrigerator for up to 3 days. Reheat in a skillet over medium heat until warm.

spinach with alliums & lemon

Serves 2 to 4 | Prep Time: 5 minutes | Cook Time: 15 minutes | Total Time: 20 minutes

1 tablespoon extra-virgin olive oil

2 cups quartered and sliced red onions (about 1 large)

4 cloves garlic, minced

1 pound spinach

1 tablespoon fresh lemon juice

1 teaspoon Worcestershire Sauce (page 106; optional)

½ teaspoon grated lemon zest

½ teaspoon fine sea salt

1. Heat the olive oil in a large pan over medium heat. Add the onions and sauté for 8 to 10 minutes, until softened and lightly caramelized, stirring every few minutes to prevent sticking.

2. Stir in the garlic and cook for 30 seconds until fragrant. Using tongs, stir in the spinach to coat it in the olive oil and alliums. Cover with a lid and cook for 4 minutes until just wilted.

3. Remove from the heat. In a small bowl, whisk together the lemon juice, Worcestershire Sauce, lemon zest, and salt and toss with the spinach. Serve warm.

Serving Suggestions
Serve with Garlic & Rosemary Crusted Pork Loin (page 208), Classic Roast Chicken (page 224), or Seared Shrimp Pasta with White Sauce (page 233).

Store & Reheat
Once cool, store in a sealed glass container in the refrigerator for up to 1 week. Reheat in a skillet or saucepan over medium-low heat until warm.

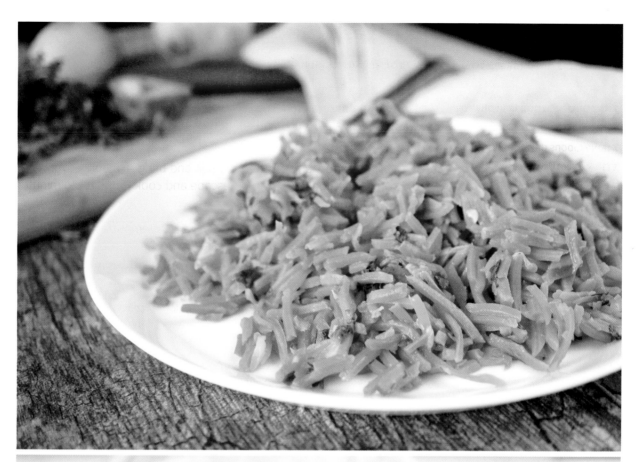

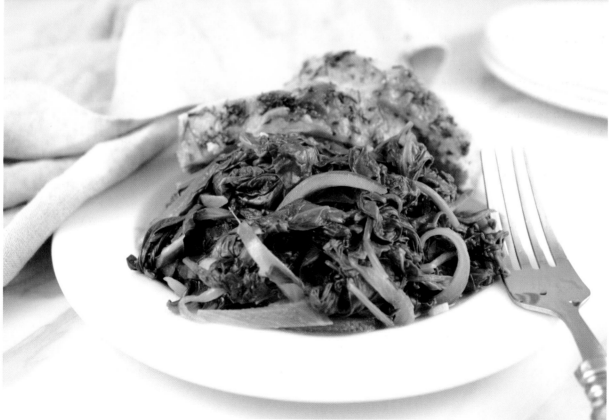

sweet potato & kale "rice" salad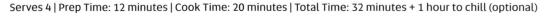

Serves 4 | Prep Time: 12 minutes | Cook Time: 20 minutes | Total Time: 32 minutes + 1 hour to chill (optional)

4 tablespoons extra-virgin olive oil, divided

¼ cup quartered and sliced red onions

1½ cups peeled and diced orange sweet potatoes

1 head cauliflower (about 1½ pounds), cored and cut into florets, or 2 (12-ounce) bags cauliflower florets

4 cups chopped kale (about 1 bunch)

½ cup raisins

1 teaspoon apple cider vinegar

½ teaspoon fine sea salt

¼ teaspoon ground cinnamon

⅓ cup chopped fresh parsley

1 tablespoon fresh lemon juice

Make Ahead

Chop the onions, sweet potatoes, cauliflower, and kale up to 3 days in advance and store in separate plastic bags or glass containers in the refrigerator until ready to use.

Store & Reheat

Once cool, store in a sealed glass container in the refrigerator for up to 5 days or in the freezer for up to 6 months. Reheat in a skillet over medium heat until warm.

1. Heat 2 tablespoons of the olive oil in a large, deep skillet over medium heat. Add the onions and sauté for a few minutes, until fragrant and softened. Stir in the sweet potatoes and cook for 5 minutes, stirring once or twice.

2. Meanwhile, place the cauliflower florets in a food processor or high-powered blender and pulse until finely chopped to the size of rice grains (work in two batches if using a blender).

3. Add the kale to the skillet with the onions and sweet potatoes and toss the vegetables continuously with tongs until the kale is wilted and very tender, about 3 minutes.

4. Stir in the riced cauliflower, raisins, vinegar, salt, and cinnamon. Cover with a lid and cook for 6 to 8 minutes, until the cauliflower and potatoes are tender.

5. Remove from the heat and stir in the parsley and lemon juice. Place in the refrigerator for 1 hour to serve cold, or serve warm.

Chicken & Sweet Potato "Rice" Salad. Add 2 cups of chopped cooked chicken at the end of Step 4.

spicy carrots

Makes 5 cups | Prep Time: 7 minutes | Total Time: 7 minutes + 2 hours to marinate

5 to 6 large carrots, peeled

¼ cup apple cider vinegar

1 tablespoon grated fresh ginger

¼ teaspoon fine sea salt

Storage

Store in a sealed glass container in the refrigerator for up to 2 weeks.

1. Shred the carrots by running them through the shredder attachment of your food processor, or shredding them with a grater. Measure out 5 cups of shredded carrots and place them in a large mixing bowl. In a small bowl, whisk together the remaining ingredients and toss with the carrots.

2. Place in the refrigerator to marinate for at least 2 hours before serving.

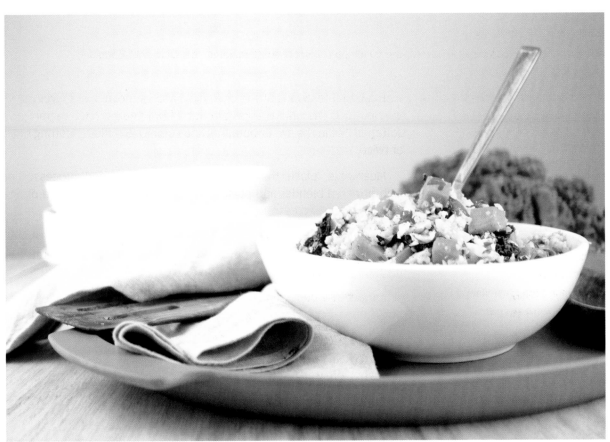

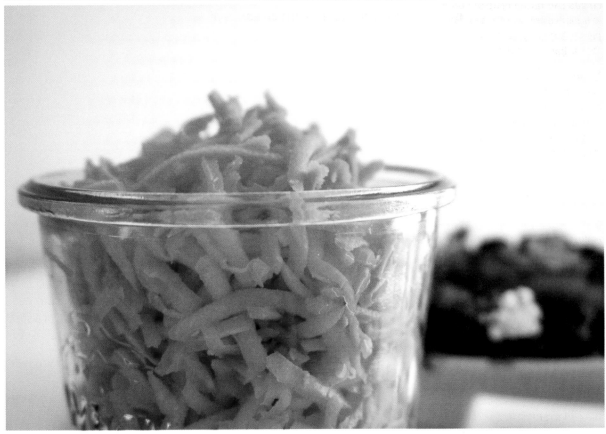

lebanese beef & rice stuffing

Serves 4 | Prep Time: 12 minutes | Cook Time: 15 minutes | Total Time: 27 minutes

1 pound lean ground beef

1 teaspoon ground cinnamon, divided

1 teaspoon fine sea salt

¼ teaspoon granulated garlic

1½ pounds parsnips, peeled and roughly chopped

1 cup diced yellow onions

½ cup Beef Broth (page 109) or water

2 tablespoons dried mint

1 tablespoon fresh lemon juice

⅛ teaspoon ground cloves

1. In a large, deep skillet over medium-high heat, cook the ground beef until browned and no longer pink. Remove from the heat and stir in ½ teaspoon of the cinnamon, along with the salt and granulated garlic. Transfer to a bowl and set aside.

2. Meanwhile, rice the parsnips by running them through the shredder attachment of your food processor or pulsing them in a blender until very finely chopped.

3. Add the parsnips, onions, and broth to the same skillet and cover with a lid. Cook for 3 to 5 minutes, until the vegetables are tender but not mushy.

4. Remove the pan from the heat and stir in the cooked ground beef, mint, lemon juice, cloves, and remaining ½ teaspoon cinnamon. Serve warm.

Serving Suggestion

Serve with Classic Roast Chicken (page 224), Grain-Free Tabbouleh (page 176), and Smoky Artichoke Baba Ghanoush (page 275) for a traditional Middle Eastern meal.

Store & Reheat

Once cool, store in a sealed glass container in the refrigerator for up to 3 days or in the freezer for up to 3 months. Reheat in a skillet over medium heat until warm.

Change It Up

Use 2 teaspoons of dried oregano in place of the 2 tablespoons of mint, or use ⅛ teaspoon of ground mace in place of the cloves.

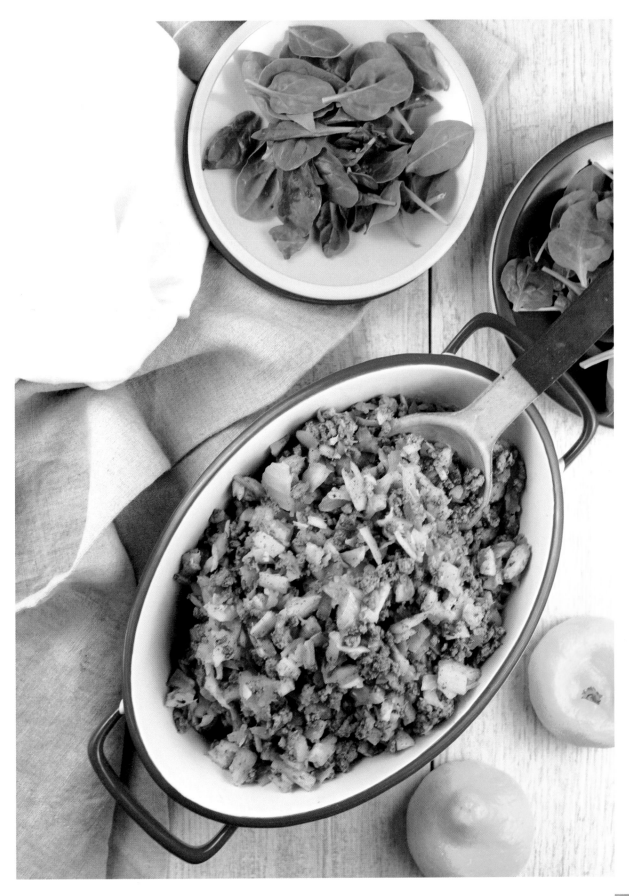

garlic-rubbed tostones

Serves 4 | Prep Time: 5 minutes | Cook Time: 15 minutes | Total Time: 20 minutes

2 green plantains

¼ cup coconut oil

1 large clove garlic, sliced in half

¼ teaspoon fine sea salt

1 recipe Cilantro Chimichurri (page 116), for serving (optional)

Make Ahead

The plantains can be sliced up to 24 hours in advance and stored in a sealed glass container in the refrigerator until ready to use.

Store & Reheat

Once cool, store in a sealed glass container in the refrigerator for up to 5 days. Reheat in a skillet greased with coconut oil over medium heat. Alternatively, place on a rimmed baking sheet under a low broil until warm.

1. Slice each plantain peel lengthwise from tip to tip without cutting into the fruit. Remove the peel by peeling it back with your fingers. Slice the plantains crosswise, on the diagonal, into 1½-inch-wide pieces.

2. Heat the coconut oil in a large, deep skillet over medium-high heat. Working in two batches to avoid overcrowding the pan, fry the plantains until golden brown, about 2 to 3 minutes per side. The centers will not be cooked through. Remove the plantains to a large cutting board with a slotted spoon.

3. Smash the plantains by pressing them with the flat bottom of a heavy glass to create ⅓-inch-thick tostones.

4. Return the tostones to the skillet to fry for 1 minute per side until crispy and golden. Transfer to a serving dish.

5. Rub the tostones with the sliced garlic clove. Sprinkle with the salt and serve immediately with Cilantro Chimichurri, if desired.

creamy herb mushrooms

Serves 4 | Prep Time: 5 minutes | Cook Time: 20 minutes | Total Time: 25 minutes

1 tablespoon coconut oil

24 ounces sliced mushrooms

1 cup sliced red onions

1 tablespoon finely chopped fresh rosemary

1½ teaspoons finely chopped fresh thyme

½ teaspoon fine sea salt

½ cup full-fat coconut milk or coconut cream

1 tablespoon balsamic vinegar

1 teaspoon dried parsley

1. Heat the coconut oil in a large sauté pan over medium-high heat. Add the mushrooms and onions and cook, stirring occasionally, for 10 minutes until the onions have softened and the mushrooms have decreased in size by half.

2. Stir the chopped herbs and salt into the vegetables. Cook uncovered to allow the liquid to evaporate. Once evaporated, stir in the coconut milk and vinegar, reduce the heat to medium, and cook for several minutes longer until thickened.

3. Remove from the heat and sprinkle with the parsley. Serve warm.

Serving Suggestions

Serve with Garlic & Rosemary Crusted Pork Loin (page 208) or Bacon-Date Crusted Salmon (page 230).

Store & Reheat

Once cool, store in a sealed glass container in the refrigerator for up to 3 days. Reheat in a saucepan over low heat until warm.

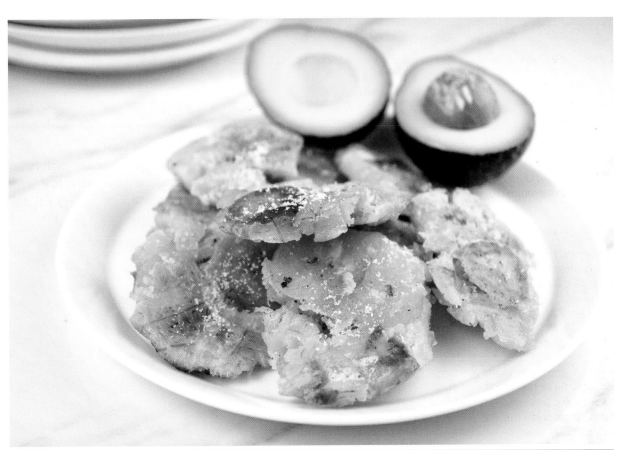

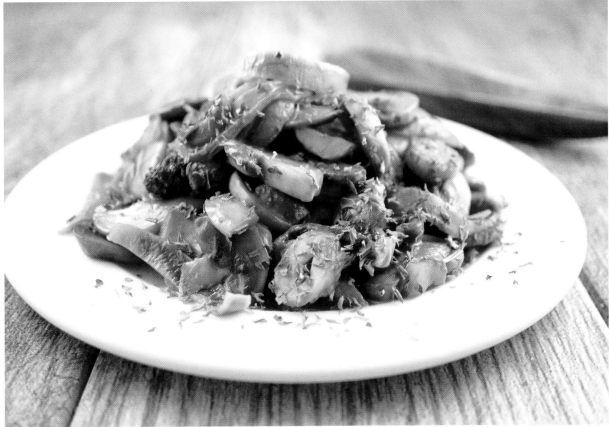

creamy bacon scalloped sweet potatoes

Serves 4 to 6 | Prep Time: 10 minutes | Cook Time: 40 minutes | Total Time: 50 minutes

2 pounds orange sweet potatoes
(about 3 medium)

6 slices bacon

2 cups chopped yellow onions

⅔ cup coconut cream

½ teaspoon garlic powder

½ teaspoon fine sea salt

1 teaspoon arrowroot starch

1 tablespoon cold water

1 tablespoon nutritional yeast

Make Ahead

*Prepare the recipe through Step 6
and store covered in the refrigerator
for up to 24 hours. Before baking,
drizzle 2 additional tablespoons
of coconut cream on top of the
potatoes to moisten them.*

Store & Reheat

*Once cool, store in a sealed glass
container in the refrigerator for up
to 5 days or in the freezer for up to 6
months. Reheat in a covered glass or
ceramic dish in a 350-degree oven
until just warm.*

1. Preheat the oven to 350 degrees.

2. Peel the sweet potatoes and cut them into ¼-inch-thick rounds. Place the potatoes in a large lidded pot, cover with salted water, and bring to a boil. Cook for 5 minutes until tender but not falling apart. Gently drain in a colander and let cool while you prepare the remaining ingredients.

3. In a large skillet over medium heat, cook the bacon until very crispy, being careful not to burn it. Transfer the bacon to a cutting board, leaving the fat in the skillet. Let the bacon cool for several minutes, then finely chop or crumble it into small pieces.

4. In the same skillet over medium heat, sauté the onions in the bacon fat for 6 to 8 minutes, until softened, fragrant, and golden brown. Add the coconut cream and bring to a low boil. Stir in the garlic powder and salt.

5. In a small bowl, whisk together the arrowroot starch and cold water to form a paste. Remove the skillet from the heat and quickly stir in the arrowroot paste until the onion mixture thickens and begins to look cheesy. Stir in the nutritional yeast.

6. Begin assembling the dish by layering half of the sweet potatoes on the bottom of a deep 8 by 8-inch glass casserole dish. Sprinkle half the crumbled bacon on top of the potatoes, then spoon half of the onion mixture evenly on top of the bacon. Repeat this step once more, using up the remaining ingredients and ending with a layer of onion mixture.

7. Bake uncovered for 20 minutes, then broil on high for 2 to 3 minutes, until bubbly. Serve warm.

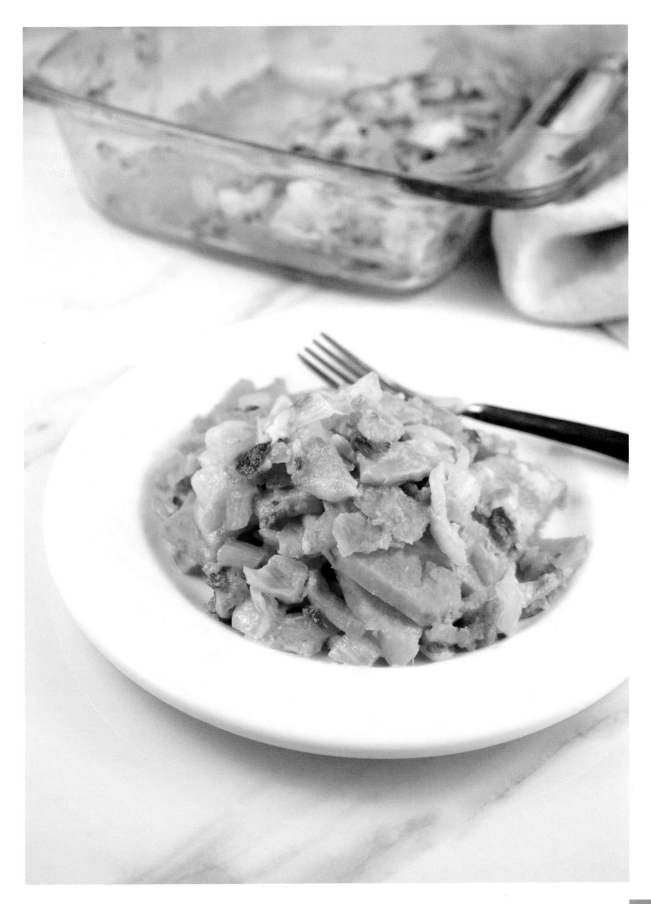

garlic-dill parsnip fries

Serves 4
Prep Time: 10 minutes
Cook Time: 25 minutes
Total Time: 35 minutes

1½ pounds parsnips

1 tablespoon extra-virgin olive oil

3 cloves garlic, pressed

1 teaspoon dried dill weed

½ teaspoon fine sea salt

¼ teaspoon garlic powder

Store & Reheat
Once cool, store in a sealed glass container in the refrigerator for up to 1 week. Reheat under a low broil until warm.

bacon five-spice sweet potato fries

Serves 4 to 6
Prep Time: 10 minutes
Cook Time: 25 minutes
Total Time: 35 minutes

2 pounds orange sweet potatoes (about 3 medium)

2 tablespoons bacon fat, melted

2 teaspoons Five-Spice Powder (page 123)

½ teaspoon fine sea salt

seasoned plantain fries

Serves 4
Prep Time: 10 minutes
Cook Time: 25 minutes
Total Time: 35 minutes

2 large green plantains

1 tablespoon extra-virgin olive oil

2 teaspoons House Rub (page 122)

1. Preheat the oven to 425 degrees. Line a rimmed baking sheet with parchment paper or grease it lightly.

2. Peel and slice the parsnips, sweet potatoes, or plantains into even fry-shape pieces about 3 inches long and ½ inch wide.

3. In a large bowl, toss the fries with the remaining ingredients until well coated. Spread the fries on the prepared baking sheet, making sure they do not overlap.

4. Bake for 25 minutes or until golden brown and crispy, flipping the fries halfway through cooking.

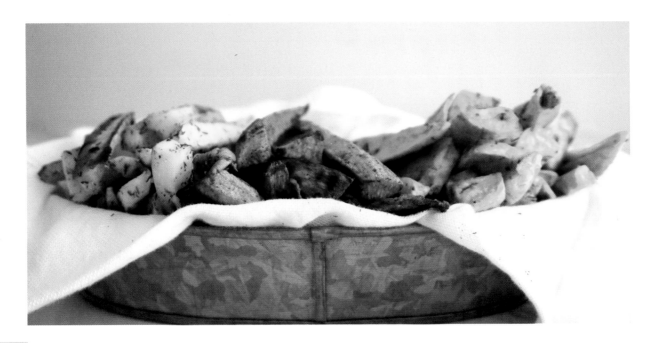

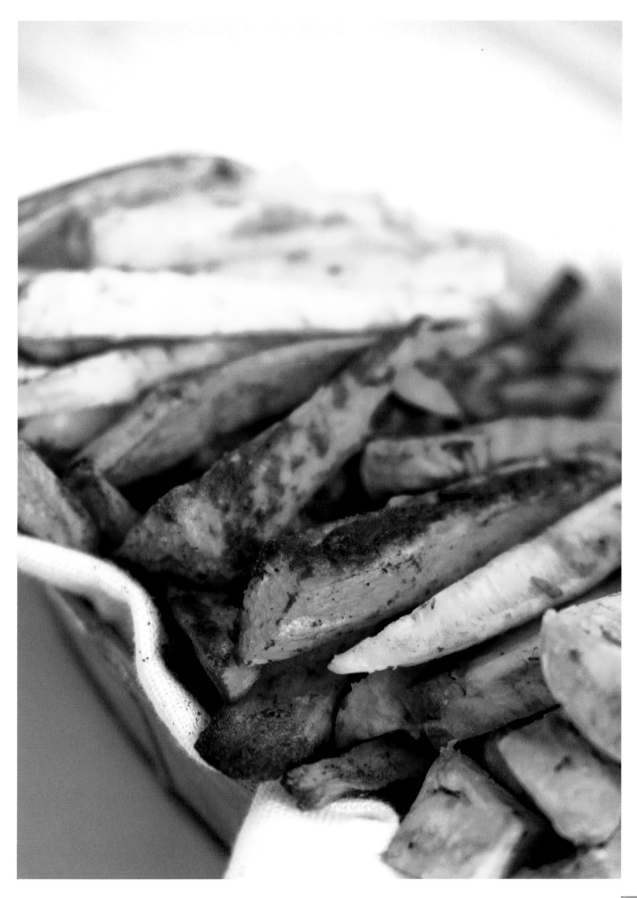

roasted brussels with bacon & cinnamon

Serves 4 | Prep Time: 7 minutes | Cook Time: 30 minutes | Total Time: 37 minutes

1 pound Brussels sprouts, halved lengthwise

1 tablespoon extra-virgin olive oil

½ teaspoon ground cinnamon

½ teaspoon fine sea salt

4 slices bacon

¼ cup raisins

1 teaspoon balsamic vinegar

Store & Reheat
Once cool, store in a sealed glass container in the refrigerator for up to 5 days or in the freezer for up to 3 months. Reheat in a skillet over medium heat until warm and crispy.

1. Preheat the oven to 400 degrees. Line a rimmed baking sheet with parchment paper.

2. In a medium bowl, toss the Brussels sprouts with the olive oil, cinnamon, and salt.

3. Roast for 25 minutes or until golden brown and crispy on the edges, stirring halfway through cooking. Add the raisins and roast for 5 minutes.

4. Meanwhile, in a skillet over medium heat, cook the bacon until crispy. Transfer to a cutting board and chop into ½-inch pieces.

5. Sprinkle the balsamic vinegar on the roasted Brussels sprouts and toss with the bacon. Serve warm.

Chicken, Bacon & Brussels Bowl. Add 2 cups of shredded cooked chicken breast to the pan at the same time as the raisins. Increase the balsamic vinegar to 2 teaspoons and serve warm as a two-person entree.

Roasted Chicken Thighs with Bacon & Brussels. On the same baking sheet with the Brussels sprouts if there is room, roast 1 pound of boneless, skinless chicken thighs sprinkled with ½ teaspoon of sea salt and ½ teaspoon of ground cinnamon. Remove the thighs from the pan after 25 minutes and let them rest while you add the raisins and finish cooking the vegetables as directed above.

cinnamon mashed carrots

Serves 4 | Prep Time: 3 minutes | Cook Time: 30 minutes | Total Time: 33 minutes

2 pounds baby carrots or slender carrots cut into 2-inch lengths

2 tablespoons coconut oil

1 teaspoon ground cinnamon

½ teaspoon fine sea salt

¼ teaspoon ground mace

¼ teaspoon dried rubbed sage

Store & Reheat
Once cool, store in a sealed glass container in the refrigerator for up to 1 week or in the freezer for up to 6 months. Reheat in a saucepan over medium-low heat until warm.

1. Place the carrots in a medium saucepan and add water to cover. Bring to a boil over medium-high heat with the lid slightly ajar. Reduce the heat to medium-low to maintain a low boil and cook for 20 to 25 minutes, until the carrots are tender and can be easily pierced with a fork.

2. Drain the water from the saucepan and transfer the carrots to a blender or food processor with the remaining ingredients. Blend until pureed, scraping down the sides of the bowl as needed. Serve warm.

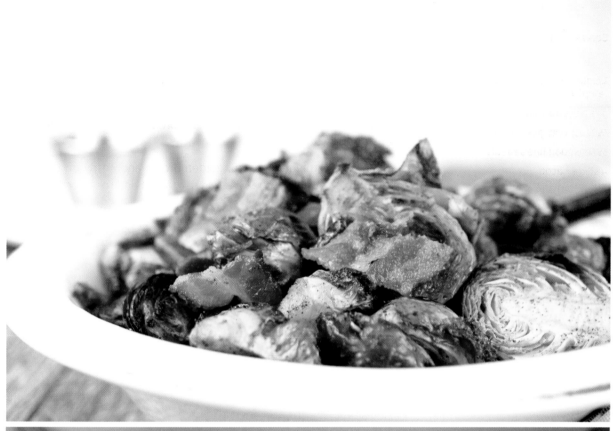

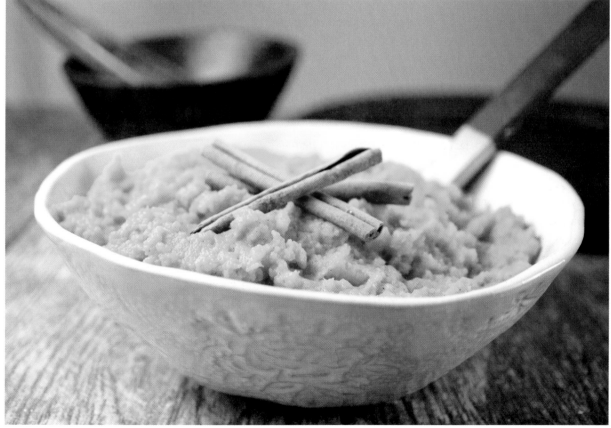

spicy african kale

Serves 4 | Prep Time: 10 minutes | Cook Time: 30 minutes | Total Time: 40 minutes

1 tablespoon coconut oil

1 cup diced onions

2 cloves garlic, minced

2 tablespoons minced fresh ginger

1 cup full-fat coconut milk

½ teaspoon Five-Spice Powder (page 123)

2 bunches curly kale, chopped (see Tip)

Tip

Curly kale is the best type of kale for this recipe because the sauce adheres to it better than it does to flatter-leafed varieties, such as lacinato.

Store & Reheat

Once cool, store in a sealed glass container in the refrigerator for up to 1 week or in the freezer for up to 3 months. Reheat in a saucepan or skillet over medium heat until warm.

1. Heat the coconut oil in a large saucepan over medium heat. Add the onions, garlic, and ginger and sauté until the onions are translucent and softened.

2. Pour the coconut milk and seasoning into the saucepan. Add the kale, cover with a lid, and cook on medium-low heat for 20 to 25 minutes, stirring halfway through cooking, until the kale is tender and wilted.

Spiced Chicken & Kale. While the kale is cooking, season 2 pounds of bone-in or boneless chicken thighs with 1 teaspoon of ginger powder, ½ teaspoon of fine sea salt, and ¼ teaspoon of ground cinnamon. Bake in a 350-degree oven for 20 to 25 minutes, until the chicken is cooked through and the juices run clear. Serve on top of the kale.

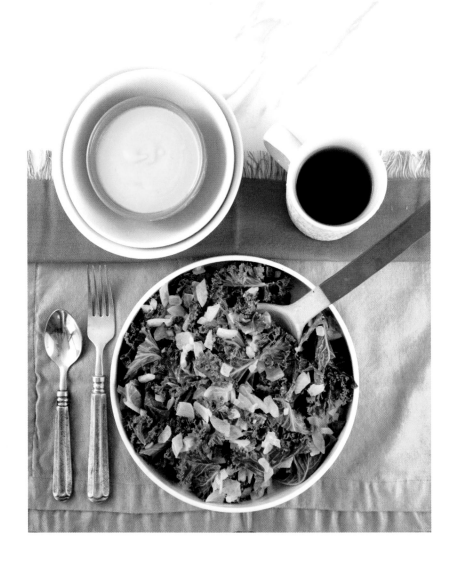

roasted sweet potatoes with tapenade

Serves 4 | Prep Time: 5 minutes | Cook Time: 30 minutes | Total Time: 35 minutes

6 cups peeled and ½-inch-diced orange sweet potatoes (about 2½ pounds)

1 tablespoon extra-virgin olive oil

1 recipe Orange & Olive Tapenade (page 276)

Make Ahead

Prepare the recipe through Step 2. When ready to serve, proceed with Step 3.

Store & Reheat

Once cool, store in a sealed glass container in the refrigerator for up to 4 days or in the freezer for up to 3 months. To reheat, warm in a 350-degree oven.

1. Preheat the oven to 400 degrees. Line a rimmed baking sheet with parchment paper.

2. Place the sweet potatoes on the prepared baking sheet and toss in the olive oil until evenly coated. Roast for 25 minutes, tossing the potatoes halfway through cooking. Remove from the oven.

3. Combine the roasted sweet potatoes and tapenade on the baking sheet and bake for an additional 5 minutes. Serve warm.

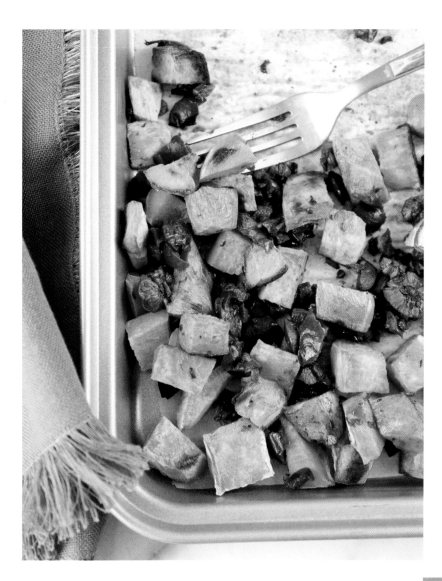

silky potato puree

Serves 6 | Prep Time: 5 minutes | Cook Time: 10 to 15 minutes | Total Time: 15 to 20 minutes

2 pounds white sweet potatoes
(about 3 medium)

1½ cups Beef Broth (page 109)

½ teaspoon fine sea salt

Serving Suggestions
Serve with Classic Roast Chicken
(page 224), Beef & Mushroom Risotto
(page 198), Bacon-Date Crusted
Salmon (page 230), or Caramelized
Onion & Herb Meatloaf (page 191).

Store & Reheat
Once cool, store in a sealed glass
container in the refrigerator for up
to 1 week or in the freezer for up to 6
months. Reheat in a small saucepan
over medium-low heat until warm,
adding extra broth if needed to thin
the puree.

1. Peel the sweet potatoes and chop them into 1-inch pieces.

2. Place the sweet potatoes and broth in the insert of a pressure cooker (see Tip, page 108), seal the lid, and cook for 10 minutes, until the potatoes can be easily broken apart with a fork. Alternatively, you can steam the potatoes by placing them in a steamer basket over a pot filled with the broth. Bring to a low boil, cover with a lid, and let the sweet potatoes steam-cook for 15 minutes until very tender.

3. In a food processor or blender, puree the cooked sweet potatoes with the broth and salt on high speed until silky smooth, at least 30 to 45 seconds.

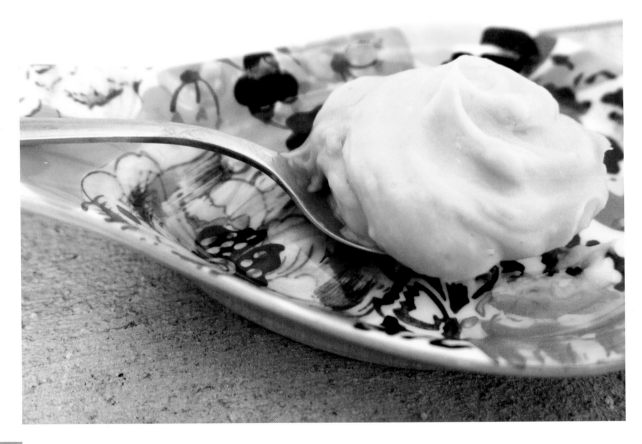

bacon-wrapped cinnamon apples

Makes 18 to 20 pieces | Prep Time: 10 minutes | Cook Time: 28 minutes | Total Time: 38 minutes

2 apples, any variety

1 teaspoon ground cinnamon

6 or 7 slices bacon

1 teaspoon chopped fresh thyme or
½ teaspoon dried thyme leaves

Make Ahead

Prepare the recipe through Step 3. Cover the baking sheet with foil or plastic wrap and store in the refrigerator for up to 1 day before baking and serving.

Store & Reheat

Once cool, store in a sealed glass container in the refrigerator for up to 5 days. Reheat under a low broil until warm.

1. Place an oven rack in the center of the oven and preheat the oven to 350 degrees. Line a rimmed baking sheet with parchment paper.

2. Core the apples and cut them into ½-inch-thick slices. Place the apples in a bowl and toss with the cinnamon to coat.

3. Cut the bacon slices crosswise into thirds. Wrap a bacon piece around each apple slice and place seam side down on the prepared baking sheet.

4. Bake for 23 to 25 minutes, then broil on high for 3 minutes until the bacon is golden brown. Sprinkle with the thyme.

5. Let cool for several minutes before serving. If serving as a party appetizer, secure with toothpicks.

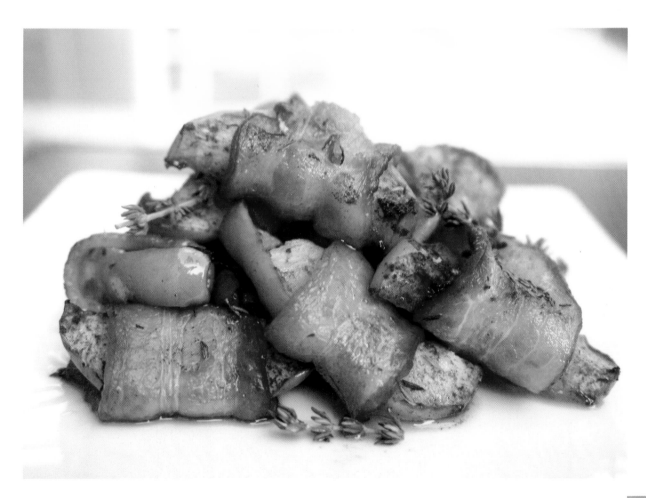

roasted roots with garlic sauce

Serves 4 | Prep Time: 8 minutes | Cook Time: 35 minutes | Total Time: 43 minutes

6 large carrots

4 large parsnips, peeled

2½ tablespoons Garlic Sauce (page 106), divided

¼ teaspoon fine sea salt

Make Ahead
Cut the root vegetables up to 5 days in advance and store in a plastic bag in the refrigerator.

Store & Reheat
Once cool, store in a sealed glass container in the refrigerator for up to 1 week or in the freezer for up to 3 months. Reheat on a rimmed baking sheet under the broiler until warm.

1. Preheat the oven to 425 degrees. Line a rimmed baking sheet with parchment paper.

2. Cut the carrots and parsnips into fry-shape pieces about 2 inches long by ¾ inch wide. Place on the prepared baking sheet and toss with 2 tablespoons of the Garlic Sauce until evenly coated.

3. Roast for 35 minutes or until golden brown, tossing halfway through cooking. Remove from the oven and use tongs to toss the roasted roots in the remaining ½ tablespoon of Garlic Sauce and salt before serving.

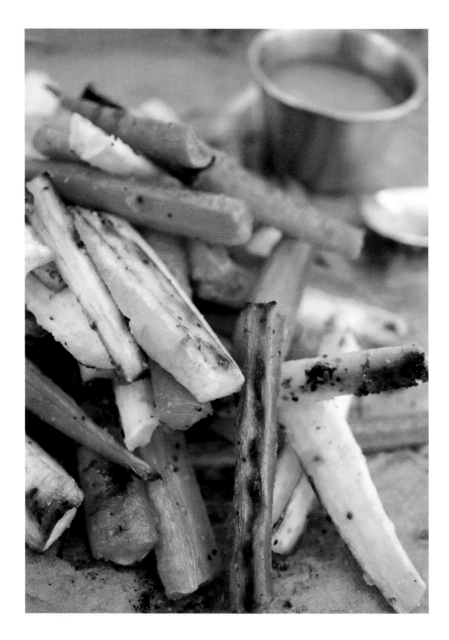

chinese stir-fried lettuce

Serves 2 to 3 | Prep Time: 5 minutes | Cook Time: 6 minutes | Total Time: 11 minutes

2 tablespoons coconut oil

2 romaine hearts, thinly sliced

2 tablespoons coconut aminos

½ teaspoon fish sauce

¼ teaspoon garlic powder

Serving Suggestion
Serve with Teriyaki Chicken & Fried Rice (page 220).

Store & Reheat
Once cool, store in a sealed glass container in the refrigerator for up to 4 days. Reheat in a greased skillet over medium heat until warm.

1. Heat the coconut oil in a large skillet over medium-high heat. Add the lettuce and stir-fry until crisp-tender, about 5 minutes.

2. Meanwhile, whisk together the coconut aminos, fish sauce, and garlic powder in a small bowl. Add to the skillet, reduce the heat to medium, and toss with the stir-fried lettuce for 1 minute. Serve immediately.

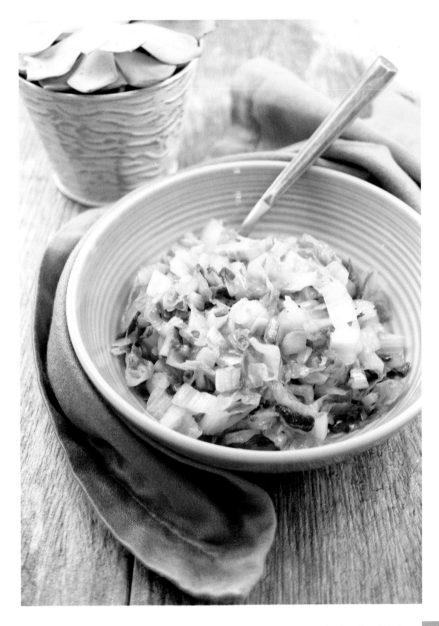

pan-roasted cauliflower with bacon & spinach

Serves 3 | Prep Time: 5 minutes | Cook Time: 30 minutes | Total Time: 35 minutes

4 slices bacon, chopped

⅔ cup sliced leeks (see Tip, page 154)

1 head cauliflower (about 1½ pounds)

1 tablespoon extra-virgin olive oil

3 cloves garlic, pressed

½ teaspoon fine sea salt, divided

3 ounces spinach

2 teaspoons fresh lemon juice

Store & Reheat

Once cool, store in a sealed glass container in the refrigerator for up to 3 days. Reheat in a skillet over medium-high heat until warm and crispy.

1. Preheat the oven to 375 degrees. Place the bacon and leeks in a large, deep, oven-safe skillet over medium heat and cook until the bacon is crispy and the leeks have softened, about 8 minutes.

2. Meanwhile, core the cauliflower and chop it into bite-size florets. Add the florets to the skillet and drizzle with the olive oil. Stir in the garlic and ¼ teaspoon of the salt and cook for 5 minutes, until the cauliflower begins to brown lightly.

3. Transfer the skillet to the preheated oven and roast for 12 to 15 minutes, until the cauliflower is cooked through and softened.

4. Remove the skillet from the oven and gently stir in the remaining ¼ teaspoon of salt and the spinach, stirring continuously until the spinach has wilted. The cauliflower will break up slightly. Sprinkle with the lemon juice and serve immediately.

Roasted Cauliflower Salad. Serve the dish slightly cooled over a large spring mix salad with a chopped avocado and Honey Balsamic Dressing (page 110).

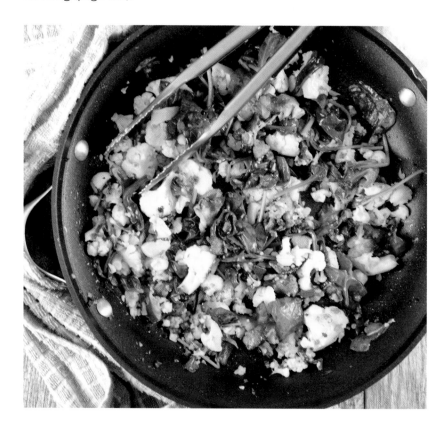

roasted cabbage
with balsamic-honey reduction ⑤ or less

Serves 4 | Prep Time: 7 minutes | Cook Time: 25 minutes | Total Time: 32 minutes

1 head green cabbage (about 2 pounds)

2 tablespoons extra-virgin olive oil

½ cup balsamic vinegar, divided

½ teaspoon dried dill weed

½ teaspoon fine sea salt

1 tablespoon honey

Serving Suggestions
Serve with Honey-Garlic Drumsticks (page 218), Bacon-Date Crusted Salmon (page 230), or Classic American Hamburgers (page 200).

Store & Reheat
Once cool, store in a sealed glass container in the refrigerator for up to 4 days. Reheat under a high broil until just warm and crispy. Drizzle with another batch of balsamic-honey reduction, if desired.

1. Preheat the oven to 450 degrees. Line a rimmed baking sheet with parchment paper.

2. Slice the cabbage through the core and stem into ½-inch-thick wedges. Place the wedges on the prepared baking sheet.

3. In a small bowl, whisk together the olive oil, 1 tablespoon of the balsamic vinegar, dill, and salt. Brush the mixture on the top of cabbage using a pastry brush or basting brush.

4. Roast for 20 to 25 minutes, until the cabbage is golden brown and tender.

5. Meanwhile, reduce the remaining balsamic vinegar in a small saucepan over medium heat until it turns into a syrup and just 1 tablespoon remains. This step will take anywhere from 7 to 12 minutes. Pour into a small bowl and whisk in the honey.

6. Drizzle the balsamic-honey reduction over the roasted cabbage and serve immediately.

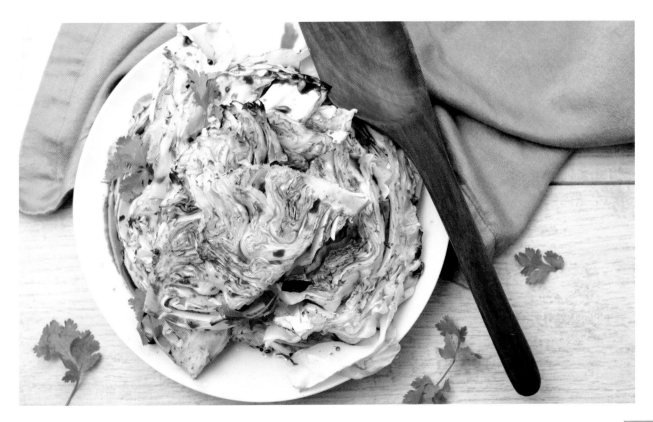

garlic roasted broccoli

Serves 3 to 4 | Prep Time: 5 minutes | Cook Time: 25 minutes | Total Time: 30 minutes

1 large head broccoli (about 2 pounds), cut into florets

3 tablespoons extra-virgin olive oil

4 cloves garlic, minced

1 tablespoon grated lemon zest

½ teaspoon fine sea salt

1½ teaspoons fresh lemon juice

1. Position an oven rack in the second-highest position and preheat the oven to 425 degrees. Line a large rimmed baking sheet with parchment paper.

2. On the prepared baking sheet, toss the broccoli with the olive oil, garlic, lemon zest, and salt and spread evenly.

3. Roast for 23 to 25 minutes, without disturbing, until crisp and browned. Sprinkle with the lemon juice and serve warm.

Serving Suggestions
Serve with Wild Salmon with Roasted Raspberries (page 234), Bacon-Date Crusted Salmon (page 230), Classic Roast Chicken (page 224), or Anti-Inflammatory Meatballs (page 194).

Store & Reheat
Once cool, store in a sealed glass container in the refrigerator for up to 5 days. Reheat under a low broil for a few minutes or gently sauté in additional olive oil over medium heat until warm.

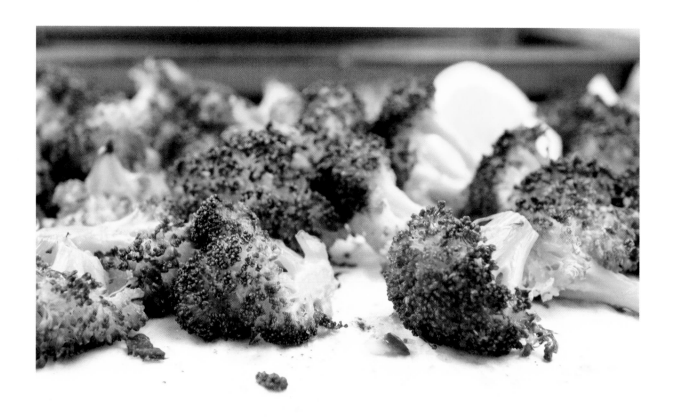

gingered asparagus

Serves 4 | Prep Time: 5 minutes | Cook Time: 15 minutes | Total Time: 20 minutes

1½ pounds asparagus, trimmed

¼ cup coconut aminos

2 tablespoons extra-virgin olive oil

2 teaspoons fish sauce

2 teaspoons ginger powder

4 cloves garlic, minced

½ teaspoon grated fresh ginger

1. Position an oven rack in the second-highest position and preheat the oven to 425 degrees. Line a rimmed baking sheet with parchment paper. Spread out the asparagus on the prepared baking sheet.

2. In a small bowl, whisk together the coconut aminos, olive oil, fish sauce, and ginger powder. Reserve 1 tablespoon of the sauce mixture and toss the asparagus with the rest of the sauce until evenly coated. Sprinkle with the garlic.

3. Roast for 15 minutes or until crisp-tender, making sure not to overcook or the asparagus will become soft and stringy.

4. Remove from the oven and toss with the remaining sauce and the grated ginger. Serve immediately.

Serving Suggestions
Serve with Speedy Shanghai Stir-fry (page 209), Wild Salmon with Roasted Raspberries (page 234), or Teriyaki Chicken & Fried Rice (page 220).

Store & Reheat
Once cool, store in a sealed glass container in the refrigerator for up to 3 days. Reheat under a low broil for a few minutes until warm.

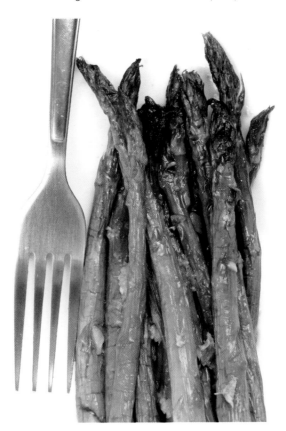

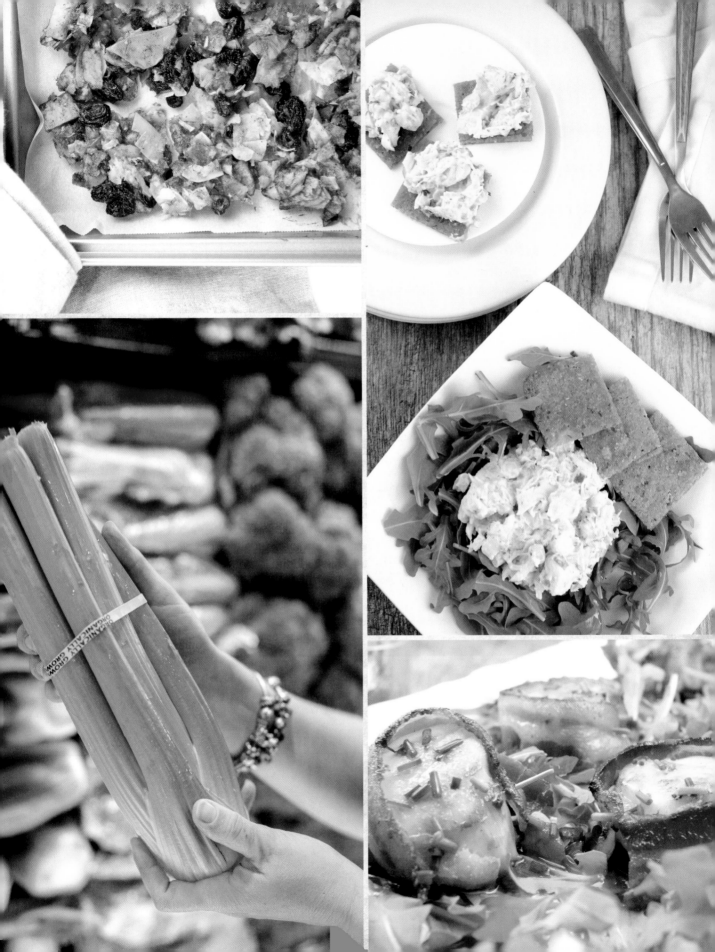

chewy trail mix granola

Serves 4 | Prep Time: 5 minutes | Cook Time: 1 hour | Total Time: 1 hour 5 minutes

2 tablespoons coconut oil

1 banana

1 cup unsweetened coconut flakes

1 cup plantain chips, chopped

½ cup chopped dried mango

⅓ cup raisins

1 teaspoon vanilla extract

½ teaspoon ground cinnamon

¼ teaspoon fine sea salt

1. Preheat the oven to 300 degrees. Line a small rimmed baking sheet with parchment paper.

2. Puree the coconut oil and banana in a blender. Alternatively, mash by hand until smooth.

3. Stir in the remaining ingredients. Spoon onto the prepared baking sheet and spread with a spatula into a layer about ¾ inch thick.

4. Bake for 55 to 60 minutes, depending on the desired texture. For a moist and chewy granola, bake for a shorter time. Let cool completely before serving.

Storage
Once cool, store in a sealed glass container in the refrigerator for up to 5 days.

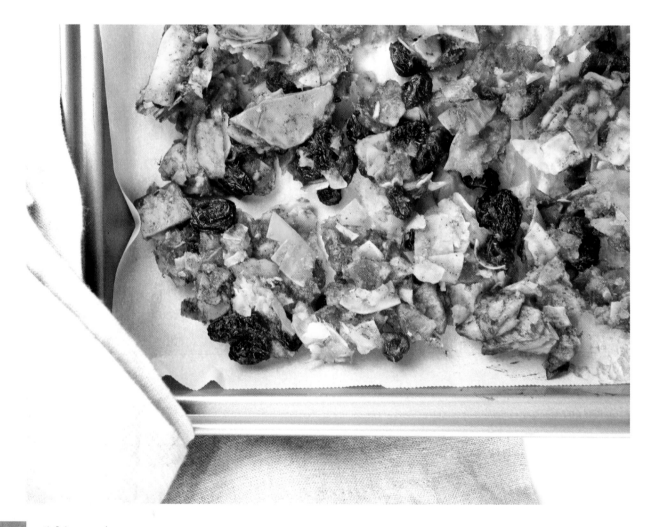

crunchy kale'nola

Serves 4 | Prep Time: 15 minutes | Cook Time: 35 minutes | Total Time: 50 minutes

1 large bunch curly kale

6 large soft Medjool dates, pitted

2 tablespoons coconut oil, melted

1 tablespoon blackstrap molasses

1 teaspoon ground cinnamon

¼ teaspoon ginger powder

¼ teaspoon fine sea salt

1 cup unsweetened coconut flakes

⅓ cup raisins

Make Ahead

Prepare the kale leaves as directed in Step 2 up to 4 days in advance and store wrapped in paper towels or a dish cloth in a sealed plastic bag in the refrigerator until ready to use.

Storage

Once cool, store in a covered glass container or sealed plastic bag at room temperature for up to 2 days.

1. Preheat the oven to 300 degrees. Line a rimmed baking sheet with parchment paper.

2. Use a knife to remove the kale stems from the leaves, then use scissors to cut the leaves into 1-inch pieces. Dry the kale in a salad spinner if you have just washed it, or it will not crisp up in the oven.

3. Soak the dates in a small bowl of just-boiled water until softened, about 10 minutes, or microwave in a bowl of water for 1 minute. Drain the water and use a fork to mash the dates with the coconut oil into a paste. Stir in the molasses, cinnamon, ginger, and salt.

4. In a large mixing bowl, coat the kale evenly with the date mixture. Stir in the coconut flakes and raisins and ensure that they are well coated.

5. Spread the kale'nola on the prepared baking sheet and bake for 15 minutes. Stir and bake for an additional 15 to 20 minutes, until the kale is crispy and the coconut is golden brown.

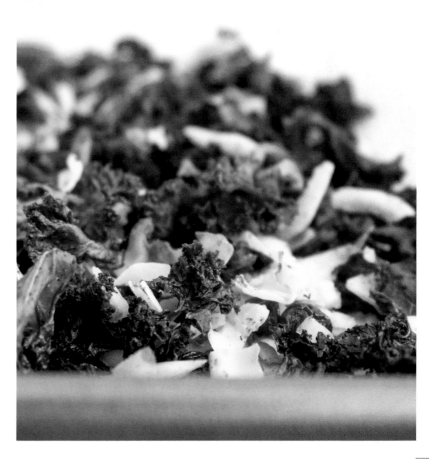

turkey jerky ⑤ 🍲

Serves 4 | Prep Time: 10 minutes | Cook Time: 4½ hours | Total Time: 4 hours 40 minutes

1 pound ground turkey

1 teaspoon fish sauce

1 teaspoon onion powder

1 teaspoon fine sea salt

½ teaspoon garlic powder

½ teaspoon dried rubbed sage

Make Ahead

Mix together all the ingredients and refrigerate overnight in a covered bowl.

Storage

The jerky must be completely cool prior to storing or moisture will build up and cause the jerky to spoil. Wrap in paper towels and store in a sealed plastic bag or glass container in the refrigerator for up to 3 weeks, or freeze for up to 6 months.

1. Preheat the oven to 170 degrees. Line a rimmed baking sheet with parchment paper.

2. Mix all the ingredients together in a large bowl. Spoon the mixture onto the prepared baking sheet and lay another sheet of parchment paper on top. Using your hands, smooth the mixture into a thin, even layer about ⅛ inch thick. Take your time to ensure uniformity, or the jerky will cook unevenly. Remove the top layer of parchment.

3. Place the baking sheet in the oven and put a wooden spoon in the oven door to keep the door slightly ajar. This will allow moisture to escape the oven for the driest jerky. Bake for 2½ to 3 hours, until the top is browned and tough. Flip over the entire sheet of jerky, leaving the parchment paper on top, and cook the underside for an additional 1 to 1½ hours, until the jerky is dried to your preference.

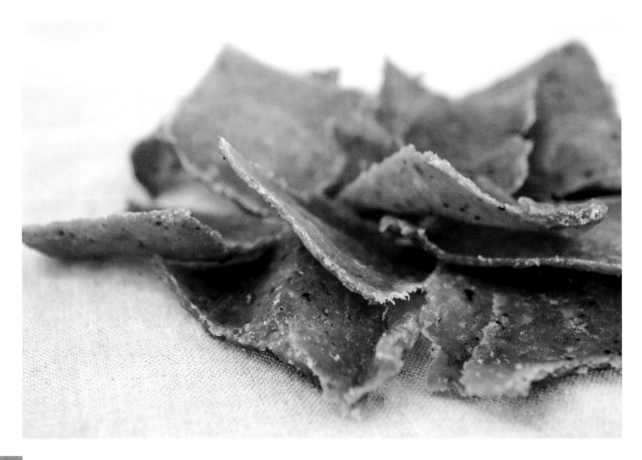

pulled pork sliders

Makes 8 to 10 sliders | Prep Time: 5 minutes | Total Time: 5 minutes

1 recipe Garlic-Rubbed Tostones (page 248; see Tip)

1 small avocado, quartered and thickly sliced

¾ cup BBQ Pulled Pork (page 206), warmed

Lime wedges, for serving

Tip
These sliders are best when the tostones have just been prepared.

Top the warm tostones with a slice of avocado and 1 to 2 tablespoons of pulled pork. Serve warm or at room temperature as a hearty appetizer or light meal, with lime wedges on the side.

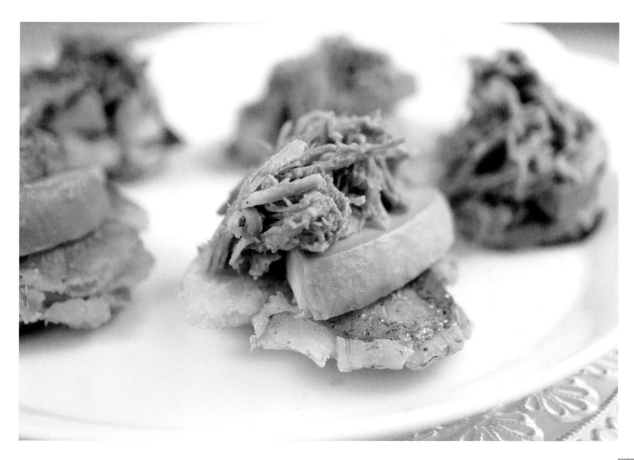

bacon-wrapped scallops with lemon-chive drizzle

Serves 5 | Prep Time: 10 minutes | Cook Time: 14 minutes | Total Time: 24 minutes

10 large sea scallops

5 slices bacon, sliced in half widthwise

½ teaspoon truffle salt (see Tip, page 122) or fine sea salt

LEMON-CHIVE DRIZZLE

2 tablespoons extra-virgin olive oil

1 tablespoon minced fresh chives

1 teaspoon lemon juice

1 teaspoon grated lemon zest

¼ teaspoon balsamic vinegar

Make Ahead

Make the Lemon-Chive Drizzle up to 3 days in advance and store in a sealed glass container in the refrigerator.

Store & Reheat

Once cool, store in a sealed glass container in the refrigerator for up to 2 days. Reheat in a skillet over medium heat until warm and crispy.

1. Rinse the scallops and dry well by patting with a paper towel. Set aside.

2. Par-cook the bacon by laying the half-slices in a large skillet over medium heat. Cook for 3 to 4 minutes per side until the bacon is partially cooked with golden brown edges but still pliable enough to wrap around the scallops. Transfer to a paper towel–lined plate until cool enough to handle. Leave the bacon fat in the skillet.

3. Sprinkle the scallops on all sides with the truffle salt.

4. Wrap a half-slice of bacon around each scallop and secure with one or two toothpicks. It's okay if it doesn't wrap around the full circumference of the scallop. Sear the scallops in the same bacon-greased skillet over medium-high heat for 3 minutes per side until golden brown and opaque throughout. Do not crowd the pan; cook in batches if needed.

5. Meanwhile, prepare the Lemon-Chive Drizzle by whisking together the olive oil, chives, lemon juice and zest, and vinegar. Drizzle over the seared scallops and serve immediately.

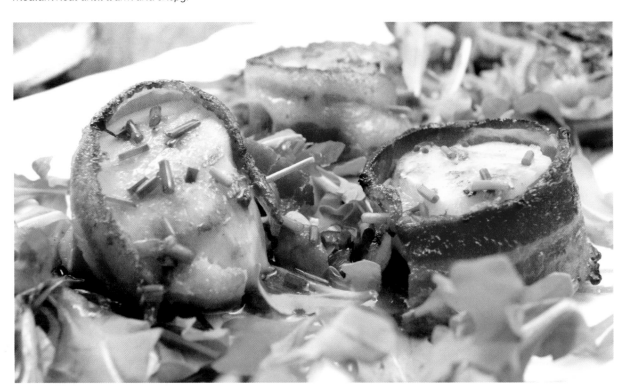

lox & everything hors d'oeuvre

Makes 12 pieces | Prep Time: 10 minutes | Cook Time: 30 minutes | Total Time: 40 minutes + 10 minutes to cool

ONION-DILL "CREAM CHEESE"

½ cup palm shortening

1 tablespoon melted coconut oil

1 teaspoon apple cider vinegar

¼ teaspoon fine sea salt

⅛ teaspoon dried dill weed

⅛ teaspoon onion powder

EVERYTHING SWEET POTATOES

1 pound white sweet potatoes

1 tablespoon melted coconut oil

1 teaspoon garlic powder

1 teaspoon onion powder

1 teaspoon dried oregano leaves

½ teaspoon dried basil

½ teaspoon fine sea salt

4 ounces lox or smoked salmon, chopped

Fresh dill, for serving

1. To make the "cream cheese": Whisk all the ingredients together in a bowl until well combined. Place in the refrigerator to set while you prepare the sweet potatoes.

2. Preheat the oven to 375 degrees. Line a rimmed baking sheet with parchment paper. Peel the sweet potatoes and slice them into ½-inch-thick rounds.

3. In a bowl, toss the sweet potato rounds with the melted coconut oil, garlic powder, onion powder, oregano, basil, and salt. Lay the potatoes on the prepared baking sheet in a single layer and bake for 30 minutes or until golden brown, flipping them halfway through cooking. Remove from the oven and let cool for 10 minutes.

4. To assemble, top each sweet potato round with a layer of lox, a dollop of "cream cheese," and a few pieces of fresh dill.

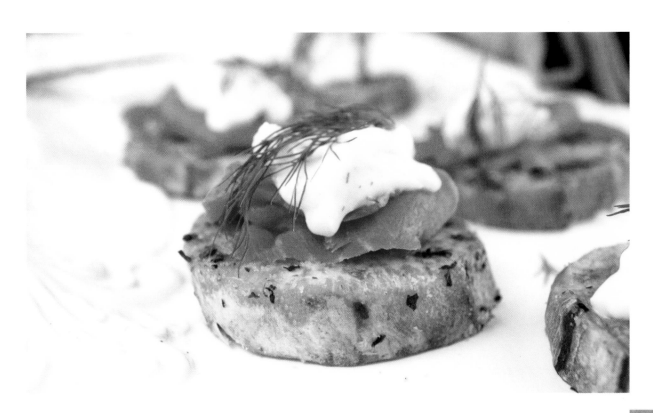

roasted garlic & pumpkin hummus

Makes 1½ cups | Prep Time: 8 minutes | Total Time: 8 minutes

1 cup canned pumpkin puree

½ cup mashed sweet potato

½ cup Roasted Garlic (page 107) or store-bought roasted garlic

2 tablespoons fresh lemon juice

½ teaspoon fine sea salt

¼ teaspoon onion powder

¼ cup extra-virgin olive oil

1. Place all the ingredients except the olive oil in a blender or food processor and blend until combined, about 30 seconds.

2. With the machine running, slowly pour in the olive oil until fully incorporated. Spoon the hummus into a serving dish and refrigerate until ready to serve.

Make Ahead
Prepare the mashed sweet potato up to 3 days in advance and store in the refrigerator until ready to use.

Storage
Store in a sealed glass container in the refrigerator for up to 3 days.

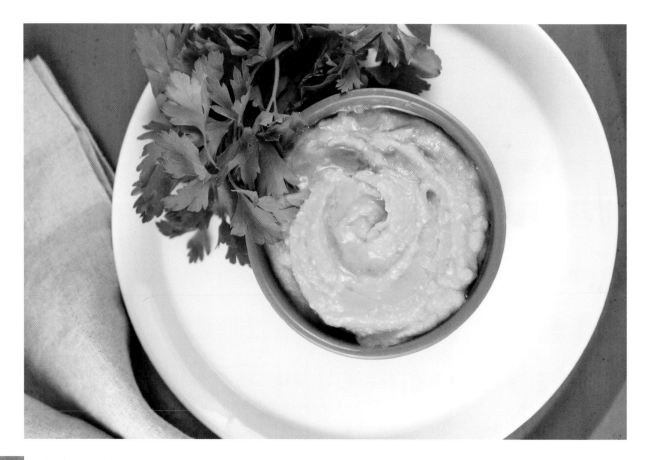

smoky artichoke baba ghanoush

Makes 1 cup | Prep Time: 7 minutes | Total Time: 7 minutes

1 (14-ounce) can artichoke hearts, drained

¼ cup extra-virgin olive oil

1½ tablespoons fresh lemon juice

2 large cloves garlic

¾ teaspoon smoked sea salt

Place all the ingredients in a blender or food processor and puree until smooth, about 1 minute.

Serving Suggestions

Serve with Classic Roast Chicken (page 224), Lebanese Beef & Rice Stuffing (page 246), and Grain-Free Tabbouleh (page 176) for a Middle Eastern feast. Or serve as part of a Greek meze appetizer plate with Orange & Olive Tapenade (page 276), Roasted Garlic & Pumpkin Hummus (opposite), plantain chips, cucumber slices, baby carrots, and olives.

Storage

Store in a sealed glass container in the refrigerator for up to 5 days.

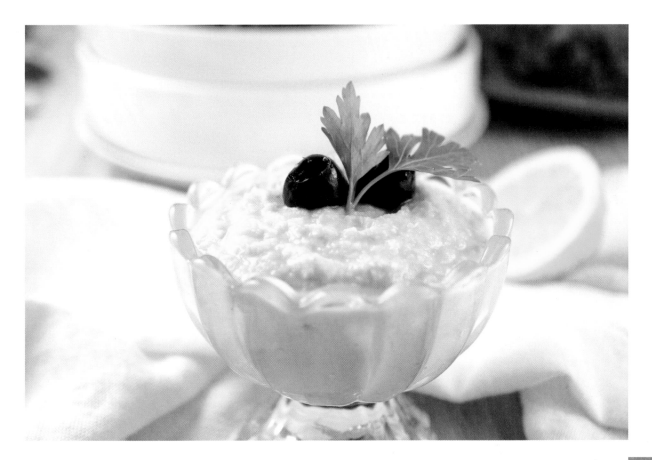

orange & olive tapenade

Makes 1 cup | Prep Time: 8 minutes | Total Time: 8 minutes

1 (6-ounce) can pitted black olives, drained

4 large Medjool dates, pitted

1 tablespoon fresh orange juice

1 teaspoon grated orange zest

1 teaspoon fresh thyme leaves

1 teaspoon balsamic vinegar

Place all the ingredients in a food processor and pulse until the desired texture is reached.

Serving Suggestions
Serve with plantain chips or as an accompaniment to Classic Roast Chicken (page 224).

Storage
Store in a sealed glass container in the refrigerator for up to 3 days.

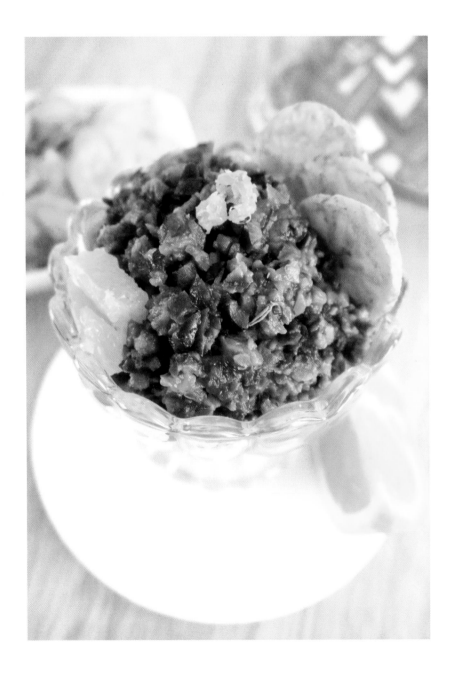

smoked salmon spread

Serves 2 to 4 | Prep Time: 10 minutes | Total Time: 10 minutes

1 (6-ounce) can wild-caught salmon, drained

4 ounces smoked salmon

2 tablespoons extra-virgin olive oil

2 tablespoons chopped fresh dill

2 tablespoons drained capers

1 tablespoon fresh lemon juice

1 teaspoon grated horseradish (optional)

Sliced cucumber or plantain chips, for serving

Make Ahead
The spread can be made up to 3 days in advance of serving.

Storage
Store in a sealed glass container in the refrigerator for up to 4 days. Do not freeze.

Place all the ingredients in a food processor and pulse until smooth. Serve with cucumber slices or plantain chips.

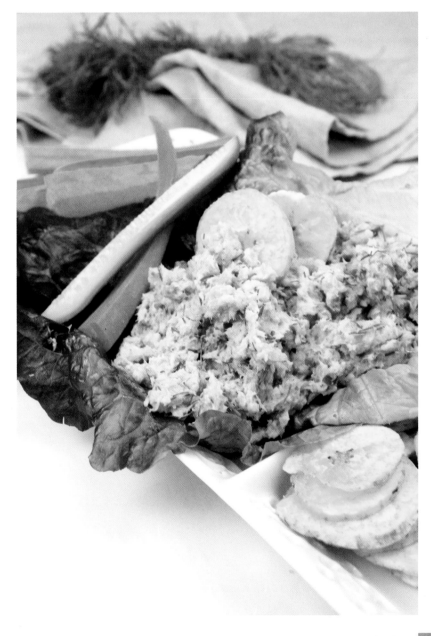

cherry balsamic pâté

Serves 4 to 6 | Prep Time: 5 minutes | Cook Time: 10 minutes | Total Time: 15 minutes + 2 hours to set

4 tablespoons coconut oil, divided

¾ pound chicken livers, rinsed and patted dry

1 (10-ounce) bag frozen cherries, thawed

1 teaspoon dried thyme leaves

1 teaspoon fine sea salt

1 tablespoon balsamic vinegar

1 recipe Garlic & Thyme Crackers (opposite) or slices of fruit, such as apple, peach, or nectarine, for serving

Storage
Once cool, store in a sealed glass container in the refrigerator for up to 4 days or in the freezer for up to 3 months.

1. Heat 2 tablespoons of the coconut oil in a large skillet over medium-high heat. Add the chicken livers and toss in the oil. Cook for 2 minutes, then add the cherries, thyme, and salt. Continue cooking for 8 more minutes until the chicken livers are cooked through and the cherries have begun to burst open and release their juices.

2. Stir in the balsamic vinegar and remove from the heat. Transfer the entire contents of the skillet to a blender or food processor with the remaining 2 tablespoons of coconut oil and blend on high speed until smooth.

3. Spoon the pâté into small serving dishes and refrigerate until cool and set, about 2 hours.

4. Serve with crackers or slices of fruit.

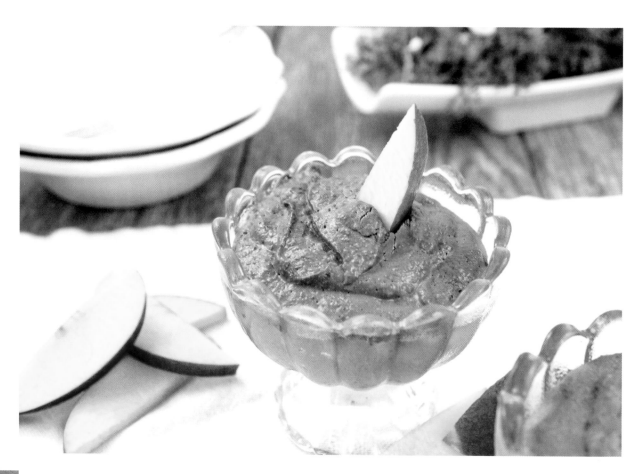

garlic & thyme crackers

Makes 12 to 15 crackers | Prep Time: 7 minutes | Cook Time: 23 minutes | Total Time: 30 minutes

1 pound green plantains (about 2 medium)

2 tablespoons extra-virgin olive oil

2 tablespoons coconut oil

3 cloves garlic, minced

1 teaspoon fresh thyme leaves

½ teaspoon fine sea salt

Storage

Once cool, store in a sealed plastic bag at room temperature for up to 3 days.

1. Preheat the oven to 400 degrees. Line a cookie sheet with parchment paper.

2. Peel and chop the plantains into large, even pieces and place in a blender or food processor. Add the oils, garlic, and thyme and puree, scraping down the sides as needed. It's okay if a few small plantain chunks remain.

3. Place the dough in the center of the prepared cookie sheet. Fold the overhanging parchment paper from the sides onto the center of the dough and use it to assist you in pressing the dough into an even ¼-inch-thick layer. Unfold the parchment paper and sprinkle the dough evenly with the salt.

4. Bake for 10 minutes, then remove from the oven and use a sharp knife or pizza cutter to score the dough in a grid pattern into 12 to 15 crackers.

5. Return to the oven for an additional 11 to 13 minutes, removing as soon as the edges begin to brown. Let cool completely before breaking apart on the scored lines. The crackers will be softer than store-bought versions.

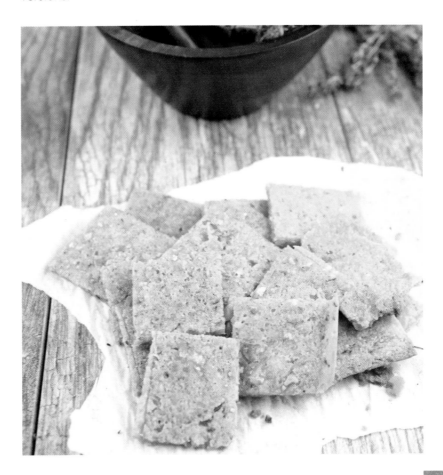

chicken ranch salad over crackers

Serves 2 | Prep Time: 5 minutes | Total Time: 5 minutes

1½ cups cooled and chopped cooked chicken

⅓ cup Garlic-Dill Ranch Dressing (page 112)

2 tablespoons minced red onion

2 tablespoons chopped green onion

1 tablespoon chopped fresh dill

¼ teaspoon fine sea salt

1 recipe Garlic & Thyme Crackers (page 279), for serving

Storage
Store the salad separate from the crackers in a sealed glass container in the refrigerator for up to 3 days.

In a medium bowl, mix together all the ingredients except the crackers. Serve the salad cold or at room temperature, with crackers, for an appetizer or a light meal.

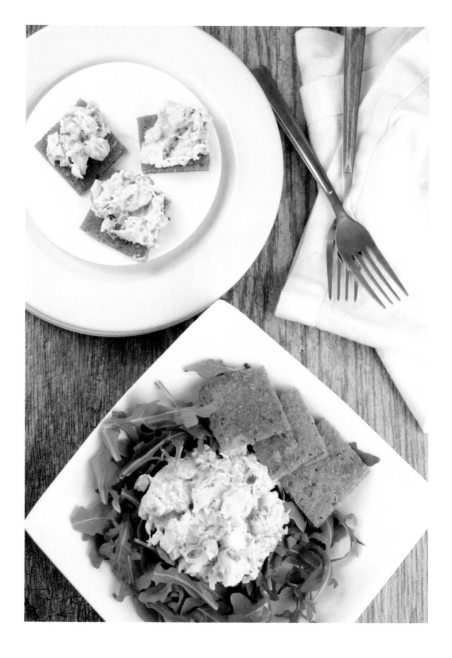

lemon-ginger energy balls

Makes 8 balls | Prep Time: 8 minutes | Total Time: 8 minutes

2 ounces crunchy apple chips (about 1 cup)

1 cup dried Turkish figs

2 tablespoons coconut oil, melted

1 teaspoon grated lemon zest

½ teaspoon ginger powder

Make Ahead
Double the recipe and store half of the balls in a freezer-safe container for up to 6 months.

Storage
Store in a sealed plastic bag or glass container in the refrigerator for up to 2 weeks.

1. Place all the ingredients in a food processor or high-powered blender and blend for 30 to 45 seconds, until the apple chips and figs are finely chopped and moistened with the coconut oil.

2. Form 8 compact balls by rolling the mixture between your palms.

3. Enjoy immediately or chill in the refrigerator before serving to allow the coconut oil to set.

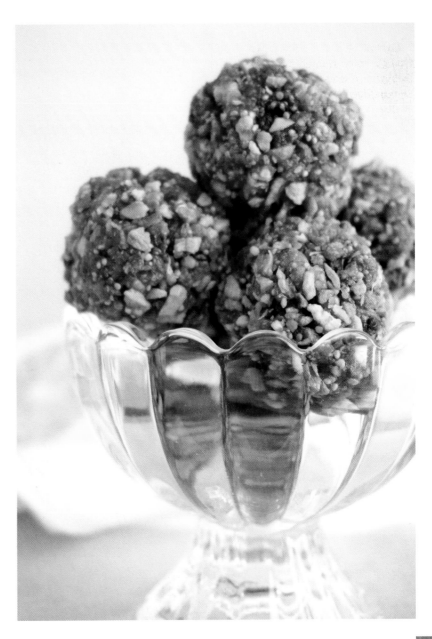

monkey bars

Makes 10 bars | Prep Time: 8 minutes | Total Time: 8 minutes + 30 minutes to set

1 cup unsweetened banana chips

1 cup unsweetened shredded coconut

⅔ cup raisins

½ teaspoon ground cinnamon

2 tablespoons coconut oil, melted

Storage

Store in a sealed glass container in the refrigerator for up to 2 weeks or in the freezer for up to 6 months. If stored in the freezer, let sit at room temperature for 5 minutes before serving.

1. Place the banana chips, coconut, raisins, and cinnamon in a food processor and process for 1½ minutes until completely broken down into a wet sand texture.

2. Add the coconut oil and process for an additional 45 seconds.

3. Place a sheet of parchment paper on a sturdy portable surface, like a cutting board. Using your hands, spread the mixture into a rectangle about 4 inches wide and 7 inches long.

4. Freeze until hardened, 20 to 30 minutes. Slice into 10 squares with a sharp knife.

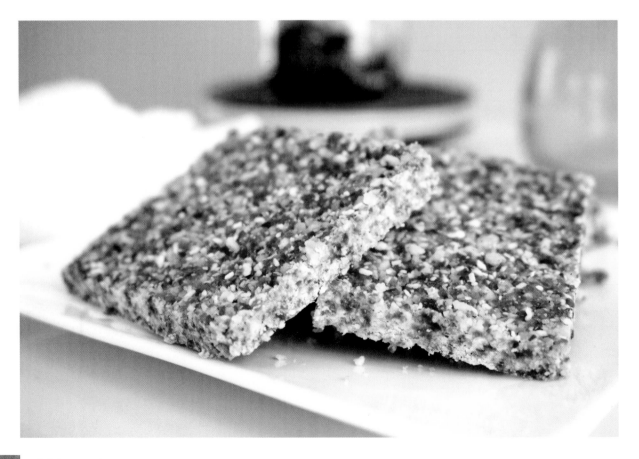

mango coconut gummies

Makes 12 gummies | Prep Time: 5 minutes | Cook Time: 10 minutes | Total Time: 15 minutes + 3 hours to set

1 (10-ounce) bag frozen diced mango

½ cup coconut water

2 tablespoons fresh lemon or lime juice

¼ cup unflavored gelatin powder

Storage
For all gummy recipes: Store the gummies in a sealed plastic bag or glass container in the refrigerator for up to 1 month.

1. In a small saucepan over medium-low heat, cook the mango until softened, about 10 minutes. Transfer to a blender.

2. Add the remaining ingredients and blend until smooth.

3. Pour into an 8-inch glass baking dish or 12 silicone molds. Refrigerate until set, about 3 hours. If a glass baking dish was used, slice into squares before serving.

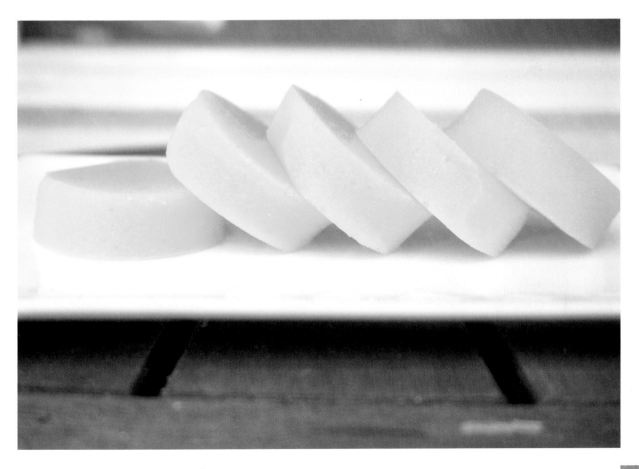

cherry lime gummies

Makes 12 gummies | Prep Time: 5 minutes | Cook Time: 10 minutes | Total Time: 15 minutes + 3 hours to set

1 (10-ounce) bag frozen cherries

¼ cup fresh lime juice

½ cup sparkling water

¼ cup unflavored gelatin powder

1. Bring the cherries and lime juice to a boil in a small saucepan over medium heat. Maintain a simmer until the cherries burst open and release their juices, 5 to 8 minutes.

2. Transfer to a blender, add the sparkling water and gelatin, and blend until smooth.

3. Pour into an 8-inch glass baking dish or 12 silicone molds. Refrigerate until set, 2 to 3 hours. If a glass baking dish was used, slice into squares before serving.

pomegranate pear gummies

Makes 12 gummies | Prep Time: 5 minutes | Cook Time: 12 minutes | Total Time: 17 minutes + 3 hours to set

1 cup pomegranate juice

1 pear, cored and chopped (leave peel on)

½ cup sparkling water

¼ cup unflavored gelatin powder

1. Place the pomegranate juice and pear in a small saucepan and bring to a boil over medium heat. Simmer for 10 minutes until the pear is tender.

2. Transfer to a blender, add the sparkling water and gelatin, and blend until smooth.

3. Pour into an 8-inch glass baking dish or 12 silicone molds. Refrigerate until set, 2 to 3 hours. If a glass baking dish was used, slice into squares before serving.

strawberry kiwi gummies

Makes 12 gummies | Prep Time: 10 minutes | Cook Time: 10 minutes | Total Time: 20 minutes + 3 hours to set

2 cups sliced strawberries (about 1½ pints)

3 kiwis, peeled and sliced

2 tablespoons fresh lemon juice

1 tablespoon honey

⅓ cup sparkling water

¼ cup unflavored gelatin powder

1. Combine the strawberries, kiwis, and lemon juice in a medium saucepan over medium-high heat. Cook for 10 minutes, stirring and mashing frequently with a wooden spoon to prevent sticking, until the fruit has cooked down to a chunky puree.

2. Stir the fruit puree and honey together until smooth. Add the sparkling water and gelatin and stir briefly until incorporated.

3. Pour into an 8-inch glass baking dish or 12 silicone molds (or more, if needed). Refrigerate until set, 2 to 3 hours. If a glass baking dish was used, slice into squares before serving.

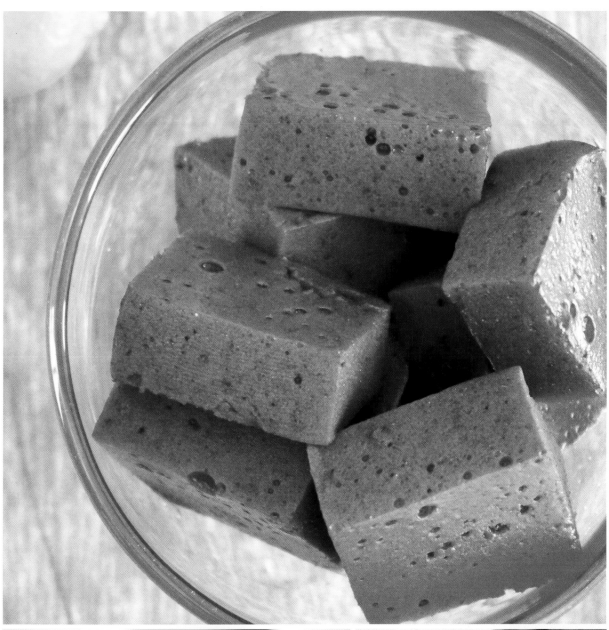

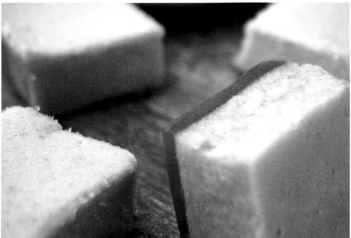

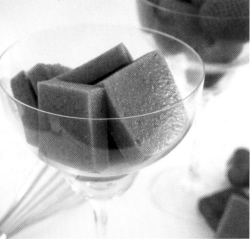

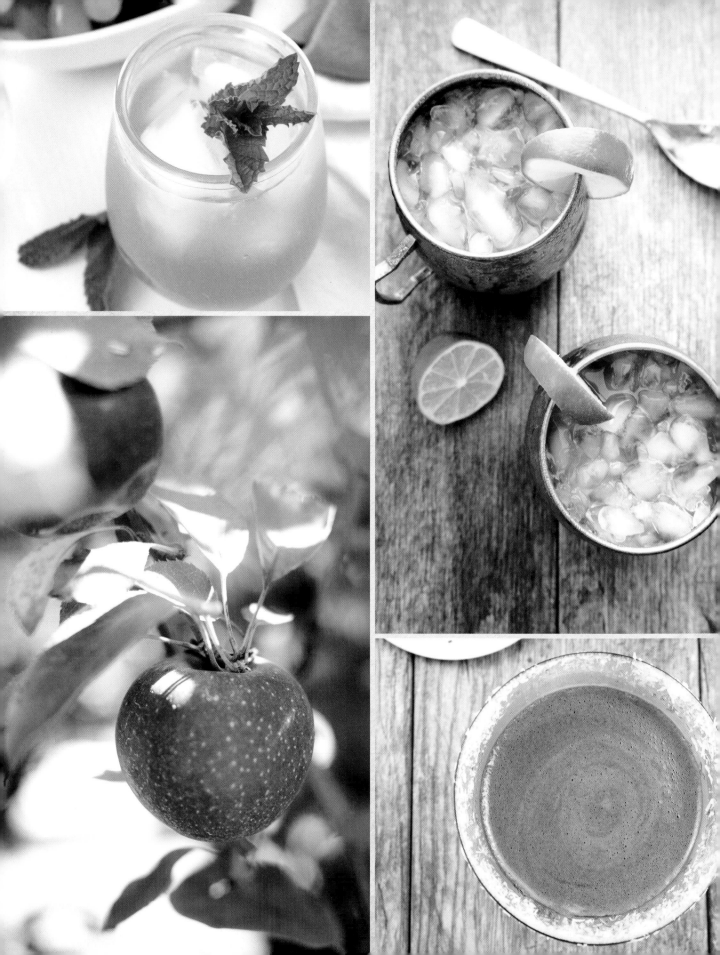

CHAPTER 11

thirst quenchers

red sangria

Serves 2 | Prep Time: 10 minutes | Total Time: 10 minutes + 8 hours to steep

1½ cups pomegranate juice

1 pear, diced

3 strips fresh orange peel

½ lemon, sliced thinly

5 whole cloves

1 cinnamon stick

1 (16-ounce) bottle unflavored kombucha, chilled

Ice, for serving (optional)

1. Combine all the ingredients except the kombucha in a large glass jar or pitcher. Place in the refrigerator to steep for 8 hours or overnight.

2. Just before serving, remove the cloves and cinnamon stick and stir in the kombucha. Serve over ice, if desired.

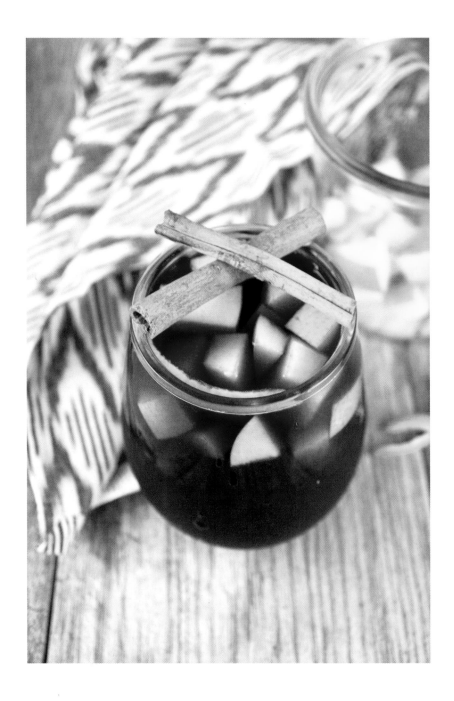

moscow mule

Serves 2 | Prep Time: 5 minutes | Total Time: 5 minutes

1 (16-ounce) bottle ginger-flavored kombucha

2 tablespoons honey

2 teaspoons fresh lime juice

½ teaspoon grated fresh ginger

Crushed ice, for serving

Make Ahead

Complete Step 1 up to 3 hours in advance. Pour over ice when ready to serve.

1. In a large glass container, stir together the kombucha, lime juice, honey, and ginger until well mixed.

2. Pour into serving glasses filled with crushed ice. Serve immediately.

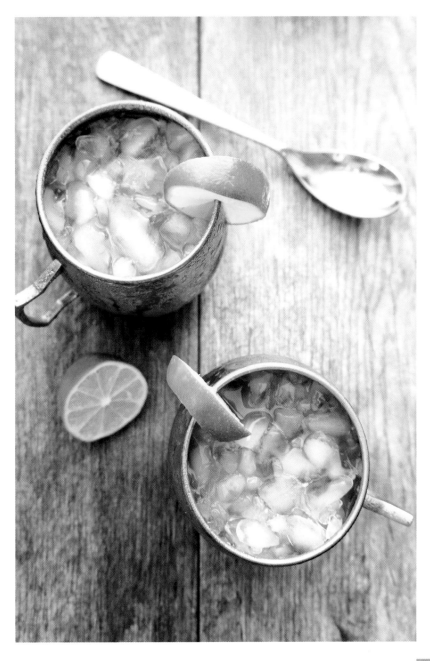

watermelon lime agua fresca

Serves 2 to 3 | Prep Time: 5 minutes | Total Time: 5 minutes

4 heaping cups chopped watermelon

½ cup water

3 tablespoons fresh lime juice

⅛ teaspoon fine sea salt

Ice, for serving

Place all the ingredients except the ice in a blender and puree. Serve immediately over ice.

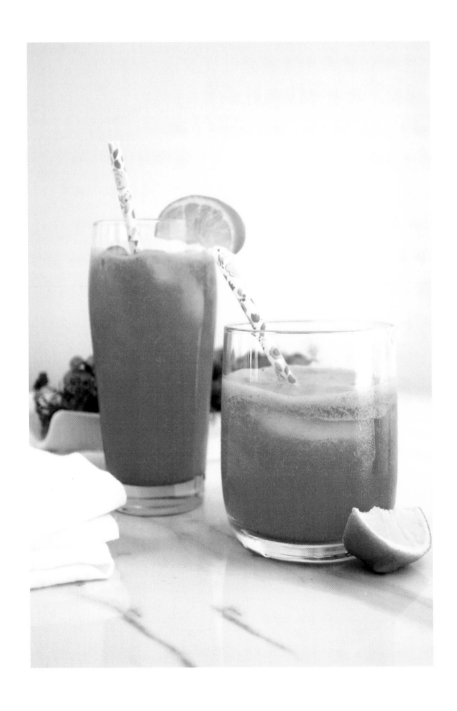

strawberry lemonade spritzer

Serves 2 | Prep Time: 5 minutes | Total Time: 5 minutes

1 cup whole strawberries, green tops removed

⅓ cup water

1 (16-ounce) bottle citrus-flavored kombucha

Ice, for serving

Lemon slices, for serving

1. In a blender, puree the strawberries with the water. Strain through a fine-mesh strainer placed over a glass measuring cup to capture ½ cup of liquid. Discard the puree.

2. Gently stir together the ½ cup of strawberry liquid and kombucha in a large glass jar. Serve at room temperature or chilled, poured over ice and garnished with lemon slices.

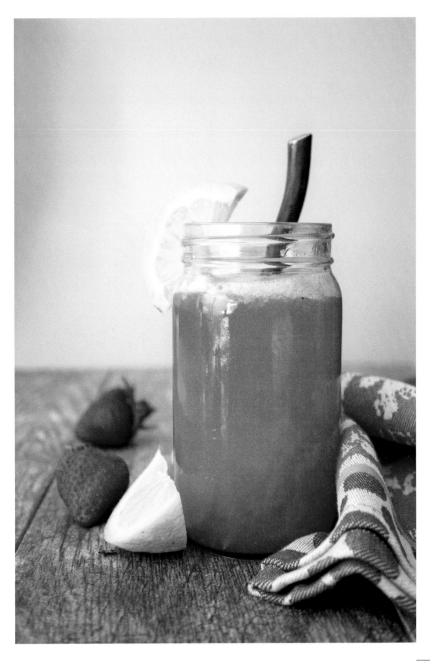

mint-ea mojito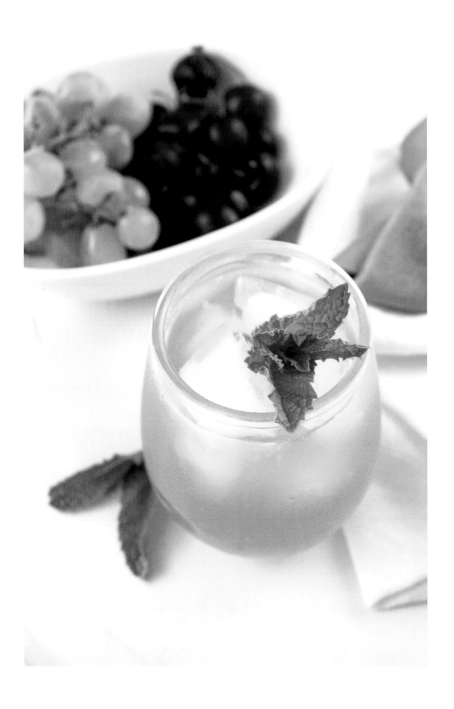

Serves 2 | Prep Time: 5 minutes | Total Time: 5 minutes + 2 hours to chill

3 cups boiling water

1 tablespoon honey

2 peppermint tea bags

Juice of 1 lime

Ice, for serving

Storage
Store the tea (without ice) in the refrigerator for up to 1 week.

1. Stir together the boiling water and honey in a large glass jar or pitcher. Add the tea bags and let steep on the countertop for 5 minutes. Place in the refrigerator (tea bags included) for about 2 hours or in the freezer for 45 minutes to 1 hour, until cold.

2. Whisk in the lime juice and pour over ice. Serve immediately.

citrus fizz

Serves 2 | Prep Time: 5 minutes | Total Time: 5 minutes

⅔ cup fresh orange juice

⅓ cup fresh grapefruit juice

1 cup unflavored kombucha or sparkling water

Mix together the juices in a large glass jar or pitcher. Stir in the kombucha, which will fizz from the carbonation, and pour into glasses.

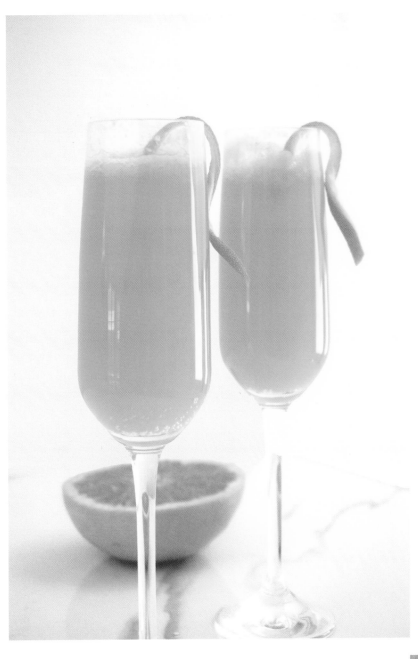

maple mocha

Serves 2 to 3 | Prep Time: 5 minutes | Cook Time: 12 minutes | Total Time: 17 minutes

2 cups full-fat coconut milk

2 cups water

4 bags roasted dandelion tea

2 tablespoons blackstrap molasses

¼ cup carob powder

2 tablespoons maple syrup

½ teaspoon ground cinnamon

⅛ teaspoon fine sea salt

1. Combine the coconut milk, water, and tea bags in a small saucepan. Bring to a boil over medium heat. Reduce the heat to medium-low and simmer covered with the lid for 8 minutes. Remove the tea bags and stir in the molasses.

2. Transfer the mixture to a blender with the remaining ingredients and blend on high speed until combined. Serve warm.

Iced Mocha. After completing Step 2, let cool to room temperature and serve over ice.

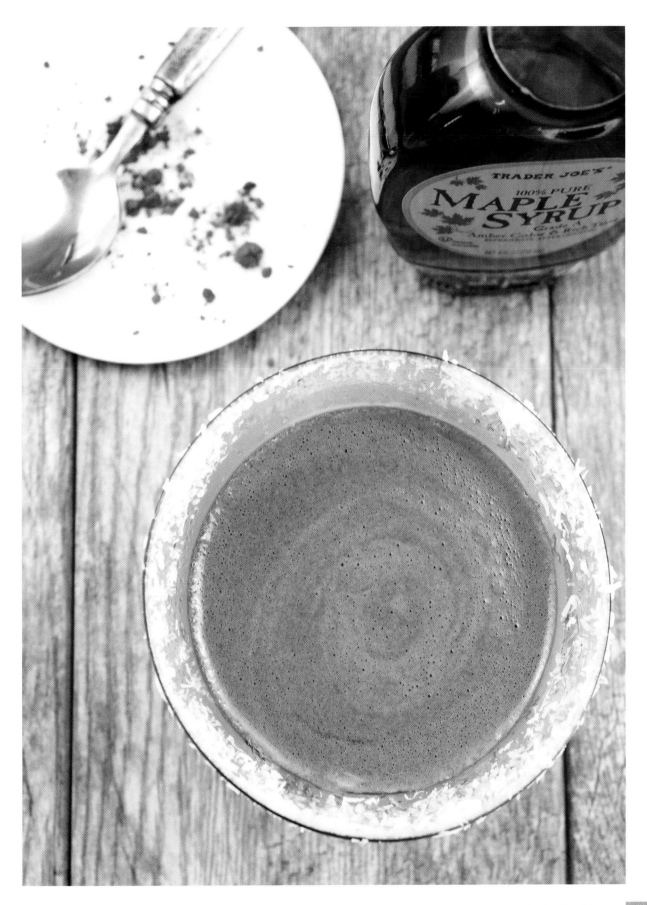

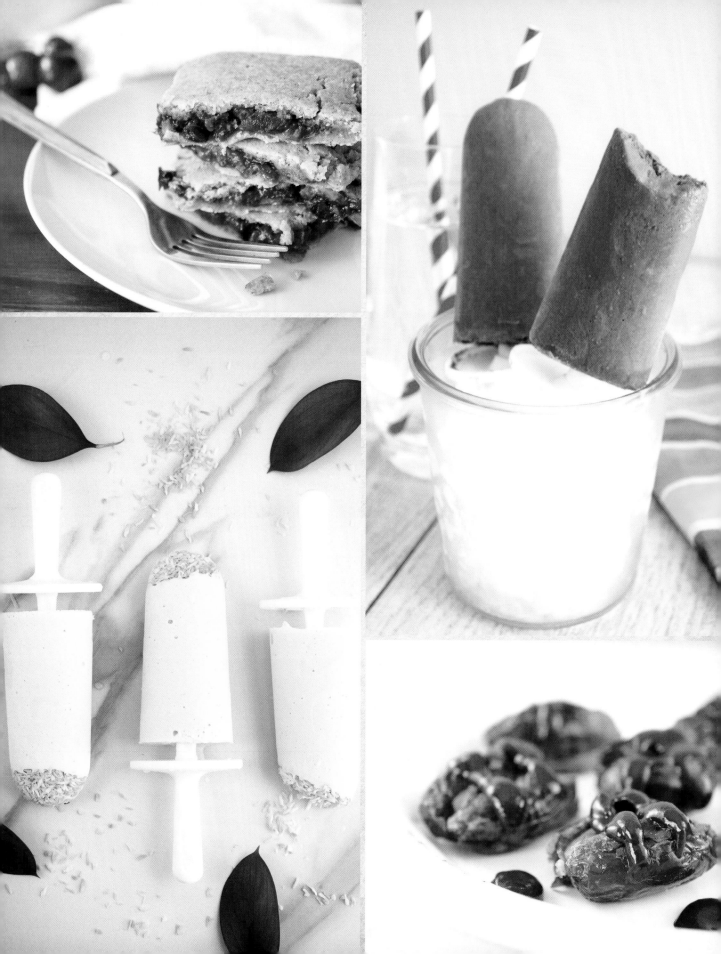

CHAPTER 12

timeless treats

ganache-stuffed dates

Makes 8 dates | Prep Time: 5 minutes | Total Time: 5 minutes + 1 hour to set

⅓ cup Hot Fudge (below), warmed

8 large Medjool dates, pitted

Storage
Store in a sealed glass container in the refrigerator for up to 1 week.

Spoon about 1½ teaspoons of hot fudge into the center of each pitted date. Place in the refrigerator for 1 hour to allow the hot fudge to set into a hardened ganache. Reserve any leftover slightly warm hot fudge to drizzle on the stuffed dates just before serving.

hot fudge & ganache

Makes 1 cup | Prep Time: 5 minutes | Cook Time: 5 minutes | Total Time: 10 minutes + 1 hour for ganache to set

6 Medjool dates, pitted

1½ cups coconut cream

½ cup carob powder

¼ cup melted coconut oil

¼ teaspoon fine sea salt

Store & Reheat
Store in a sealed glass container in the refrigerator for up to 1 month or in the freezer for up to 6 months. For hot fudge, reheat in a small saucepan over medium-low heat until it returns to a thick liquid.

1. Place the dates in a small microwave-safe bowl and cover with water. Microwave for 1 minute until very soft. Drain the water and place the dates in a blender.

2. Add the remaining ingredients to the blender and blend until very smooth, scraping down the sides as needed to ensure that the dates break down completely.

3. Transfer the mixture to a small saucepan over medium heat. Stir continuously until smooth and shiny. Remove from the heat before the fudge comes to a boil.

4. To make ganache: Pour the fudge mixture into a medium heatproof glass container and refrigerate until set, about 1 hour.

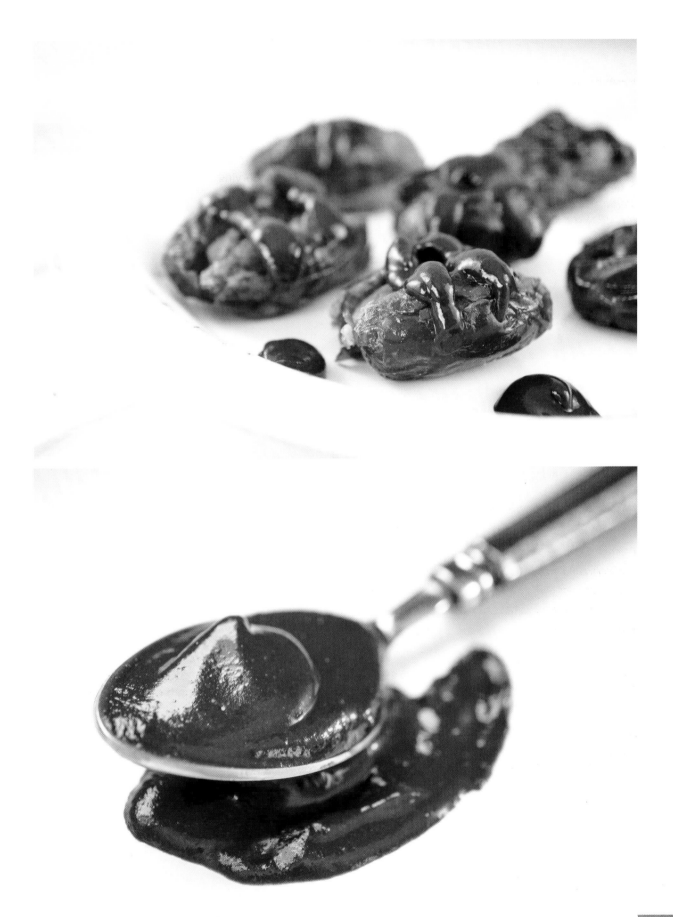

no-bake lemon macaroons

Makes 15 macaroons | Prep Time: 10 minutes | Total Time: 10 minutes + 1 hour to set

2 cups unsweetened shredded coconut

¼ cup melted coconut oil

2 tablespoons honey

1 tablespoon grated lemon zest or 10 drops lemon oil (see Tip), or more as desired

⅛ teaspoon fine sea salt

1. Place all the ingredients in a food processor and process until a large ball forms, about 30 seconds. Taste and add more lemon zest or oil if a stronger lemon flavor is desired.

2. Using firm pressure, scoop tablespoon-size macaroons onto a parchment-lined plate. Refrigerate until set, about 1 hour.

Tip
Make sure to purchase food-grade lemon oil (not extract), which can be found online. Using lemon oil in this recipe gives the macaroons a stronger lemon flavor, but lemon zest is a great easy-to-find alternative.

Storage
Store in a sealed glass container in the refrigerator for up to 2 weeks or in the freezer for up to 4 weeks.

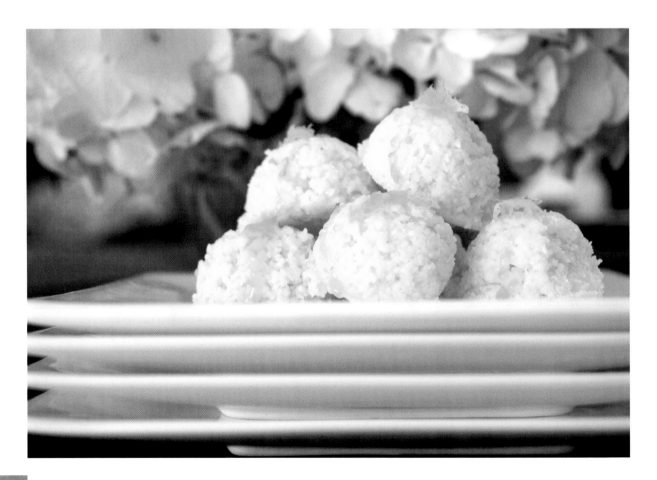

warm bananas with date caramel sauce

Serves 2 | Prep Time: 7 minutes | Cook Time: 3 minutes | Total Time: 10 minutes

CARAMEL SAUCE

¾ cup pitted Medjool dates, divided

¾ cup full-fat coconut milk, warmed

½ teaspoon vanilla extract

¼ teaspoon fine sea salt

CRUMBLE TOPPING

2 tablespoons crushed unsweetened banana chips

2 tablespoons unsweetened shredded coconut, toasted

2 medium-yellow bananas (see Tip)

1 tablespoon coconut oil

Tip
For a less-sweet dessert, use green bananas, which will not caramelize. If you prefer a sweeter treat, use fully ripe yellow bananas with some brown spots.

Make Ahead
The caramel sauce can be made up to 3 days in advance and stored covered in the refrigerator until ready to use.

Store & Reheat
Once cool, store in a sealed glass container in the refrigerator for up to 3 days. Reheat in a small saucepan over medium-low heat just until warm.

Change It Up
For a coconut-free dessert, cook the bananas in lard instead of coconut oil and use warm water in place of the coconut milk in the caramel sauce.

1. To make the sauce: Place the dates, warmed coconut milk, vanilla, and salt in a high-powered blender and blend until smooth. If you do not own a high-powered blender or your dates are not soft, soak the dates in a small bowl of just-boiled water until softened, about 10 minutes, or microwave in a bowl of water for 1 minute before blending to prevent a chunky sauce. Set aside.

2. In a small bowl, mix together the ingredients for the topping.

3. Slice the bananas lengthwise into ⅓-inch-thick planks, then crosswise into thirds to make long, flat pieces.

4. Heat the coconut oil in a medium skillet over medium heat. Add the bananas and cook for 2 minutes. Flip and cook for 1 minute to warm the undersides. Gently stir in the caramel sauce and cook for 30 seconds until the sugars have started to caramelize. Sprinkle with the crumble topping and serve immediately.

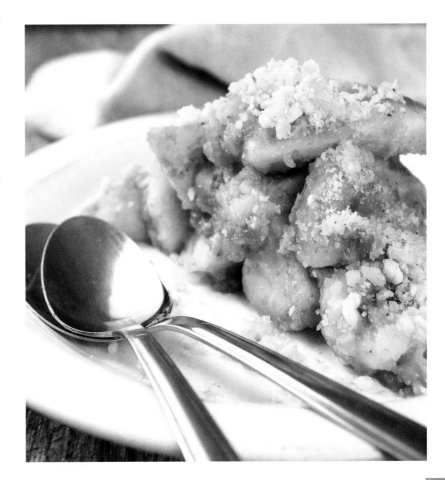

strawberry milkshake

Serves 1 to 2 | Prep Time: 5 minutes | Total Time: 5 minutes

1 (10-ounce) bag frozen strawberries

1⅓ cups full-fat coconut milk

1½ tablespoons honey

⅛ teaspoon fine sea salt

Place all the ingredients in a high-powered blender and puree until smooth. Serve immediately while still cold or refrigerate for up to 1 day before serving.

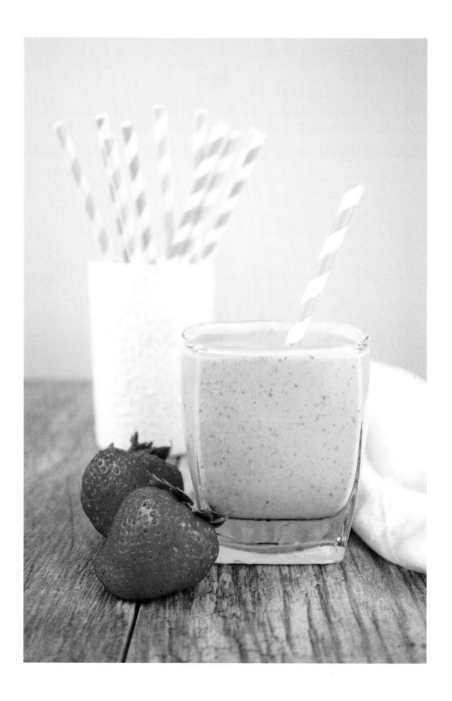

cinnamon banana ice cream

Serves 2 | Prep Time: 5 minutes | Freeze Time: 2 hours + 1 hour (optional) | Total Time: 3 hours 5 minutes

3 large bananas, sliced

½ teaspoon ground cinnamon

⅛ teaspoon fine sea salt

Serving Suggestions
Serve with Roasted Strawberries (page 321) and/or Hot Fudge (page 298). If serving with Hot Fudge, freeze the ice cream for 1 hour after blending or it will melt too quickly.

Storage
Store in a sealed glass container in the freezer for up to 1 month.

1. Place the sliced bananas on a parchment-lined plate and freeze for 2 hours or until solid.

2. Place the frozen bananas, cinnamon, and salt in a blender and blend on high speed for 30 to 60 seconds, until the mixture thickens to the texture of ice cream.

3. Serve immediately for soft-serve ice cream, or scoop into a glass container and return to the freezer for at least 1 hour for harder ice cream.

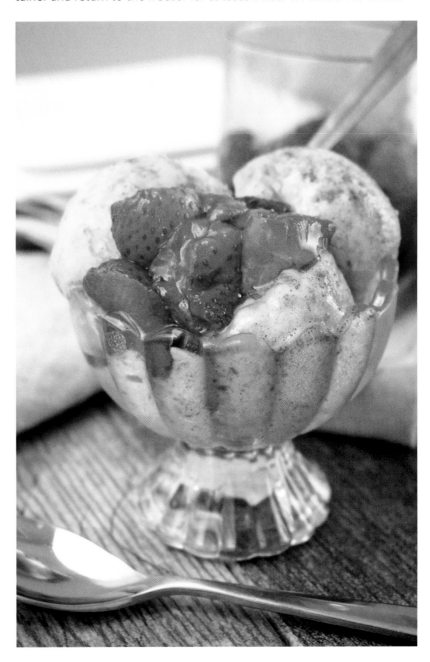

sweet potato ice cream

Serves 4 | Prep Time: 5 minutes | Freeze Time: 35 minutes or 6 hours, depending on method | Total Time: 40 minutes or 6 hours 5 minutes, depending on method

1 (13½-ounce) can full-fat coconut milk, chilled

1 cup well-mashed cooked sweet potato, chilled

½ packed cup pitted soft Medjool dates

1 tablespoon blackstrap molasses

1½ teaspoons ground cinnamon

¼ teaspoon ground mace

¼ teaspoon fine sea salt

1 teaspoon unflavored gelatin powder

Storage

Store in a sealed glass container in the freezer for up to 3 months. To serve, let sit at room temperature for 10 to 20 minutes until soft enough to scoop.

Ice cream maker instructions: Place all the ingredients in a blender and puree until smooth. Pour the mixture into an ice cream maker and follow the manufacturer's instructions for churning.

Blender instructions: Place all the ingredients in a blender and puree until smooth. Place the blender jar in the freezer for 2 hours. Remove from the freezer and scrape down the sides of the jar to release any frozen pieces. Blend for 10 to 15 seconds, until the mixture has the consistency of soft-serve ice cream. Place back in the freezer for 3 to 4 hours, until completely frozen. Before serving, defrost at room temperature until scoopable.

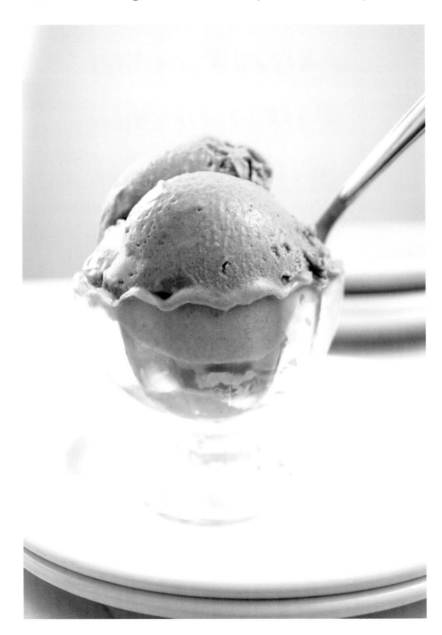

truffle fudge pops

Makes 4 pops | Prep Time: 5 minutes | Freeze Time: 6 hours | Total Time: 6 hours 5 minutes

2 cups full-fat coconut milk

¼ cup carob powder

2 tablespoons honey

1 teaspoon unflavored gelatin powder

½ teaspoon truffle salt (see Tip, page 122)

Storage
Store in the molds in the freezer for up to 2 months.

1. Place all the ingredients in a food processor or blender and blend until smooth. Pour into 4 molds and freeze until solid, 4 to 6 hours.

2. To remove the pops from the molds, run the molds briefly under warm water until the pops loosen from the sides.

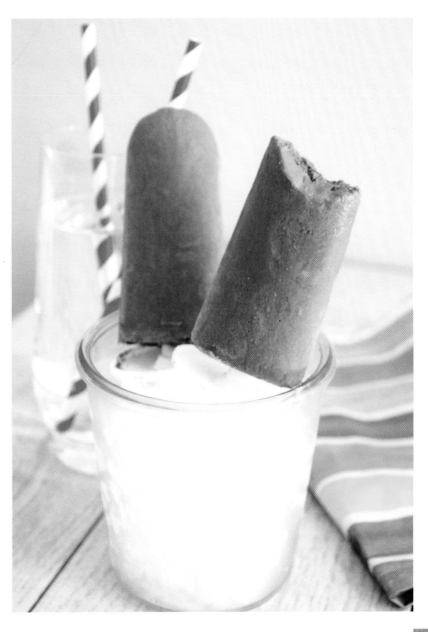

toasted coconut cream pops

Makes 4 pops | Prep Time: 5 minutes | Cook Time: 5 minutes | Freeze Time: 4 hours | Total Time: 4 hours 10 minutes

2 cups unsweetened shredded coconut

1 (14-ounce) can coconut cream (see Tip)

2 tablespoons honey

2 teaspoons unflavored gelatin powder

¼ teaspoon fine sea salt

1. Preheat the oven to 350 degrees. Lay the coconut on a rimmed baking sheet in a thin layer. Toast for 4 to 5 minutes, until very lightly browned. Watch it carefully, as coconut can burn quickly.

2. Reserve 3 tablespoons of the toasted coconut and pour the rest into a blender with the remaining ingredients. Blend for 15 seconds until a thick, slightly grainy mixture forms.

3. Pour immediately into the desired molds. The reserved toasted coconut can be added to either the top, middle, or bottom of the molds. Freeze until solid, 3 to 4 hours.

4. To remove the pops from the molds, run the molds briefly under warm water until the pops loosen from the sides. The pops are extra creamy when left out at room temperature for a few minutes before serving.

Tip
If you can't find canned coconut cream, place 3 (13½-ounce) cans of full-fat coconut milk in the refrigerator overnight. Carefully open the cans and scoop out the thick cream that has risen to the tops of the cans. Avoid purchasing "cream of coconut," which tends to be sweetened. I prefer the Savoy and Aroy-D brands of coconut milk and coconut cream.

Make Ahead
Complete Step 1 up to 2 weeks in advance. Store the cooled toasted coconut in a plastic bag at room temperature until ready to use.

Storage
Store in the molds in the freezer for up to 6 months.

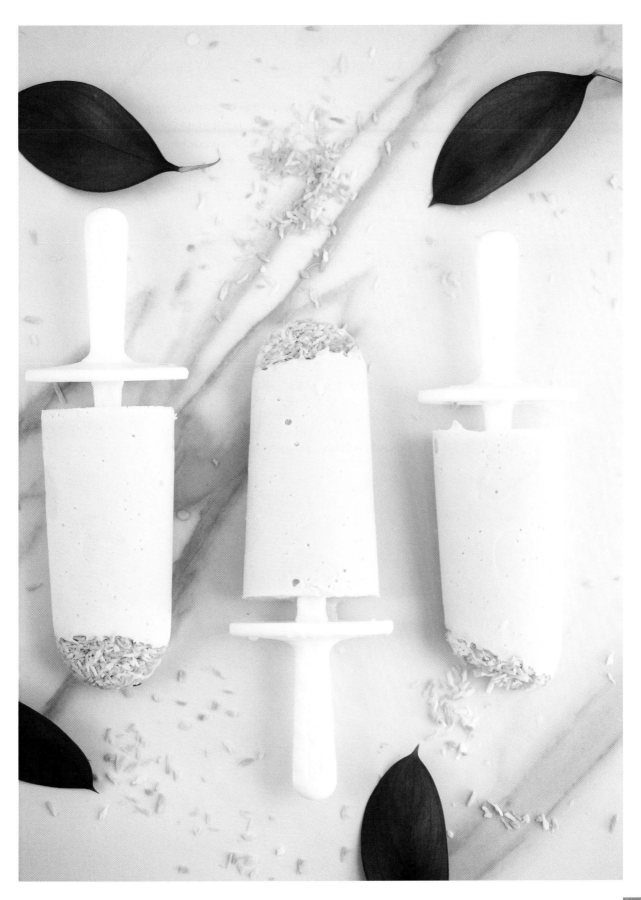

friendship cake
with whipped cinnamon honey frosting

Makes one 9 by 5-inch cake, serves 8 | Prep Time: 15 minutes | Cook Time: 55 minutes | Total Time: 1 hour 10 minutes

2 cups chopped green plantains (about 1¼ pounds or 2 medium)

½ cup unsweetened applesauce

1 (8-ounce) can pineapple chunks, drained

¼ cup honey

2 teaspoons vanilla extract

1 teaspoon apple cider vinegar

1 Gelatin "Egg" (below)

¾ cup coconut flour

¼ cup arrowroot starch

2 teaspoons ground cinnamon

1 teaspoon baking soda

½ cup unsweetened shredded coconut

½ cup raisins

1 recipe Whipped Cinnamon Honey Frosting (page 310)

1. Preheat the oven to 350 degrees. Grease a 9 by 5-inch loaf pan with coconut oil.

2. Place the plantains, applesauce, pineapple, honey, vanilla, and vinegar in a food processor or blender and puree until smooth.

3. Prepare the gelatin "egg" as directed. Add to the machine and blend until just incorporated.

4. Add the coconut flour, arrowroot starch, cinnamon, and baking soda to the machine and pulse to combine evenly. Stir in the shredded coconut and raisins.

5. Pour the cake batter into the prepared loaf pan and pack it down gently with a spatula. Bake for 50 to 55 minutes, until the cake begins to pull away from the sides of the pan and the edges are golden brown.

6. Let cool to room temperature before cutting into 8 slices and spreading with Whipped Cinnamon Honey Frosting. The cake is best served the same day it is baked.

Storage
Once cool, store in a sealed glass container in the refrigerator for up to 2 days, or wrap the unfrosted cake in plastic wrap, seal in a freezer bag, and freeze for up to 6 months. Bring the cake to room temperature before frosting and serving. Do not store at room temperature, as the cake will dry out and lose its flavor.

gelatin "egg"

Makes 1 egg | Prep Time: 5 minutes | Total Time: 5 minutes

1 tablespoon unflavored gelatin powder

1 tablespoon lukewarm water

2 tablespoons hot water

1. Whisk together the gelatin and lukewarm water in a small bowl to allow the gelatin to bloom.

2. Immediately whisk in the hot water and let the gelatin "egg" sit for 2 minutes prior to incorporating into your recipe as directed.

Tip
This gelatin "egg" can be used as a replacement for 1 large egg.

Make Ahead
Gelatin "eggs" should not be made ahead unless you plan on prebaking a dish and reheating it for leftovers.

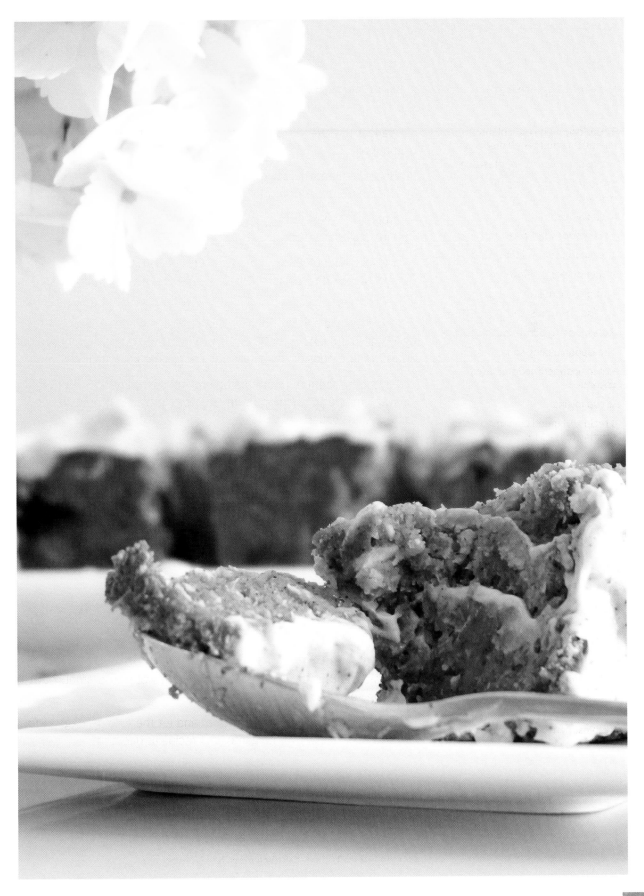

whipped cinnamon honey frosting

Makes ¾ cup | Prep Time: 5 minutes | Total Time: 5 minutes

1 cup palm shortening, room temperature

3 tablespoons honey

½ teaspoon ground cinnamon

¼ teaspoon fine sea salt

Storage
Store in a sealed glass container at room temperature for up to 1 month.

In a high-powered blender or food processor, blend all the ingredients together until whipped, 30 to 45 seconds, scraping down the sides as needed. Alternatively, you may place the ingredients in a medium mixing bowl and whip with a hand mixer for 1 minute.

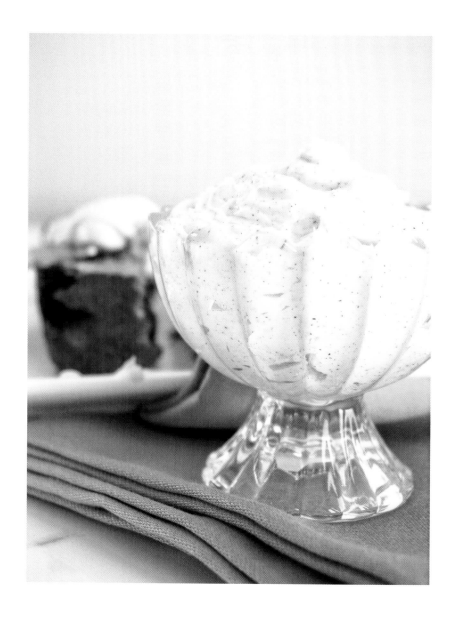

carob mousse frosting

Makes 1 cup | Prep Time: 5 minutes | Total Time: 5 minutes

1 cup coconut cream (see Tip, page 306), chilled overnight

¼ cup carob powder

1 teaspoon unflavored gelatin powder

¼ teaspoon fine sea salt

Make Ahead
The frosting can be made up to 1 day in advance. Give it a quick whip with a hand mixer just before using.

Storage
Store in a sealed glass container in the refrigerator for up to 1 day.

1. Ensure that the coconut cream has solidified and thickened.

2. Using a hand mixer or stand mixer, whip the cold coconut cream in a medium mixing bowl for 2 to 3 minutes, until fluffy and soft peaks form. Stir in the carob, gelatin, and salt until smooth. Keep the frosting cold until ready to pipe or spread.

Carob Mousse Stuffed Strawberries. Pipe the Carob Mousse Frosting into hulled strawberries and chill until ready to serve.

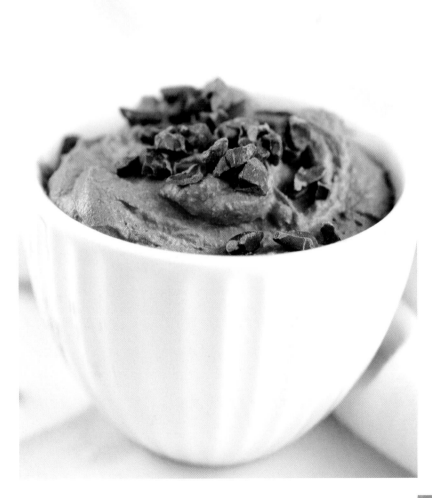

pumpkin roll with clementine cream

Serves 7 | Prep Time: 20 minutes | Cook Time: 20 minutes | Total Time: 40 minutes + 50 minutes to cool and set

PUMPKIN CAKE

1 (15-ounce) can pumpkin puree

2 tablespoons honey

1 tablespoon palm shortening

½ cup plus 1 teaspoon coconut flour

2 tablespoons tapioca starch

2 teaspoons ground cinnamon

1 teaspoon ginger powder

¾ teaspoon ground mace

1 teaspoon baking soda

1 teaspoon apple cider vinegar

CLEMENTINE CREAM

1 cup fresh clementine segments (4 to 5 clementines)

1 cup palm shortening

3 tablespoons honey

½ teaspoon grated clementine zest

½ teaspoon ground cinnamon

¼ teaspoon fine sea salt

Storage

Store in a sealed glass container in the refrigerator for up to 1 week. To freeze, wrap each slice or the entire roll tightly in plastic wrap and store sealed in a freezer bag for up to 3 months.

1. Preheat the oven to 350 degrees. Line a cookie sheet with parchment paper.

2. In a medium bowl, whisk together the pumpkin puree, honey, and palm shortening until smooth. Stir in the remaining ingredients for the cake to form a wet and fluffy dough.

3. Spoon the dough onto the center of the prepared cookie sheet and use your hands to spread it into an 8 by 12-inch rectangle, making sure that it is an even thickness.

4. Bake for 20 minutes or until the cake is golden brown with cracks on top. Place directly in the refrigerator until cool to the touch, about 30 minutes.

5. While the cake cools, make the clementine cream: Place all the ingredients for the cream in a blender and blend on high speed until pureed into a smooth, light-orange cream, scraping down the sides of the blender jar with a spoon if needed to keep the mixture going.

6. Once the cake is cool, use a spatula to spread the clementine cream over the entire surface of the cake.

7. Starting at the wide end of the cake, use the parchment paper to assist you in rolling the cake gently and tightly away from you, ensuring that it does not break. Place the roll seam side down and refrigerate for 10 to 20 minutes to firm up, which will make slicing easier.

8. Using a sharp knife, carefully slice the pumpkin roll into 7 even pieces. Turn each slice on its side and reshape into a circle with your hands, if needed. Serve cold.

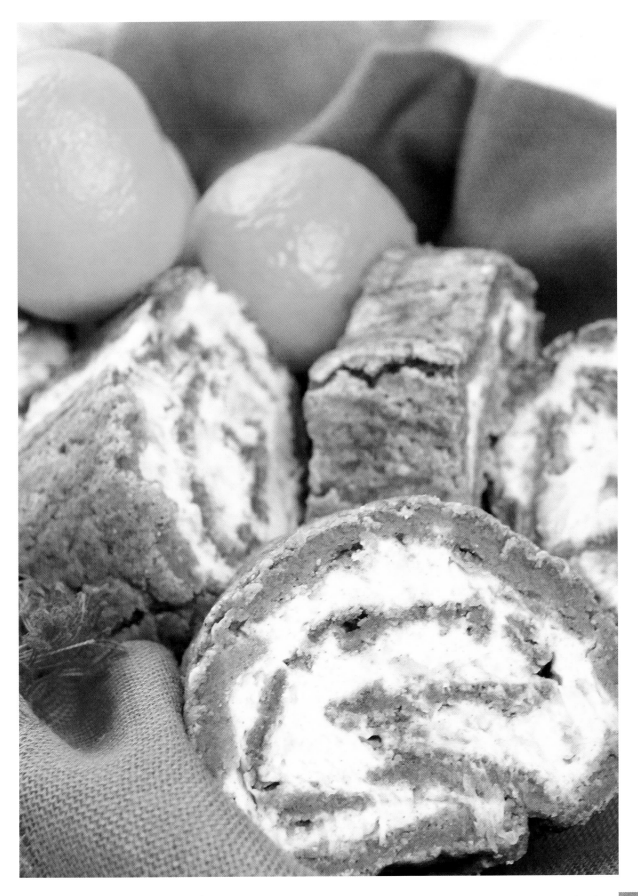

cherry pie bars

Makes 6 bars | Prep Time: 15 minutes | Cook Time: 40 minutes | Total Time: 55 minutes + time to cool

CHERRY FILLING

1 heaping cup pitted and chopped cherries (about 1 pound)

1 teaspoon fresh lemon juice

5 pitted Medjool dates

1 teaspoon arrowroot starch

¼ teaspoon ground cinnamon

DOUGH

1½ cups peeled and chopped white sweet potatoes (about 1 large)

2 tablespoons coconut oil

2 tablespoons coconut flour

¼ teaspoon ground cinnamon

¼ teaspoon fine sea salt

Storage

Once cool, store in a sealed glass container in the refrigerator for up to 5 days, or wrap tightly in plastic wrap, seal in a freezer bag, and freeze for up to 3 months.

1. To make the filling: Bring the cherries and lemon juice to a simmer in a small saucepan over medium-low heat. Continue cooking for 5 to 7 minutes to allow the cherries to soften and release their juices as you break them up with a wooden spoon.

2. Meanwhile, place the dates in a small bowl, cover with water, and microwave for 1 minute to soften. Add the dates to the saucepan with 2 teaspoons of the date water. Stir continuously for 1 to 2 minutes as the mixture thickens.

3. Remove from the heat and stir in the arrowroot starch and cinnamon until the mixture has thickened to a paste.

4. As the cherries are cooking, make the dough: Steam the sweet potatoes in a lidded steamer basket set over a pot of boiling water for 10 to 12 minutes, until fork-tender. This will ensure that the potatoes can be mashed smoothly. Transfer the cooked potatoes to a mixing bowl with the coconut oil. Mash using a potato masher or fork until smooth and no lumps remain. Stir in the coconut flour, cinnamon, and salt. The dough should be moist but still workable.

5. To assemble the bars: Preheat the oven to 350 degrees. Line a cookie sheet with parchment paper.

6. Divide the dough into two equal portions. On the prepared cookie sheet, use your hands to smooth the dough into a 4 by 5-inch rectangle. Top with the cherry filling and smooth with a spatula so that only a ¼-inch edge is left uncovered.

7. Place another sheet of parchment paper on a separate flat surface and form a second 4 by 5-inch rectangle of dough. Use the parchment paper to assist you in turning the dough on top of the filling. Remove the top sheet of parchment and use your fingers to seal the edges gently.

8. Bake for 25 minutes or until the top is light golden brown. Let cool completely in the refrigerator, then slice into 6 bars and serve.

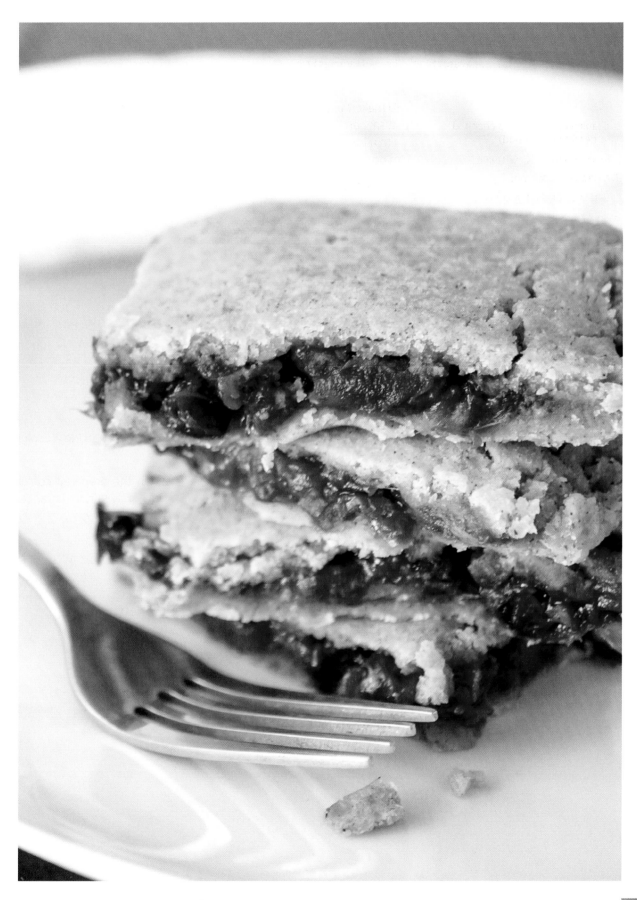

apple crumble

Serves 2 to 3 | Prep Time: 10 minutes | Cook Time: 20 minutes | Total Time: 30 minutes

3 apples, any variety

½ teaspoon ground cinnamon

1 tablespoon coconut oil

¼ teaspoon fine sea salt

CRUMBLE

2 tablespoons melted coconut oil or lard

½ cup crushed unsweetened apple chips

½ teaspoon ground cinnamon

¼ teaspoon ground mace

Whipped Cinnamon Honey Frosting (page 310), for serving (optional)

Make Ahead

Slice the apples and toss with ½ teaspoon ground cinnamon and 2 teaspoons fresh lemon juice to prevent browning. Store in a sealed plastic bag until ready to cook.

Store & Reheat

Once cool, cover and store at room temperature for up to 1 day or in the refrigerator for up to 1 week. Reheat in a 350-degree oven until warm.

1. Preheat the oven to 350 degrees.

2. Peel and slice the apples into ⅓-inch-thick slices. In a large bowl, toss the apples in the cinnamon.

3. In an oven-safe 8-inch skillet over medium heat, sauté the apples in the coconut oil until softened but not mushy, 8 to 10 minutes. Stir in the salt and remove from the heat.

4. Make the crumble: In a small bowl, whisk together the crumble ingredients.

5. To make skillet apple crumble: Spoon the crumble on top of the cooked apples in the skillet.

   To make individual servings (as shown opposite): Divide the cooked apples among three 4-inch tart pans or three 6-ounce ramekins. Spoon the crumble on top of the cooked apples, dividing it evenly among the pans or ramekins.

6. Bake for 10 minutes or until the crumble is crispy. Serve topped with Whipped Cinnamon Honey Frosting, if desired.

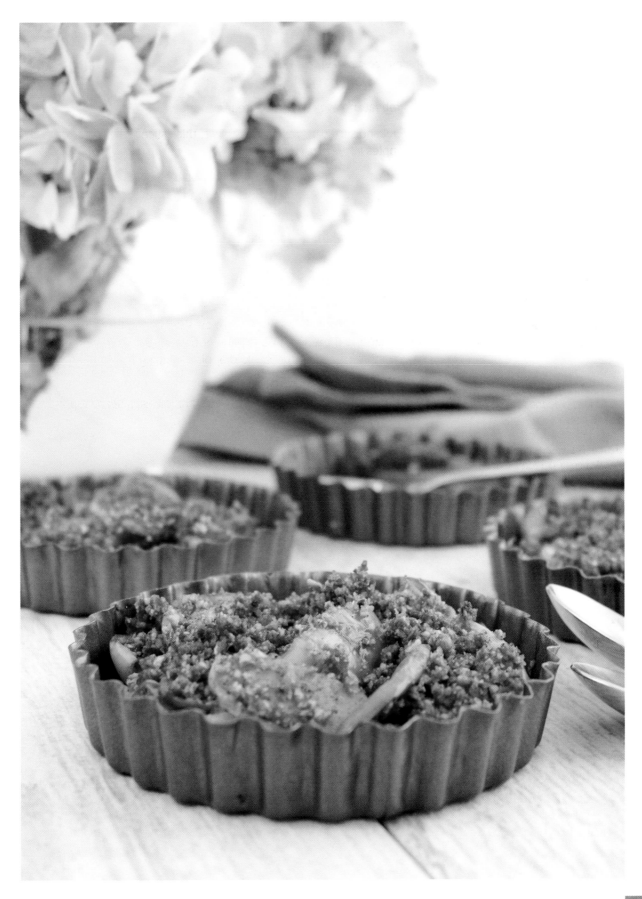

caramelized figs with lemon & vanilla

Serves 4 to 6 | Prep Time: 5 minutes | Cook Time: 25 minutes | Total Time: 30 minutes

¾ pound fresh black figs, any variety

1 teaspoon balsamic vinegar

1 teaspoon grated lemon zest

1 teaspoon vanilla extract

⅛ teaspoon fine sea salt

Store & Reheat
Once cool, store in a sealed glass container in the refrigerator for up to 1 week or in the freezer for up to 1 year. Reheat on a rimmed baking sheet on the top rack of the oven under a low broil for a few minutes until warm.

Change It Up
Use 1 teaspoon grated orange or grapefruit zest in place of the lemon zest.

1. Place an oven rack in the center of the oven and preheat the broiler to high.

2. Remove the stems from the figs. Halve the figs if they are small or quarter them if they are large, ensuring that all the pieces are the same size. Toss the figs with the vinegar, lemon zest, vanilla, and salt in a medium glass baking dish. Arrange in a single layer.

3. Broil for 20 to 25 minutes, until the figs have caramelized.

coconut panna cotta with caramelized figs

Serves 2 to 3 | Prep Time: 5 minutes | Cook Time: 5 minutes | Total Time: 10 minutes + 3 hours to set

1 (14-ounce) can coconut cream (see Tip, page 306)

1 tablespoon honey

¼ teaspoon fine sea salt

1 tablespoon unflavored gelatin powder

¼ cup warm water

½ cup Caramelized Figs with Lemon & Vanilla (above)

Make Ahead
Prepare the Caramelized Figs up to 1 week in advance and reheat using the instructions above.

Storage
Store in a sealed glass container in the refrigerator for up to 5 days.

1. In a small saucepan over medium heat, whisk together the coconut cream, honey, and salt and allow to come to a simmer.

2. Meanwhile, whisk together the gelatin and warm water in a small bowl. Set aside for 5 minutes to allow the gelatin to thicken and bloom.

3. Once the coconut cream mixture begins to simmer, remove it from the heat. Give the gelatin another good stir, then whisk it into the coconut cream until completely dissolved and no small clumps remain.

4. Pour the mixture into small serving dishes, such as ramekins. Chill for 2 to 3 hours, until set.

5. When ready to serve, warm the Caramelized Figs under the broiler or in the microwave. Spoon on top of the panna cotta and serve immediately.

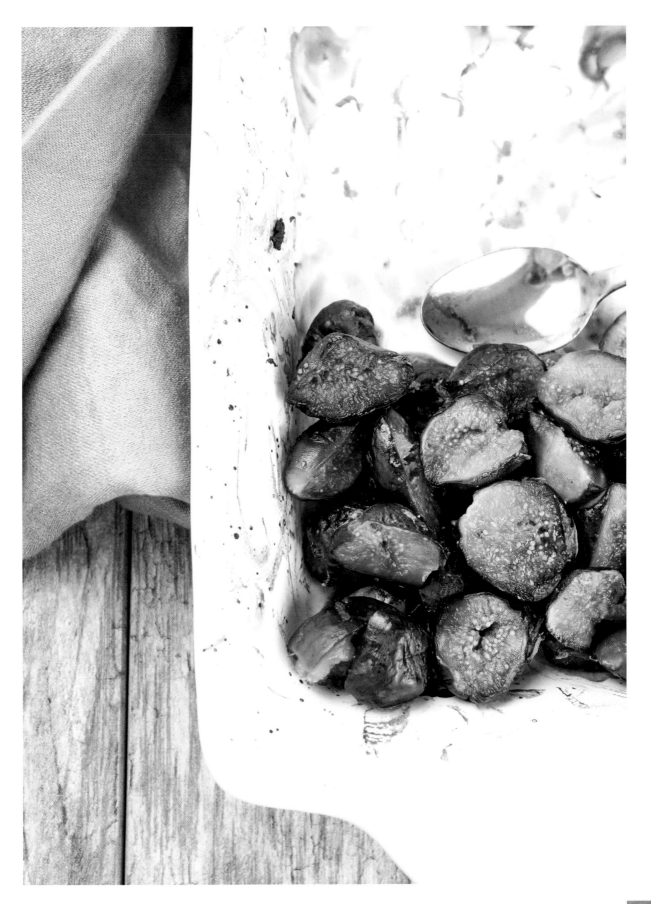

"chocolate"-ginger pudding

Serves 2 | Prep Time: 5 minutes | Total Time: 5 minutes

2 avocados, ripened to the consistency of room-temperature butter

2 tablespoons honey

1 tablespoon water

¼ cup carob powder

½ teaspoon ginger powder

½ teaspoon fine sea salt

Coarse sea salt, for garnish (optional)

Storage

Once cool, store in a sealed glass container in the refrigerator for up to 2 days. Stir before serving.

1. In a blender, puree the avocados with the honey and water. Add the carob, ginger, and salt and blend until shiny and smooth.

2. Transfer to individual serving bowls, garnish with coarse sea salt (if using), and either serve immediately or refrigerate until cold.

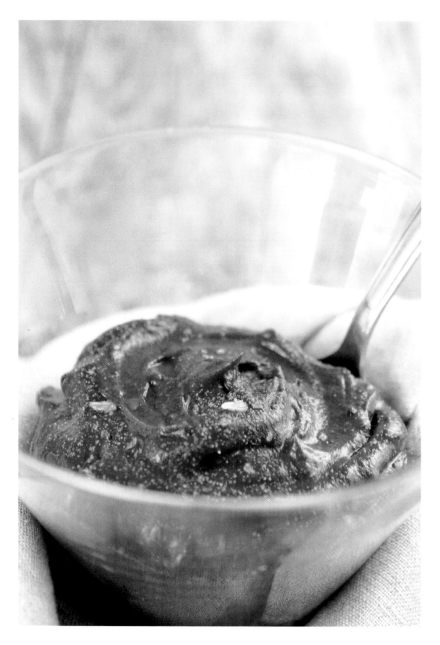

roasted strawberries

Makes 1 cup | Prep Time: 8 minutes | Cook Time: 35 minutes | Total Time: 43 minutes

1 pound strawberries

1 teaspoon honey

½ teaspoon vanilla extract

Make Ahead

Slice the strawberries, wrap in paper towels, and store in a sealed plastic bag in the refrigerator for up to 2 days prior to roasting.

Serving Suggestions

Serve over Cinnamon Banana Ice Cream (page 303) or over a bowl of coconut cream for a low-sugar treat.

Store & Reheat

Once cool, store in a sealed glass container in the refrigerator for up to 1 week or in the freezer for up to 6 months. Reheat in a small saucepan over medium-low heat until warm.

1. Preheat the oven to 350 degrees. Line a rimmed baking sheet with parchment paper.

2. Remove the green tops from the strawberries and slice the berries in half lengthwise. Large strawberries may need to be sliced into thirds to ensure they are all equal sizes. Toss the strawberries with the honey and vanilla on the prepared baking sheet.

3. Roast for 30 to 35 minutes until the berries have softened and the juices have thickened. Let cool slightly before serving.

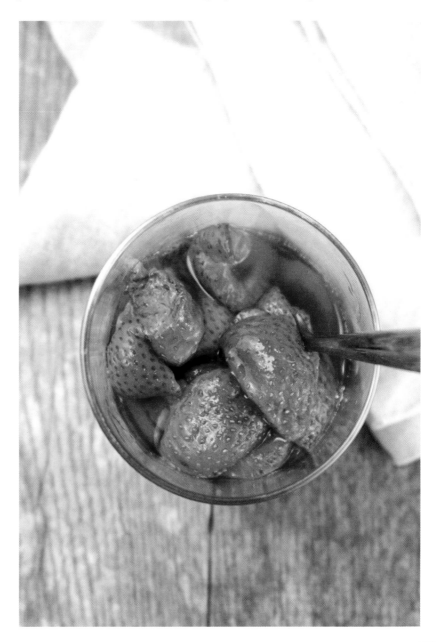

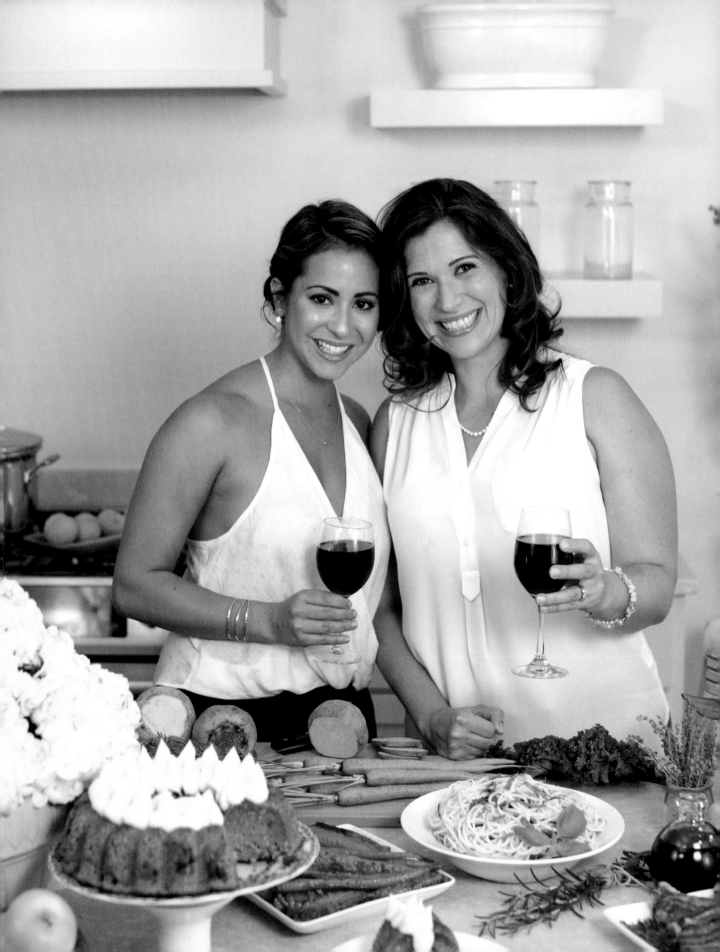

appendix

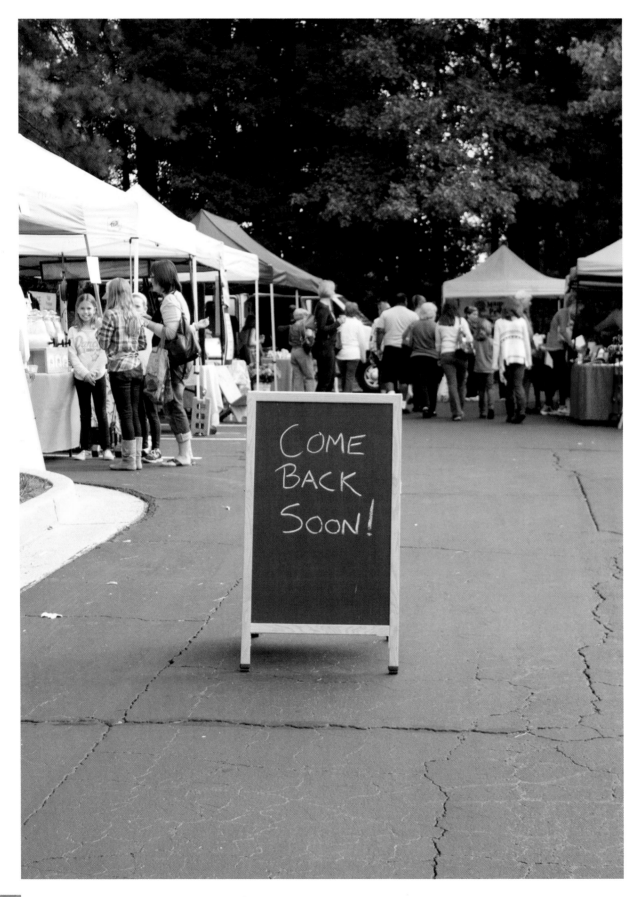

resources

additional references

- *The Paleo Approach,* by Sarah Ballantyne, PhD
- *Gluten Freedom,* by Alessio Fasano, MD
- *Perfect Health Diet,* by Paul Jaminet, PhD, and Shou-Ching Jaminet, PhD
- *Death by Food Pyramid,* by Denise Minger
- *Eating on the Wild Side,* by Jo Robinson
- *Primal Connections,* by Mark Sisson
- *The Wahls Protocol,* by Terry Wahls, MD
- *Eat the Yolks,* by Liz Wolfe

recommended informational cookbooks

- *The Paleo Approach Cookbook,* by Sarah Ballantyne, PhD
- *The Homegrown Paleo Cookbook,* by Diana Rodgers, NTP
- *Real Life Paleo,* by Stacy Toth and Matthew McCarry
- *The Autoimmune Paleo Cookbook,* by Mickey Trescott, NTP

online shopping

meat, seafood & vegetables

- Farmbox Direct, farmboxdirect.com
- Grass-Fed Traditions, grassfedtraditions.com
- Massa Natural Meats, massanaturalmeats.com
- US Wellness Meats, grasslandbeef.com
- Vital Choice, vitalchoice.com
- Wild Planet, wildplanetfoods.com

pantry items

- Amazon.com
- Barefoot Provisions, barefootprovisions.com
- Fatworks, fatworksfoods.com
- Kasandrinos, kasandrinos.com
- One Stop Paleo Shop, onestoppaleoshop.com
- Tropical Traditions, tropicaltraditions.com

5 ingredients or less recipes

20 minutes or less recipes

- worcestershire sauce *(page 106)*
- garlic sauce *(page 106)*
- greek dressing *(page 110)*
- strawberry lime dressing *(page 110)*
- honey balsamic dressing *(page 110)*
- caesar dressing *(page 110)*
- garlic-dill ranch dressing *(page 112)*
- avocado mayo *(page 113)*
- make it bolognese! *(page 114)*
- tzatziki sauce *(page 115)*
- pronto pesto *(page 116)*
- mango guacamole *(page 116)*
- cilantro chimichurri *(page 116)*
- tangy carolina bbq sauce *(page 118)*
- cauli'fredo sauce *(page 119)*
- thin pizza crust *(page 120)*
- plantain wraps *(page 121)*
- seasoning mixes *(page 122)*
- antioxidant morning smoothie *(page 126)*
- pumpkin spice smoothie *(page 127)*
- garlic & herb breakfast sausage *(page 130)*
- country herb gravy *(page 134)*
- biscuits & gravy *(page 135)*
- cinnamon & raisin porridge *(page 137)*
- garlicky greek lamb skillet *(page 142)*
- crispy salmon hash *(page 144)*
- "cheesy" broccoli soup *(page 158)*
- caesar salad *(page 165)*
- antipasto salad *(page 166)*
- sweet & smoky spa salad *(page 166)*
- roasted root, arugula & balsamic salad *(page 168)*
- fennel mandarin slaw *(page 170)*
- chunky tuna salad *(page 172)*
- peach & kale summer salad *(page 174)*
- grain-free tabbouleh *(page 176)*
- thai green mango salad *(page 178)*
- west coast burritos with cucumber pico de gallo *(page 183)*
- grilled steak cucumber noodle bowl *(page 190)*

- burgers *(page 200)*
- speedy shanghai stir-fry *(page 209)*
- ham & pineapple pizza *(page 212)*
- prosciutto & fig bistro pizza *(page 213)*
- pesto chicken pasta *(page 217)*
- mojo-mango stuffed sweet potatoes *(page 219)*
- pesto chicken pizza *(page 227)*
- spinach & garlic lover's pizza *(page 228)*
- lamb with olive-butternut rice *(page 229)*
- seared shrimp pasta with white sauce *(page 233)*
- wild salmon with roasted raspberries *(page 234)*
- spaghetti squash noodles *(page 238)*
- caribbean plantain rice *(page 239)*
- mac n' cheese *(page 240)*
- spinach with alliums & lemon *(page 242)*
- garlic-rubbed tostones *(page 248)*
- silky potato puree *(page 258)*
- chinese stir-fried lettuce *(page 261)*
- gingered asparagus *(page 265)*
- pulled pork sliders *(page 271)*
- roasted garlic & pumpkin hummus *(page 274)*
- smoky artichoke baba ghanoush *(page 275)*
- orange & olive tapenade *(page 276)*
- smoked salmon spread *(page 277)*
- chicken ranch salad over crackers *(page 280)*
- lemon-ginger energy balls *(page 281)*
- moscow mule *(page 289)*
- watermelon lime agua fresca *(page 290)*
- strawberry lemonade spritzer *(page 291)*
- citrus fizz *(page 293)*
- maple mocha *(page 294)*
- hot fudge & ganache *(page 298)*
- warm bananas with date caramel sauce *(page 301)*
- strawberry milkshake *(page 302)*
- gelatin "egg" *(page 308)*
- whipped cinnamon honey frosting *(page 310)*
- carob mousse frosting *(page 311)*
- "chocolate"-ginger pudding *(page 320)*

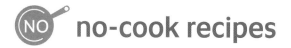

no-cook recipes

- garlic sauce (*page 106*)
- greek dressing (*page 110*)
- strawberry lime dressing (*page 110*)
- honey balsamic dressing (*page 110*)
- caesar dressing (*page 110*)
- garlic-dill ranch dressing (*page 112*)
- avocado mayo (*page 113*)
- tzatziki sauce (*page 115*)
- pronto pesto (*page 116*)
- mango guacamole (*page 116*)
- cilantro chimichurri (*page 116*)
- seasoning mixes (*page 122*)
- antioxidant morning smoothie (*page 126*)
- pumpkin spice smoothie (*page 127*)
- watermelon gazpacho (*page 160*)
- caesar salad (*page 165*)
- sweet & smoky spa salad (*page 166*)
- roasted root, arugula & balsamic salad (*page 168*)
- fennel mandarin slaw (*page 170*)
- chunky tuna salad (*page 172*)
- peach & kale summer salad (*page 174*)
- grain-free tabbouleh (*page 176*)
- thai green mango salad (*page 178*)
- tropical broccoli salad (*page 179*)

- spicy carrots (*page 244*)
- pulled pork sliders (*page 271*)
- roasted garlic & pumpkin hummus (*page 274*)
- smoky artichoke baba ghanoush (*page 275*)
- orange & olive tapenade (*page 276*)
- smoked salmon spread (*page 277*)
- chicken ranch salad over crackers (*page 280*)
- lemon-ginger energy balls (*page 281*)
- monkey bars (*page 282*)
- red sangria (*page 288*)
- moscow mule (*page 289*)
- watermelon lime agua fresca (*page 290*)
- strawberry lemonade spritzer (*page 291*)
- citrus fizz (*page 293*)
- ganache-stuffed dates (*page 298*)
- no-bake lemon macaroons (*page 300*)
- strawberry milkshake (*page 302*)
- cinnamon banana ice cream (*page 303*)
- sweet potato ice cream (*page 304*)
- truffle fudge pops (*page 305*)
- toasted coconut cream pops (*page 306*)
- gelatin "egg" (*page 308*)
- whipped cinnamon honey frosting (*page 310*)
- carob mousse frosting (*page 311*)
- "chocolate"-ginger pudding (*page 320*)

leftovers reinvented recipes

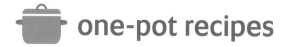

one-pot recipes

acknowledgments

Thank you to my biggest supporters who cheered me along from the sidelines during the creation of this book. I don't think I would have survived the making and remaking (and remaking and remaking) of 175 recipes without you amazing crew of people. The world would be so lucky to have each and every one of you in their lives, but I'm going to selfishly hoard all of you on my team because I don't think it could get any better.

Jeff, your positivity, honesty, and encouragement when I wanted to give up were what kept me going. Thank you for being my #1 taste-tester, dishwasher, and tear-wiper. Without you and Rafael, life wouldn't be nearly as bright and exciting. I owe my success in healing to you and your undying belief that I would get better. I love you more than anything, husband. Here's to many more decades of traveling, laughing, bickering, and loving together!

Mom and Dad, thank you for always allowing me to explore what makes me happy and supporting me along the way. Knowing you are always only a phone call away has made me feel close to home even when I'm a thousand miles away. Stay vibrant, happy, and selfless because there's no better way to ensure a long and healthy life.

Olivia and Scott, half of this cookbook happened in your kitchen! You are saints for putting up with my endless messes and sink full of dishes. Your feedback on the recipes was taken to heart and I know you'll enjoy cooking from the book as a family (Archie included!). I love you guys and know that we'll be back in Florida growing old together before we know it.

Alexis, you're my big sister and the most hard-working, fun-loving woman I know. Always go after what you want no matter how far-fetched it seems. Yes, I am talking about that event-planning business that you would be insanely successful at—you have a talent that the world (or at least North America) needs to see! I love you, Lexi!

Andrea, you left this world far too soon, and I wish we could have spent many more nights laughing over how silly and obsessed with each other the boys are. I write this on your two-year anniversary, and I want you and your family to know that your passing inspired me to go after what I've always wanted but never thought possible because life is meant to be LIVED. And from all the stories I've heard, you lived it up, woman! Your bright eyes shine down on Ava, Hartley, and Jadyn each day. Always thinking of you.

Kathy, Jim, Kristi, Todd, Page, Lauren, Cole, and Gus, my second family! You didn't think I had forgotten you, did you? Our families combined over a year ago, and even though we've been so far, I keep each of you very close to my heart. Thank you for raising such a good man who is an absolute angel in my life. Tell the kids Aunt Laena wrote about them in her book, and now they're famous! Or you can just give them all a big kiss from me instead.

Nanny, I miss you every day. I wish you were here to celebrate with me, but I know you're saying "Go get 'em, Peanut" from above ... even though you may be too busy dancing and laughing with Dedo and Uncle Gary to notice (I hope you are). You lived every one of your healthy days on earth with vibrancy to be admired and an infectious "I do what I want" attitude. I am not offended when Mom says we are so much alike. I love you, Mickey.

Teta, so many recipes from this book are inspired by you and all of our family meals together. My love for food developed in childhood thanks to the fresh Lebanese dishes you and Auntie Katie slaved all day over to make us happy. I miss your simple nods of wisdom and tight hugs, but I know you are finally in a pain-free and restful state. I hope I did you proud with this one.

Hannah, Nicole, McKenzie, Heidi, and Jessica, your friendships are a source of light, laughter, and healing in my life. I can always count on each of you to lend an ear and offer honest advice. You are a strong, compassionate, and successful group of women who are going to conquer everything that life hands you, and I admire each of you immensely.

Victory Belt, the entire team has been so welcoming and supportive. I couldn't be more grateful to work with all of you and be a part of the VB family. Keep spreading the word of good health.

Sarah, thank you for agreeing to go on the wild ride that is collaborating on a book from across the country together. If our friendship can withstand four-hour conversations about meal plans, I think we're in it for the long haul. All jokes aside, you play many roles in my life aside from friend. I appreciate each and every one of them. Thank you for inviting me into your home so many times (and feeding my crazy appetite) and letting me into your family. Cheers to many more years of health for both of us!

Love,
Alaena

Nothing I write would have any meaning without people willing to read it. More than that, though, my devoted readers and followers are a source of inspiration, motivation, encouragement, connection, appreciation, and meaning that would be missing from my life without them. Thank you for all your support and enthusiasm, and for making all the hard work worthwhile. And thank you for inspiring the people in your lives to make changes to improve their health. By sharing your success and helping your friends and family learn more and implement better choices, you create a momentum that no amount of books, websites, or news articles could generate. You are the reason this movement is growing so rapidly, you are why millions of people are reclaiming their health, and you are how positive and lasting change happens.

Grandad, I miss you every day, and when I complete a project like this, I always wonder what you would say when you saw it. Okay, I know what you'd say (you'd cry and tell me you're proud of me), but I wish you were here to actually say it. Thank you for showing me what science can do.

Adele and Mira, watching you two grow up is truly my greatest joy. There are no better cheerleaders in life than you, no better companions or motivators, no better reflections of me, my efforts, and my accomplishments. Everything I do, I do it for you and because of you. Thank you for making every day magical, for wanting to help, and for compelling me to find balance in life.

Mom, I am who I am because of you. You are my best friend, my confidant, my inspiration, my kick-in-the-pants, my shoulder to cry on, and my rock to lean on. Thank you for instilling in me my passion for science, my love of cooking, my talent for art, my curiosity for all things, and my drive to make my dreams come true.

David, I finally figured out an adequate way to celebrate 20 years together: dedicate a book to you! In all seriousness, though, you are the reason I have been able to accomplish so much. Without your support and inexorable love throughout university, the post-doc years, those bleary-eyed, sleep-deprived first few years of parenthood, the challenging-yet-rewarding, slightly less sleep-deprived years that parenthood has been ever since, and the roller-coaster ride that has been my career transition to author, I would not have succeeded, or maybe even survived, any of it.

My team: Charissa, Christina, Claire, Denise, Katie, and Brooke, you are the reason I can do something like this and stay sane and healthy. I am better and what I create is better because of your hard work, ideas, enthusiasm, support, and cheerleading. I cherish each and every one of you and feel blessed to have you on my team.

Dawn, I'm going to keep coming up with ideas for projects I can bring you in on and fun things for us to do together. Thank you for sharing my passion for healthy food and my general dorkiness and for always making me laugh! Your artistic eye and magic shutter-release-button finger are an asset to yet another one of my books. Plus, we got to hang out! Woot!

Heritage Sandy Springs Farmer's Market, thank you for being such a welcoming and friendly place and a great supporter of our local farmers, food vendors, and artisans. Saturday morning at the market is truly the highlight of my week. Thank you also to Fry Farm, Bray Family Farm, Yve's Garden, Mama J's Produce, Skylight Farm, Owl Pine Farm, Heritage Farm, Cultured Traditions, Wholly Pops, Georgia Grinders, Mercier Orchards, and Rev Coffee for feeding my family so well every week! It is truly a privilege to be part of this amazing local food community.

CrossFit Dwala, I don't think I could stay sane or healthy through a project like this without you. Anne Marie, Jake, and Corynne, thank you for making me do burpees (there, it's in writing!), insisting I squeeze my butt during lifts, installing a PR bell, all the running jokes, and generally being willing to share TMI. You've made me stronger and tougher, not just physically, but emotionally and mentally as well—and that might be even more important.

Red Door Playhouse, thanks to you, Seth and Leah, I am far more successful at finding work-life balance. Thank you for making my brain do somersaults, challenging my creativity, laughing with me (and sometimes at me), and never again mentioning the thing with the thing.

Victory Belt, your support and passion for every project never ceases to astound me. Thank you for making our visions come to life, letting our books be truly ours but still helping to make them better, putting your authors ahead of their books, and all of your contributions to this community. Thank you, Erich, Michele, Susan, Pam, Erin, Holly, the design team, and everyone who has a hand, big or small, in making each book a reality.

Alaena, writing a book together was either going to secure our BFF status or destroy our friendship irreparably, and I'm sure glad it was the former! Working with you on this project was a joy. I loved watching how our ideas could build on each other to form something amazing, sharing this passion for helping people, creating a resource unlike anything else out there, and genuinely having fun every step of the way. Shall we start brainstorming for *The Healing Kitchen 2*?

Love,
Sarah

breakfast favorites

126 antioxidant morning smoothie

127 pumpkin spice smoothie

128 chicken hash brown patties

130 garlic & herb breakfast sausage / american breakfast sausage

132 bacon-wrapped apple & cinnamon sausage

133 bacon-herb biscuits

134 country herb gravy

135 biscuits & gravy

136 oven-baked pancakes

137 cinnamon & raisin porridge

138 baked carrot-banana bread n'oatmeal

139 spiced candied bacon

140 comforting breakfast casserole

141 creamy caesar beef skillet

142 garlicky greek lamb skillet

144 crispy salmon hash

146 ollie's diy sunrise hash

soups & salads

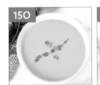
150 vibrant healing soup base

152 hamburger stew

154 bacon & salmon chowder

156 roasted fennel & parsnip soup with citrus drizzle

157 pumpkin chili

158 chicken "tortilla" soup

158 "cheesy" broccoli soup

160 watermelon gazpacho

161 hearty healing beef stew

162 new england clam chowder

164 lettuce soup

165 caesar salad

166 antipasto salad

166 sweet & smoky spa salad

168 grilled chicken souvlaki salad

168 roasted root, arugula & balsamic salad

170 fennel mandarin slaw

171 honey-lime chicken & strawberry salad

172 chunky tuna salad

172 toasted coconut, fig & kale salad

174 peach & kale summer salad

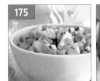
175 smoked salmon potato salad

176 grain-free tabbouleh

178 thai green mango salad

179 tropical broccoli salad

easy-peasy mains

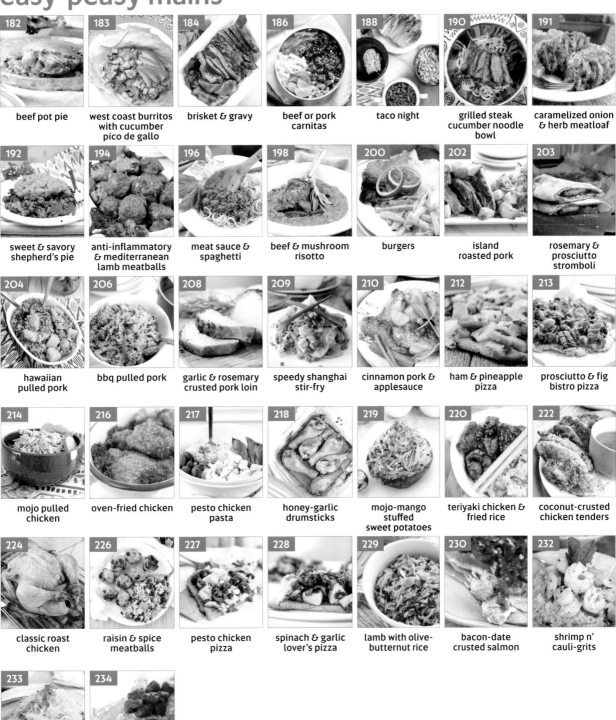

182 beef pot pie

183 west coast burritos with cucumber pico de gallo

184 brisket & gravy

186 beef or pork carnitas

188 taco night

190 grilled steak cucumber noodle bowl

191 caramelized onion & herb meatloaf

192 sweet & savory shepherd's pie

194 anti-inflammatory & mediterranean lamb meatballs

196 meat sauce & spaghetti

198 beef & mushroom risotto

200 burgers

202 island roasted pork

203 rosemary & prosciutto stromboli

204 hawaiian pulled pork

206 bbq pulled pork

208 garlic & rosemary crusted pork loin

209 speedy shanghai stir-fry

210 cinnamon pork & applesauce

212 ham & pineapple pizza

213 prosciutto & fig bistro pizza

214 mojo pulled chicken

216 oven-fried chicken

217 pesto chicken pasta

218 honey-garlic drumsticks

219 mojo-mango stuffed sweet potatoes

220 teriyaki chicken & fried rice

222 coconut-crusted chicken tenders

224 classic roast chicken

226 raisin & spice meatballs

227 pesto chicken pizza

228 spinach & garlic lover's pizza

229 lamb with olive-butternut rice

230 bacon-date crusted salmon

232 shrimp n' cauli-grits

233 seared shrimp pasta with white sauce

234 wild salmon with roasted raspberries

simple sides

238
spaghetti squash noodles

239
caribbean plantain rice

240
mac n' cheese

242
carrot pilaf with lemon & parsley

242
spinach with alliums & lemon

244
sweet potato & kale "rice" salad

244
spicy carrots

246
lebanese beef & rice stuffing

248
garlic-rubbed tostones

248
creamy herb mushrooms

250
creamy bacon scalloped sweet potatoes

252
fries

254
roasted brussels with bacon & cinnamon

254
cinnamon mashed carrots

256
spicy african kale

257
roasted sweet potatoes with tapenade

258
silky potato puree

259
bacon-wrapped cinnamon apples

260
roasted roots with garlic sauce

261
chinese stir-fried lettuce

262
pan-roasted cauliflower with bacon & spinach

263
roasted cabbage with balsamic-honey reduction

264
garlic roasted broccoli

265
gingered asparagus

satisfying snacks

268
chewy trail mix granola

269
crunchy kale'nola

270
turkey jerky

271
pulled pork sliders

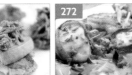
272
bacon-wrapped scallops with lemon-chive drizzle

273
lox & everything hors d'oeuvre

274
roasted garlic & pumpkin hummus

275
smoky artichoke baba ghanoush

276
orange & olive tapenade

277
smoked salmon spread

278
cherry balsamic pâté

279
garlic & thyme crackers

280
chicken ranch salad over crackers

281
lemon-ginger energy balls

282
monkey bars

283
mango coconut gummies

284
gummies

thirst quenchers

 288
red sangria

 289
moscow mule

 290
watermelon lime
agua fresca

 291
strawberry
lemonade spritzer

 292
mint-ea mojito

 293
citrus fizz

 294
maple mocha

timeless treats

 298
ganache-stuffed
dates

 298
hot fudge &
ganache

 300
no-bake lemon
macaroons

 301
warm bananas
with date caramel
sauce

 302
strawberry
milkshake

 303
cinnamon banana
ice cream

 304
sweet potato
ice cream

 305
truffle fudge pops

 306
toasted coconut
cream pops

 308
friendship cake with
whipped cinnamon
honey frosting

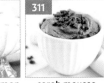 310
whipped cinnamon
honey frosting

 311
carob mousse
frosting

 312
pumpkin roll with
clementine cream

 314
cherry pie bars

 316
apple crumble

 318
caramelized figs
with lemon &
vanilla

 320
"chocolate"-ginger
pudding

 321
roasted
strawberries

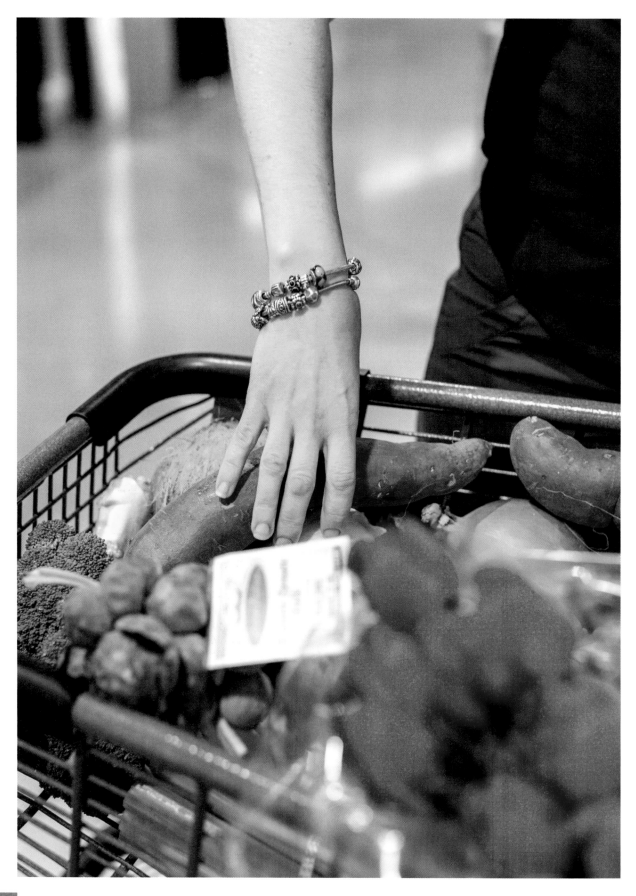

index